Physical Education Programming for Exceptional Learners

M. Rhonda Folio

Tennessee Technological University
Cookeville, Tennessee

AN ASPEN PUBLICATION®
Aspen Systems Corporation

1986

Rockville, Maryland
Royal Tunbridge Wells

Library of Congress Cataloging in Publication Data

Folio, M. Rhonda.
Physical education programming for exceptional learners.

"An Aspen publication."
Bibliography: p.
Includes index.
1. Physical education for handicapped children. 2. Physical education for handicapped children—Study and teaching. 3. Physical fitness—Testing. 4. Handicapped children—Nutrition. 5. Recreational therapy. I. Title.

GV445.F65   1985   371.9'044   85-19965
ISBN: 0-87189-243-X

Editorial Services: Carolyn Ormes

Library of Congress Catalog Card Number: 85-19965
ISBN: 0-87189-243-X

Printed in the United States of America

1 2 3 4 5

IN MEMORIAM

R. Curtis Whitesel, Editorial Director of the
Rehabilitation and Special Education Divisions of
Aspen Systems

and

My father, Sam Albert Folio

This book is dedicated to my mother, Ruby G. Folio,
for her love, understanding, and encouragement
of my professional development.

Table of Contents

Preface

To move is to achieve, communicate, express one's self, and become all that one can physically be. Motor and physical development are often taken for granted in nondisabled children and youth. These important skills, however, may lag behind, or never develop, in disabled children and youth. All children, handicapped or not, have the right to develop to their maximum potential motorically and physically.

Physical and motor skills develop sequentially and intervention should be applied in the same fashion. This approach is best suited to meet the needs of handicapped students. How we help them meet those needs through strategies, techniques, adaptations, and modifications of activities is the core of effective program development.

Professionals concerned with the motor and physical development of handicapped individuals are able to assist them in reaching their maximum potential when they have knowledge and resources to develop individualized and meaningful instructional programs. The purpose of this book is to provide information, consisting of programming ideas, methods, strategies, and adaptations of the learning environment, for implementing physical education programs for handicapped students.

A balance between theoretical and practical issues is stressed. The professionals for whom this book is intended include those who choose to be or are responsible for the handicapped student's individualized physical education program. The text has applications at both the preprofessional and professional levels.

Physical Education Programming for Exceptional Learners is based on several years of experience with a model physical education program for handicapped students. Many of the techniques suggested were implemented and refined as we evolved an approach that emphasized individualized programming, adaptation of the learning environment, mainstreaming, and methods so that every child, no matter how disabled, was able to participate in a rewarding physical education program.

This book contains six parts. Part I, "Legislation and the Challenge," (Chapters 1 and 2) introduces the reader to P.L. 94–142, The Education for All Handicapped Children Act, its mandates and procedures for implementing individualized educational programs. The role of the physical education service provider is explained and discussed. Chapter 2 discusses the general learning and psychomotor characteristics of particular types of disabilities and the implications for physical education.

Part II, "The Psychomotor Domain and Motor Skill Acquisition," (Chapters 3 through 6), stresses the learning of motor skills and the sequential order in which they develop. It includes numerous teaching strategies for basic fundamental patterns and skills, perceptual motor integration, and health and related physical fitness. A unique feature of this part is the inclusion of information on weight management and the nutritional health of handicapped children and youth.

Part III, "Program Development," (Chapters 7 through 9), emphasizes assessment techniques for determining psychomotor strengths and weaknesses, testing instruments, interpretation of test results into recommendations, IEP development, and methods of achieving the least restrictive environment. A unique feature of this section is the inclusion of a model assessment report with recommendations. Also, a sample IEP is provided. Methods and techniques for including handicapped students in the regular physical education program are suggested.

Part IV, "Methods and Strategies of Good Teaching," (Chapters 10 and 11) focuses on noncategorized and categorized approaches to teaching methods for developing psychomotor skills. Noncategorized methods include task analysis, behavior management, and classroom organization. Categorized methods include those that should be practiced with particular types of disabilities. When used in combination, categorized and noncategorized methods and strategies can foster the success of handicapped students in physical education activities.

Part V, "Specific Skill Areas and Modifications," (Chapters 12 and 13), addresses games and lead-ups to team sports with techniques and adaptations suggested for effective programming with handicapped students. This section should be implemented when fundamental and perceptual skills have been developed. These skill areas are more for older elementary students or those at the secondary level, who are functioning below their chronological age.

Part VI, "Therapeutic Approaches," (Chapters 14 and 15), stresses understanding the value of therapeutic activities combined with the physical education program. It is hoped that this section will provide an introduction and overview of these approaches so the value of including them as part of the handicapped student's total physical education program can be recognized. A unique feature of this section is the inclu-

sion of the extension of physical education and leisure into the community.

The practicing professional is encouraged to use the text as a guide for implementing physical education programs for disabled youngsters. Preprofessionals should use the text to familiarize themselves with the global aspect of physical education program development with handicapped students. The fact that the methods and strategies suggested have been implemented in an actual program should entice students to learn and want to implement the strategies. *Physical Education Programming for Exceptional Learners* will help you put theoretical issues into practice.

Acknowledgments

Several individuals have provided me with the inspiration for writing this text. Those who stand out most are all the handicapped students and peer tutors who participated in Project PERMIT, the model mainstreaming program in physical education for which I served as coordinator. These children have demonstrated that the strategies, methods, and adaptations included in this text can provide successful physical education experiences.

The teachers who participated in Project PERMIT have shown me that when teachers care and are open to new methods and strategies for physical education, exciting and successful experiences result with handicapped students. My thanks to those teachers, Eunice Avriett, Beth Bell, Sherry Clark, Will England, Karen Farley, Janet Green, Betty Grissom, Louise Judd, Sarah Khlief, Wayne Lewis, Onilia Maxwell, Ruth Redus, Beyrl Reid, and Brenda Vickers. Also, to Margaret Allison, graduate assistant, for her good ideas and optimism, and to Anne Norman, the model program teacher who helped develop methods and put them into practice.

Several individuals have provided me with personal encouragement in professional development. To those persons I am grateful: Dr. Cecil Morgan, Paula Goodroe, Dr. Connie McIntyre, and my professional colleagues at Tennessee Tech University, Dr. David Dean Richey, Dr. Tom Willis, Dr. Marion Madison, and Dr. Bill J. Willis.

Special friends offered much support and encouragement during this project. I am grateful for the friendship of Gail and Robert Ring, Scott MacLeod, Marilyn Rackard, and Chris Coflin.

I am very appreciative of the editorial efforts of Aspen Systems Corporation. My thanks to Ms. Anne Gousha for supporting this project and for her encouragement, to Ms. Margaret Quinlin for her editorial assistance, comments, and advice in the development of this work, and to Ms. Carolyn Ormes for editorial comments.

Part I

Legislation and the Challenge

Chapter 1

P.L. 94–142 and Its Physical Education Requirements

Focus

- Defines Public Law 94–142, The Education of All Handicapped Children Act.
- Describes specific components of the law related to special education and physical education.
- Discusses the role of the physical education teacher in carrying out the mandate of the law regarding physical education programs for handicapped students.

This chapter is designed to define the legislative requirement for providing an appropriate education for handicapped students. With the advent of public attention to the needs of students with disabilities, educational practices, policies, and procedures have seen dramatic improvements within the last 20 years. In formulating the regulations of Public Law 94–142, legislators found it significant to include physical education as part of the federal mandate to meet the educational needs of exceptional students. Never before have disabled individuals had so many opportunities to be a part of the educational environment.

PUBLIC LAW 94–142

Public Law 94–142, The Education for All Handicapped Children Act, has and will continue to have profound effects on the educational provisions and opportunities for handicapped children. The major purpose of P.L. 94–142 is to ensure that all handicapped children have a free appropriate public education. The law issues explicit guidelines that have a significant impact on physical education and the efforts of those responsible for implementing such programs.

Teachers of physical education, or others responsible for this part of the handicapped student's curriculum, must comply with the guidelines of P.L. 94–142. At the time that President Gerald Ford signed P.L. 94–142 into effect in 1975, many handicapped students were being denied educational provisions, in some cases because of the severity of their handicaps, and were isolated from their peers whenever educational services were provided. Consequently, P.L. 94–142 has many broad-range purposes and provisions. The general content and provisions of the law include the following as cited in the August 1977 *Federal Register*:

- All handicapped children shall have a free appropriate public education designed to meet their unique needs. Handicapped children include the following:
  mentally retarded
  hard of hearing, deaf
  speech impaired
  visually handicapped
  seriously emotionally disturbed
  orthopedically impaired or other health impaired
  children with specific learning disabilities
- The law is concerned only with children who, because of their handicap, need special education and related services in order to learn.
- All handicapped children needing special education shall have an individualized educational plan based on their unique needs.
- Whenever and wherever possible, handicapped children shall be educated along with their regular peers, to

the maximum extent possible, within the least restrictive environment.

- Procedural safeguards are provided to assure the rights of parents and their handicapped children.
- Due process hearings are guaranteed to parents who may not be satisfied that a free appropriate education is being provided.
- Special education is defined as specially designed instruction which may include placement in a special class or program in the regular classroom. Special education may also refer to homebound and hospital instruction or in institutional settings.

Special Education and Physical Education

Special education, as defined by P.L. 94–142, also includes instruction in physical education. This is the one curriculum specified as an integral part of special education. Physical education is further defined as the development of the following:

physical and motor fitness
fundamental motor skills
motor development and movement education
instruction in aquatics and dance
individual and team games
sports that include intramural and lifetime sports

Exceptional students, receiving special education, must be educated within the regular physical education program unless specially designed physical education is otherwise indicated. However, it is still the local education agency's responsibility to either implement the handicapped child's specially designed physical education program or contract with other agencies to provide such services.

Related Services

Related services specifically defined by P.L. 94–142 can include social services, speech therapy, transportation, recreation, and physical and occupational therapy. Other types of services may be included as deemed necessary. However, physical educators must be aware that physical therapy is not to be a replacement for physical education services. Physical therapy is a related service and should be used in conjunction with physical education where needed. Physical therapy, in most instances, involves a corrective medical approach on an individual basis, whereas physical education includes the development of many skills related to sports, games, aquatics, dance, and motor and fitness skills. When physical education is replaced by a physical therapy program, the parent has a right to initiate a due process hearing. Handicapped students must not be denied the broad range of activities provided in the physical education program.

THE LEAST RESTRICTIVE ENVIRONMENT

P.L. 94–142 mandates that handicapped children be educated, to the maximum extent possible, with their non-handicapped peers. Only when handicapping conditions are so severe that they prevent successful participation in the regular classroom should handicapped children be placed in special or separate classes. This is why a continuum of service options must be made available for physical education. A continuum of service options in physical education would provide opportunities for partial and progressive interaction with regular peers.

Mainstreaming is the popular term educators use to refer to the least restrictive environment. Actually, P.L. 94–142 never mentions mainstreaming. Regular classroom and physical education teachers often lack a clear understanding of the concepts of mainstreaming and the least restrictive environment. Not every student with a handicapping condition can be placed or mainstreamed into a regular classroom. P.L. 94–142 clearly states that the educational placement and procedures must be based on the student's individual needs. A separate physical education class may very well be the most appropriate placement and the least restrictive environment for some handicapped students. Some schools tend to operate at the extremes. Either handicapped students are dumped into the regular physical education class or they are totally segregated. Neither may be appropriate for some handicapped students. In some cases, partial placement in the special or adapted physical education classroom, with part-time placement in the regular class, is possible.

By providing a variety of service alternatives, it is possible for progressive mainstreaming to take place. However, such a system is not easily developed. This requires trained personnel, concern, cooperation, and commitment. Unless dialogue and interaction occur at all levels, the least restrictive environment may be in portable buildings behind the main school building where all special education students are left and usually forgotten. Such separation creates negative attitudes and further segregation. Every effort must be made to give handicapped students opportunities to interact with their peers.

THE INDIVIDUALIZED EDUCATION PROGRAM (IEP)

All handicapped students receiving special education must have had developed for them an individualized education pro-

gram or plan, usually referred to as an IEP. A team made up of representatives of the public agency, the student's teacher, parents, and the student, where appropriate, shall formulate the IEP. When used appropriately and effectively, the IEP can be a valuable document that fosters communication about the handicapped student's needs. The IEP further ensures that the most appropriate educational experiences are being provided.

Unfortunately, many educators view the IEP as additional paperwork. An IEP is not as difficult to develop or as time consuming as most teachers perceive it to be. When developed through team effort, it is not difficult to put together and implement. The IEP is not a document to be developed by the special education teacher, who secures all the necessary signatures and then files it in a drawer, retrieving it only if the state department decides to monitor a local school district. The IEP is a vehicle by which educational services shall be delivered based on the needs of each handicapped student. It should be an ongoing process of commitment to the handicapped student's progress and achievement.

P.L. 94–142 specifies the content of the individualized educational program as follows:

- A statement of the handicapped student's *present levels of performance*.
- A statement of *annual goals* and *short term objectives* for instruction.
- A statement of the *special education* and *related services* to be provided and the extent to which participation will occur in the regular classroom.
- Appropriate *objective criteria* and *evaluation procedures* to be followed.
- Schedule for determining, *at least annually*, whether the goals and objectives are being achieved. (*Federal Register*, 1977, August)

Physical education personnel should take part in the IEP development process to provide input into the establishment of goals and objectives related to physical education. It may be necessary only to decide if placement in the regular class is possible. On the other hand, a physical education specialist may be involved to provide special physical education goals and objectives.

Figure 1–1 indicates the roles of the special education and physical education professional in developing the IEP. This takes a cooperative effort.

The IEP Committee

The IEP committee must follow certain guidelines, particularly with regard to participants and procedures. Turnbull,

Figure 1–1 Physical Educator's Role in IEPs

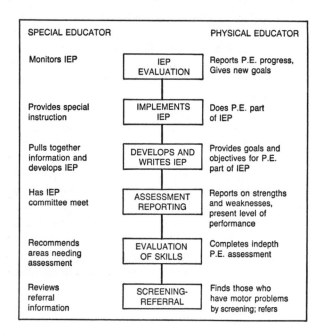

Strickland, and Brantly (1978) state that IEP participants should include the following persons:

- a representative of the public agency, other than the student's teacher, who has the qualifications to supervise the provisions of special education
- the handicapped student's teacher/teachers
- one or both of the parents/guardian
- the student, whenever appropriate
- other individuals at the request of the parent or public agency

The main purpose of the IEP committee is to develop the student's individualized educational program. It is during the IEP committee meeting that the type of physical education program is determined. Physical education may often be the weakest part of the handicapped student's IEP. Dunn (1979) reported that this area of the IEP often frustrates the IEP committee because of the lack of trained personnel with expertise in special or adapted physical education. The majority of the time the special education teacher ends up developing physical education goals and objectives for the handicapped student.

Parent Involvement

P.L. 94–142 provides parents with the opportunity to participate in the planning of their handicapped child's indi-

vidualized education program. In fact, public agencies must document their efforts to involve parents in the formulation of the IEP. The following concerns must be addressed:

- Written notification must be given in the parent's native language of the time and location of the IEP committee meeting.
- The IEP committee meeting must be scheduled at a mutually agreed on time and place.
- The public agency must ensure that the parent understands the proceedings of the IEP meeting.
- Parents must be provided with a copy of the student's IEP upon request.

If parents cannot attend the meeting, phone calls must be made to ensure their participation. Documentation of efforts to arrange meetings with the parents must be made. This includes records of phone calls and copies of all correspondence. If after all this parents reject all efforts, the IEP committee meeting may be held without the parents being present (Turnbull et al., 1978).

Due Process

Due process may be considered as a system to monitor the assurances that appropriate educational placement and experiences are being provided to each handicapped student. If parents are not satisfied with their handicapped child's educational placement, procedures, or the IEP, they may initiate a *due process hearing*.

P.L. 94–142 specifies due process safeguards. These include the following:

- The due process hearing must be conducted by someone not employed by the public agency responsible for the handicapped child's educational program.
- Parents, or any party to the hearing, have a right to be provided with and accompanied by counsel. Those with expertise concerning the child's handicapping condition may also be present.
- A verbatim record of the hearing, either written or recorded, must be available to anyone involved.
- If parents or anyone is aggrieved by the hearing's decisions at the local education district level, they may appeal such decisions at the local education district agency.
- Parents may obtain independent evaluations at the expense of the public agency if they do not agree with the agency's findings or if they feel the evaluation was unfair.
- Parents must be given written notice before any evaluations or changes in the student's educational placement are made.

ASSESSMENT AND EVALUATION

P.L. 94–142 provides safeguards concerning any evaluations of handicapped students. According to the law, all testing and evaluation materials used for evaluation and placement of handicapped students must be selected and administered in a way that does not racially or culturally discriminate. No single testing procedure may be used as the sole criterion for developing the IEP for handicapped students. Evaluation must occur in all areas of suspected disability. These areas shall include, where appropriate:

- health
- vision and hearing
- social and emotional levels.
- general intelligence
- academic performance
- communicative status
- motor abilities

The evaluations must be made by the IEP committee members, including at least a teacher or other specialist with knowledge in the area of the suspected disability. This may be interpreted as a person with expertise in adapted physical education when motor problems are suspected as part of the handicapped student's disability. However, in many public schools there are no specialists with knowledge about motor disabilities of handicapped students. This is particularly true in rural areas.

SERVICE DELIVERY OPTIONS

Special education has developed a cascade system of service delivery based on the location of services from the least restrictive to the most restrictive environment. A hierarchy of services developed by Reynolds (1977) would include the following service delivery options, listed from the most restrictive to the least restrictive environment:

- hospitals and homebound instruction
- hospital school
- residential school
- special day school
- full-time special education class
- part-time special education class
- regular classroom in addition to part-time resource room
- regular classroom with supplementary learning aids
- regular classroom

In the past, adapted physical education programs were located in special schools and some training was provided in self-contained classrooms. Only recently have special physical education programs become more readily available in public schools. In some states entire school districts have well-designed special physical education programs. However, there are still school districts that do not adequately provide special physical education programs that comply with P.L. 94–142. The negative results are often related to lack of financial support and not enough trained personnel. Since physical education is a part of special education, it should be implemented within the same service delivery structure. The two professions of special and physical education must work closely together to provide successful programs for handicapped students.

Aufsesser (1981) suggested a modified service delivery system used in special education to implement physical education. Listed from the most restrictive to the least restrictive environment, Aufsesser's model includes:

- adapted physical education in a special school
- full-time self-contained physical education in a regular school
- self-contained physical education class with partial regular physical education class
- part-time self-contained adapted resource physical education with regular physical education
- regular physical education class with consultation from the special physical education consultant
- full-time regular physical education.

A full system of service delivery for physical education is not as widely implemented as the services for special education. Each should be delivered in the same manner since physical education is included as part of special education under P.L. 94–142.

By examining a service delivery model in special physical education, one can understand various levels of the least restrictive environment. As previously noted, not every child with a handicapping condition can function within a regular classroom setting; a variety of service options must be made available so that the concept of the least restrictive environment is realized.

Adapted physical education in a special school or other type of residential facility would be concerned with special needs students with a particular type of handicapping condition. Groups might include those who are blind, severely mentally retarded, deaf, multiply handicapped, or emotionally disturbed. Usually, such residential schools and centers are located in major regional areas. Buildings are designed to be barrier free, and teachers are employed who have expertise in the type of handicapped person served. The special physical education instructor should also be trained in providing physical education instruction to the particular handicapped persons in residence. In this instance, the special physical education instructor needs to work closely with other professionals serving students in this setting. These might include physical therapists, occupational therapists, psychologists, physicians, and vocational and career directors. In addition, in residential centers and special schools, the special physical education instructor may be asked to develop and supervise special events and field day programs.

A full-time self-contained physical education class within a regular school would have students with similar handicapping conditions. These may be moderately retarded, behavior disordered, or multiply handicapped. The special physical education teacher in self-contained classes may work with a variety of students who have similar physical and motor deficits. These students may not have developed many of the basic skills required to participate in simple games. A large part of the instruction would concern the development of basic motor skills, physical development, social behavior, and cooperative activities.

In self-contained classes with partial regular physical education placement, the special physical education teacher would provide the major part of the individualized program. However, the specialist would work closely with the regular physical education teacher to develop an ongoing program where self-contained students could participate in the regular physical education class for some activities that skill levels would allow. Activities must be carefully analyzed and selected. Also, the regular class should be prepared for the arrival of the special needs students so that a positive and accepting environment can be established.

Part-time self-contained adapted resource physical education with part-time regular physical education would occur if special needs students could manage several components of the regular physical education curriculum. Generally, any type of disability could be managed. For example, a mentally retarded student may be able to manage some of the less complicated gymnastics skills. However, in advanced gymnastics, placement may not be possible in the regular education setting. Also, mentally retarded students may be able to handle games of lower organization but may not be able to take part in those of high complexity. During those phases of the curriculum, placement within the self-contained physical education class may be necessary. An example of placement might include two days per week in the regular physical education class and three days per week in the self-contained class. This approach works well in the elementary school. An activity-by-activity method may have to be used at the secondary level.

Placement in the regular physical education class with consultation from a special physical education teacher would be suitable for special needs students with mild handicapping conditions. These might include students with mild visual perceptual problems, mild behavior disorders, or mild hear-

ing impairments. Students with mild orthopedic disabilities could also be included. The regular teacher may need assistance with particular teaching strategies and materials. Aid in modifying equipment is often necessary. Even though consultation on a regular basis may be necessary, it is the regular physical education teacher who is responsible for the majority of the special needs student's program.

Full-time regular physical education placement would include special needs students who, in spite of their handicapping condition, can participate in the regular physical education program. Generally, students with mild handicapping conditions are placed full time in the regular physical education class. This placement must meet the individual needs of the special student. Meyen (1978) suggests that the regular teacher should have training in the management of special needs students. Training should include the modification of teaching strategies and materials. Access to a special teacher, as well as resource materials, should be available to the regular teacher.

Another concept not used frequently in physical education is the resource room. This is probably the most widely used service delivery option for special education in the public schools. This concept has some interesting implications for special physical education. The resource room in special physical education would be the level between placement in the regular physical education class and the part-time self-contained physical education class. This service option would be designed for the special needs student who could function in the regular physical education class but more individualized instruction might be needed related to problems resulting from a particular handicapping condition. For example, learning-disabled students who have visual perceptual problems may also have poor eye-hand and eye-foot coordination. Intense individualized remedial and developmental programming may be necessary in these areas beyond the amount that the regular physical education teacher can give. Thus, these students may need to attend a resource room in physical education where a specialist can provide intensive individualized training for an hour each day.

With a variety of service delivery options in physical education, the needs of special students can be met more effectively. Many schools have, at most, two options in physical education. These include either self-contained programs or regular programs.

ISSUES AND CONCERNS

P.L. 94–142 has many implications for the field of physical education. The law clearly states that physical education is an integral part of special education and that it be made available to every handicapped child. Physical educators must be aware of their responsibility for providing an appropriate physical education experience whether the handicapped student is mainstreamed or requires specially designed physical education services. If no specially designed instruction is required in physical education, the student may participate in whatever physical education program is offered to regular students.

Geddes (1981) reported that some special education and regular classroom teachers may use some motor and physical activities as supplements to their classroom instruction. These should in no way be used to replace the physical education needs of the handicapped student, just as physical therapy and recreation may not be substituted for physical education when specially designed instruction is required for the handicapped student.

The issue of who shall provide physical education services is not addressed by P.L. 94–142. However, the law does state that handicapped children must have programs designed to meet their needs. Thus, if a local school district does not have specific personnel trained in physical education, then the regular classroom teacher, if knowledgeable in physical education, may provide such services. If, on the other hand, the appropriate program is not being provided, the local education agency must see that the handicapped student's physical education needs are being met. Local agencies may contract for such services when they are unable to provide adequately trained personnel.

Trained personnel with adequate knowledge concerning the implementation of physical education programs for students with special needs are sorely needed. P.L. 94–142 requires that every state establish and implement a comprehensive system of personnel development. This system shall include the preservice and inservice training of general and special education personnel. The state agency must be responsible for carrying out such plans. Many states have developed inservice training strategies that have been relatively effective in providing a general awareness of P.L. 94–142. Unless inservice is comprehensive and ongoing, it is not effective in giving teachers the skills, materials, and resources for teaching handicapped students.

Folio and Durley (1981) reported that teachers seem to prefer ongoing inservice training with consultation within their classrooms related to methods, procedures, and materials for working with handicapped students. Teachers also indicated that they prefer to see a model in practice. School systems should at least provide a consulting specialist to give assistance to the regular classroom physical education teacher who has students in the regular class.

POINTS TO REMEMBER

1. P.L. 94–142 assures that a free appropriate public education shall be provided to all handicapped students needing special education.

2. The law contains procedural safeguards related to testing, placement, and parental rights.

3. Students with disabilities must be educated within the least restrictive environment.

4. The IEP is developed by a designated IEP committee with parents involved in the process.

5. Physical education is defined as an integral part of special education.

6. Related services, such as physical therapy, cannot be substituted for instruction in physical education.

7. Physical education services must follow the same regulations as those for delivering special education services.

REFERENCES

Aufsesser, P.M. (1981). Adapted physical education; A look back, a look ahead. *Journal of Health, Physical Education, Recreation and Dance, 52,* 28–31.

Dunn, J.M. (1979). *Adaptive physical education: A resource guide for teachers, administrators, and parents.* Eugene, OR: Oregon State University.

Folio, M.R., & Durley, M. (1981). *A resource guide outline for mainstreaming in physical education.* Unpublished manuscript, Tennessee Technological University, Cookeville, TN.

Geddes, D. (1981). *Psychomotor individualized educational programs for intellectual, learning and behavioral disabilities.* Boston: Allyn & Bacon.

Federal Register. 96th Congress, Rules and regulations on P.L. 94–142, August 23, 1977.

Meyen, E.L. (1978). *Exceptional Children and Youth: An Introduction.* Denver: Love Publishing Co.

Reynolds, M.C. (1977). *Teaching exceptional children in all America's schools.* Reston, VA: Council for Exceptional Children.

Turnbull, A.P., Strickland, B.B., & Brantly, J.C. (1978). *Developing and implementing IEP's.* Columbus, OH: Charles E. Merrill.

Chapter 2

Psychomotor and Learning Characteristics of Exceptional Students

Focus

- Defines handicapping conditions.
- Provides an overview of learning and psychomotor characteristics of students with disabilities.
- Discusses the general implications for physical education based on characteristics of disabling conditions.

If one approaches teaching from the total child concept, then it is significant to understand the learning and motor characteristics of exceptional students. A general understanding of these characteristics will enable the physical education service provider to be more effective in dealing with exceptional populations.

By understanding the characteristics and motor development needs of exceptional students, educators can see that many characteristics may cut across different categories of exceptionalities, particularly if one focuses on skill strengths and deficits. For example, mentally retarded students as well as behavior-disordered children can have behavioral problems. The approaches to changing the behavior may be similar, if there is not a large discrepancy in intelligence.

Care must be taken, however, not to stereotype handicapped students. They are a heterogeneous group and deserve individual consideration. If behaviors are targeted, sometimes similar teaching methods can be used that will generalize to several different handicapped students.

This chapter focuses on the psychomotor and learning characteristics of exceptional students, providing a background for the chapter dealing with teaching methodology. For more in-depth information related to causes, nature, incidence, and prevalence, references should be made to the readings listed at the end of this chapter.

MENTAL RETARDATION

Current definitions of mental retardation include both intelligence and adaptive behavior. P.L. 94–142, in fact, protects individuals from being classified as mentally retarded on the basis of intellectual deficits alone. The most widely used and accepted definition for educational purposes is the one established by the American Association on Mental Deficiency (AAMD).

According to Grossman (1983), the AAMD definition of mental retardation includes the following:

> Mental retardation refers to significantly subaverage general intellectual functioning, that result in, or are associated with impairments in adaptive behavior, manifested during the developmental period (p. 7).

Each individual must meet all three established criteria before being classified as mentally retarded.

Subaverage general intellectual functioning to a significant degree is measured by standardized individually administered intelligence tests. Significant subaverage general intellectual functioning by the AAMD definition refers to an intelligence test score that is greater than two standard deviations below the average score on a standardized intelligence test. Approximately 3 percent of the population falls into the category of two standard deviations below the mean on standardized intelligence tests. Thus, if the mean is 100 on an IQ test and one standard deviation below the mean is a minus 15 points, two standard deviations would be 30 points. Consequently, to be considered mentally retarded, a person would have to score 69 or less on the intelligence test.

Associated impairments in adaptive behavior refer to the effectiveness or degree to which the child meets the standards of personal independence and social skills expected of peers of the same age and social group (Grossman, 1983). Adaptive behavior may also refer to the ability to make appropriate adjustments to environmental demands. Thus, adaptive behavior is different for specific age levels. Crowe, Auxter, and Pyfer (1981) relate deficits in adaptive behavior to the lack of or delay in acquiring perceptual motor skills, the lack of motor skills to socially interact at a young age, and the lack of general experiences.

It is well to include adaptive behavior as a part of the classification of individuals as mentally retarded. If the IQ is used alone, far more individuals would be classified as mentally retarded. There are many individuals who cannot function successfully in school and who cannot score above 69 on an intelligence test but function within their social environment. As a result, some individuals may be retarded as far as academic work is concerned, but succeed quite well in their homes and surrounding communities.

The developmental period portion of the AAMD definition refers to the first 18 years of life. As a result, someone who met the other criteria of mental retardation after age 18 would not be considered mentally retarded according to the AAMD standards.

Educators classify mentally retarded individuals by the degree of educability and the specific skill levels of a particular individual (Smith, 1971). The educational classifications closely correspond to the AAMD classifications. (See Table 2–1.)

Mentally retarded students can be better understood by looking at their general learning characteristics and motor development levels and potential. The intent is not to stereotype mentally retarded individuals, but to discuss in a broad sense characteristics that are generally found in different levels of this population. This will produce some general

Table 2–1 Educational Levels of Retardation Compared with AAMD Levels

AAMD Level	Educational Level
Mild retardation	Educable mentally retarded (EMR)
Moderate retardation	Trainable mentally retarded (TMR)
Severe and profound retardation	Severely mentally retarded (SMR)

guidelines for providing physical education activities. Later, the information can be used as a background for the chapter discussing specific methodology.

MILD RETARDATION

Jerome

Jerome is a mildly retarded 9-year-old receiving his academic program in a regular classroom for half a day and a resource room for the other half day. Academically, Jerome functions at about 7 years in some academic areas, math and reading, but social skills are at almost his age level. Motor skills are more like that of a 6-year-old. Jerome enjoys simple motor games and skills but has difficulty with coordinated and more complex tasks such as hopping, jumping, and simple adaptations of basic skills. Physically, Jerome looks more like a second grader. He receives most of his physical education with a regular second grade class and has special instruction on skill deficits with the help of a peer tutor three days per week.

General Learning Characteristics

Heward and Orlansky (1984) emphasize that mildly retarded or educable retarded persons will generally acquire social, communication, and motor skills that are similar to those of their nonretarded peers. Mildly retarded individuals will develop a repertoire of basic skills in math, reading, writing, and vocational courses. Usually, if given proper educational intervention, they can become productive members of society. Most of their difficulty in learning relates to higher cognitive thought processes and abstract thinking. Geddes (1981) reports that difficulty is often associated with reasoning and critical evaluation of problems. Leadership roles are not often assumed by mentally retarded individuals. The physical educator should carefully explore the student's ability before placing a mentally retarded student in a leadership role. MacMillan (1982) suggests that mentally retarded students have poor self-esteem as a result of being labeled and not accepted by their peers.

Academic skills up to the sixth grade can be acquired by mildly retarded persons. MacMillan (1982) further suggests that mentally retarded children who are mainstreamed tend to have higher academic achievement than those who are not, if the mainstreaming situation is appropriate.

Psychomotor Characteristics

Numerous investigations of motor skill levels of mildly retarded subjects have been completed. These studies have included the areas of physical fitness, coordination, flexibility, running speed, balance, reaction time, and movement time.

Measures of Physical Fitness

One of the major studies regarding physical fitness performance of mentally retarded was conducted by Rarick, Widdop, and Broadhead (1970). Their study investigated physical fitness levels of mildly retarded boys and girls compared with levels of normal boys and girls. They found that mildly retarded boys and girls followed the same fitness patterns as normal children, however, both sexes in the mentally retarded group were substantially behind standards of fitness and motor performance levels established on normal children. Other findings demonstrated that mildly mentally retarded boys were significantly better in sit-ups than the mildly retarded girls.

As ages increased, mildly retarded boys were found to be better at sit-ups than mentally retarded girls. Also, mildly retarded boys were found to be stronger than moderately and severely retarded subjects (Rarick & McQuillan, 1977).

Speed studies by Rarick, Dobbins, and Broadhead (1976) found that measures on the 50-yard dash among retarded and normal children differed. Nonretarded youngsters were able to run faster than retarded children. In fact, the gaps were greater as age increased.

When comparisons of mildly retarded children were made with lower-functioning retarded children, the mildly retarded were found to be superior in running speed.

Cardiovascular endurance measures have also been found to be different between retarded and nonretarded groups. Sengstock (1966) found that mildly retarded youngsters had lower levels of cardiovascular proficiency than normal children. Mildly retarded youngsters were found to have greater levels of cardiovascular proficiency than lower-functioning mentally retarded subjects.

Shuttle run performances were compared between mildly retarded children and their nonretarded peers. Sengstock (1966) demonstrated that mildly retarded children were slower in performing the shuttle run than normal children of the same age.

Francis and Rarick (1959) compared the physical performance of over 200 mentally retarded boys and girls classified as educable. The main trend in their findings indicated that educable mentally retarded boys were generally better on several measures. The researcher used specific measures that could be easily understood and administered. The measures included grip strength, 35-yard dash, dynamic strength (broad jump and vertical jump), tennis and softball throw for distance, balance beam walk, agility run, and squat thrust.

Specific Motor Skills

Cratty (1974) also measured levels of specific motor skills between mildly retarded and moderately retarded youngsters. Skills included body perception, throwing, tracking, balance, and locomotor agility. In all skill areas, mildly retarded youngsters were found to be superior to lower functioning mentally retarded children on these measures.

Cratty (1974) also investigated differences in accuracy and precision while performing motor skills between educable mentally retarded and normal peers. For example, accuracy and precision were lower among the mentally retarded group than the normal group when performing hopping and jumping skills. Cratty (1980) also noted that mentally retarded children generally have delayed reactions to stimuli. Thus, their reaction times tend to be slower than those of their normal peers.

Geddes (1981) makes a major point related to the findings that mentally retarded children are inferior in motor performance when compared with their normal peers:

> Teachers should not make overt generalizations about how mentally retarded students will perform motorically. Each student's motor skills must be viewed individually!

Physical Education Intervention

When given the opportunity to receive physical education programming, mentally retarded students in the educable category respond well and can receive most of their physical education instruction with their nonretarded peers in most cases. Positive effects on self-concept and increases in motor performance have been documented, particularly when attention was paid to individual needs. These trends have been confirmed by researchers with preschool mildly retarded and adolescents (see for example, Chasey & Wyrick, 1970; Corder, 1969; Folio, 1975; Goodwin, 1970).

Implications for Physical Education

Mentally retarded children in the educable category need an all-around physical education program that offers opportunities to practice a variety of skills in many different situations. Sherrill (1981) notes that when working with a skill, providing many different experiences such as throwing many different objects in different activities helps the mildly retarded learn and transfer the task.

Mildly retarded children can benefit from being educated in settings with their nonretarded peers. This teaches play skills and good social development for younger mildly retarded children. Older mildly retarded children need to learn leisure activities that will assist them as adults in their reactional experiences. Most of the leisure activities of mildly retarded persons may take the form of individual and dual type sports such as swimming, bowling, dancing, and skating.

MODERATE RETARDATION

Andrea

Andrea is an 11-year-old considered to be trainable mentally retarded. All of her academic programming occurs in a self-contained classroom. Physical education activities are also provided with her group of eight other students functioning on a similar level as Andrea. Andrea's primary goals in physical education include the development and some refinement of basic fundamental movements, physical fitness, social interaction, the development of some group activities that consist of simple games, and training for the Special Olympics. Andrea entered the bowling events in the fall Olympics and completed the standing long jump and softball throw in the spring events. Andrea is beginning to like to participate in small group activities that are of the low organized type. She enjoys simple dances and keeping time to music. She understands short, simple commands.

General Learning Characteristics

Another term used to identify moderately retarded is *trainable*. In most instances, moderately retarded students will not benefit from traditional academic programs offered in traditional regular classrooms.

Learning deficits in moderately retarded children can be seen before school age, whereas in mildly retarded youngsters, evidence of retardation or developmental lags may not be noticed until school age (MacMillan, 1982).

Many moderately retarded children will have some form of brain damage. Neisworth and Smith (1978) report the incidence of brain damage in about 50 percent of individuals classified as moderately retarded. Broader discrepancies in skills are noted between moderately retarded and nonretarded youngsters as they grow older.

The learning potential of moderately retarded students will include basic language concepts such as common daily words used in familiar surroundings, self-help skills, and simple number concepts.

Social skills can also be developed so that appropriate social behaviors can be expected, though on an elementary level. Reminders may have to be given regarding the social skills desired, since generalizations from one situation to another are difficult for mentally retarded persons at this level.

Moderately retarded students may have problems with attention, memory, recognition, and generalization of learned skills. Motor skill development of the mentally retarded student in the moderate category is important since many of the kinds of self-help and vocational skills will be heavily weighted with motor processes and responses rather than more abstract processing. Employment for moderately retarded individuals will be primarily in a sheltered environment. Skills that are required may involve sorting, tying, and other manipulative movements with the hands. Modifications can be built into the system for learning the task; however, the motor skill is very important.

Psychomotor Characteristics

As the degree of mental retardation increases, so do the deficits in psychomotor skill levels. Studies of the motor characteristics of moderately retarded individuals reveal wider margins of motor skill deficits than among mildly retarded youngsters when compared to nonretarded peers.

Geddes (1981) reported increased deficits in fitness levels, balance, general body coordination, muscular strength and endurance, locomotor skills, and reaction time. Sherrill (1981) reported that moderately retarded youngsters, up to age 9, will be still in need of basic motor skill development. Motorically, students at this level, will be very similar to preschool children.

Down's Syndrome

Since Down's Syndrome individuals make up a significant segment of the moderately retarded category, their motor characteristics will be discussed separately. The motor and physical attributes of Down's Syndrome subjects have been studied, comparing them with normal children.

Cratty (1980) reports several motor patterns found in Down's children and their differences from normal children. Cratty found that Down's children have immature throwing patterns and are usually three or four years behind normal peers of the same chronological age.

Locomotor skills are also immature, with the body not well coordinated when trying to perform skills such as running, hopping, jumping, and skipping. Timing in motor performance is poor.

Balance, according to Cratty (1980), is also poor among Down's children, particularly for standing on one foot. Balance with eyes closed is significantly more difficult for Down's children compared with balance with the eyes open.

Perceptual motor integration is more delayed in Down's children than mildly retarded subjects of the same chronological age. Knight, Hyman, and Wozny (1965) found Down's persons to have more difficulty with tactual and kinesthetic discrimination than other perceptual areas. Visual perception is more developed among Down's children than other forms of perception.

Flexibility among Down's children is greater than that of other mentally retarded children. Generally, ligaments and supporting tissue may be weak and the musculature is somewhat flabby. Down's children and adults tend to have more problems with overweight and obesity.

Susceptibility to respiratory infections is common since the respiratory system is weak. Folio (1981) reported that Down's children were extremely low in zinc and iron. Zinc is known to aid in strengthening the body's immune system. When Down's children are infected, they may have a slower recovery time.

Congenital heart defects are also found among Down's persons. In most cases surgical procedures can correct septum defects. Fatigue may be more common among Down's children compared with other retarded children and should be considered when having them participate in endurance activities.

Physical Education Intervention

Moderately retarded children, including Down's Syndrome subjects, respond favorably to physical education programming. Several investigators have demonstrated through research that improvements do occur in performance of motor development and physical fitness.

Taylor (1969) found that a program of physical fitness activities administered over a six-month period was successful in increasing skills of trainable mentally retarded children based on measures with the Krauss-Weber Physical Fitness Test.

Another study by Sharpe (1968) revealed that a physical education program of fitness activities and basic motor skills proved to be successful with trainable mentally retarded children, particularly on measures with the Hayden Physical Fitness Test for Mentally Retarded.

Morrison (1972) found that with a physical education program based on diagnostic prescriptive instruction, trainable mentally retarded subjects improved in basic fundamental motor skills and patterns. The subjects were preschool trainable retarded children. Morrison's training program, although based on each child's needs, consisted of sensory motor training and skills that normally occur at the preschool level, such as walking, climbing, jumping, throwing, etc. This study is different from the other intervention studies cited in that Morrison stressed that a detailed analysis of each subject's skills be completed prior to initiating the physical education program.

Implications for Physical Education

Moderately retarded youngsters will require more individualized programming related to motor skill development than mildly retarded youngsters. These students will, on the average, have to have physical education within a self-contained setting. However, after some degree of social ability and motor skill achievement is acquired, moderately retarded youngsters can be educated within the regular physical education class if specific procedures and guidelines are followed that will allow for peer instruction, good behavior management techniques, and a curriculum of basic skills. Younger moderately retarded youngsters, ages 6–9, most likely can function with nonretarded peers ages 4–6, provided that social and behavioral skills are somewhat acceptable. Older moderately retarded youngsters will have more success in physical education activities that place less emphasis on team sports and more emphasis on individual and dual type activities such as swimming, bowling, dancing, track and field, and recreational games.

SEVERE MENTAL RETARDATION

Michael

Michael is ten years old and severely mentally retarded. His educational program is delivered in a public school self-contained classroom with eight other students who have similar educational needs and abilities. Michael has some receptive language and only responds to one-word commands, such as "Eat," "Drink," "Look." Motor skills are limited at this point. A few basic skills are present such as walking, but the pattern is immature with a wide base and no arm integration. He does attempt to throw a ball, but without directionality. Assistance is needed to climb steps, and he must be totally aided in descending stairs. There is no continued purposeful movement to interact with the environment. Movements are more for self-stimulation, such as rocking, swaying, and banging objects. Physical education is delivered on a one-to-one basis by an adapted specialist. Michael's program is designed to fill in gross motor gaps, sensory motor training, balance, body awareness, and tracking.

General Learning Characteristics

Severe delays and deficits in learning may be noted in severely and profoundly mentally retarded individuals. In addition, there are usually accompanying disorders such as neuromuscular and medical problems. In some cases, multiply handicapped persons may fall into the severely retarded category.

Accompanying disorders such as visual defects, hearing and speech problems, growth retardation, and delayed maturation are also found. Communication disorders make it more difficult to teach these individuals than those who are less impaired. Fortunately, advanced technology is making communication and teaching more easily accomplished with this population.

Behavioral Characteristics

Inappropriate behaviors are found frequently in persons who are severely retarded. The behaviors are more severe when intervention begins at later ages. Self-stimulating behaviors occur such as rocking and head banging. Body patting and spinning are also evident.

Self-injurious behaviors have also been observed within this category of retardation. Examples include biting, scratching, and pinching one's own body. Some of these behaviors can also be seen in children who are severely emotionally disturbed. In cases of severe mental retardation, many are dually diagnosed as being mentally retarded and emotionally disturbed. Individuals within this category may be in constant motion or exhibit very little movement responses at all. There is little development of self-help, motor, or language skills in children with severe and profound retardation.

Psychomotor Characteristics

Motor skills may be very limited or, if developed, gaps may exist. Mobility may be limited as a result of accompanying neurological impairments and structural deformities. Even simple movements such as holding up the head, rolling over, and sitting are impossible without an assistive device. However, technology is also advancing in mechanical aids for assisting with body positioning and movement for severely handicapped individuals. Even as teenagers and adults, severely mentally retarded youngsters will function motorically like preschool children. Meaningful movement and interaction with objects may be much like that of an infant under one year of age. The severely retarded student may mouth a tennis ball, rather than throw it. Or the severely retarded child may bang two tennis balls together.

Sensory motor integration is limited among this population. Motor responses may be inappropriate to the sensory input, no matter what sensory modality is used. Some children may not like to be touched or may even be tactually defensive, withdrawing from touching objects or being touched.

Physical deformity, such as hip dislocation and postural deviation, is present in some cases of severely retarded children. Muscle tone can vary from very little tone to hypertonic musculature.

Physical Education Intervention

A basic approach to physical education for this level of retardation would involve the development of fundamental movement that is also integrated with sensory input. Another approach is to eliminate unwanted and inappropriate movement.

Webb (1969) suggests that physical education activities for severely retarded groups concentrate on improving four psychomotor components. These include:

- awareness and arousal levels
- purposeful movement
- manipulative skills
- posture and motor transport skills

Webb and Koller's program enables some skill to be developed as positive responding to environmental stimuli. The implication is to provide a variety of sensory stimuli using a structural procedure.

Another approach that is successful with mentally retarded children is that developed by Ayres (1972). Sensory integration is the basic theme. Ayres' program is heavily weighted with sensory integration activities as well as nonlocomotor and locomotor activities. Also included are activities to foster vestibular and balance functions. Ayres includes a thorough developmental assessment with her program and has developed several of her own tests: the *California Kinesthesia and Tactile Perception Tests* and the *Southern California Motor Accuracy Tests.*

Physical therapy is used extensively with severely retarded youngsters, particularly when neurological impairments accompany retardation. The aim is to offer programming that will provide the student with developmental skills of movement and prevent postural deformities from occurring within the structure of the body. Other goals of physical therapy are to facilitate the development of normal reflexes and inhibit primitive reflexes in children with neurological problems. While it is not the physical educator's role to provide or initiate physical therapy, there may be occasions when the adapted specialist in physical education will work closely with the physical therapist to assist in implementing the routine exercises established by the therapist.

Some of the motor skill areas that may be included in the curriculum are

- prelocomotor skills: sitting, rolling, standing
- manipulative skills: grasping, and object exploration
- locomotor skills, with or without assistive devices

Other curriculum considerations need to be included for the older severely retarded individual. Sherrill (1981) suggests that older severely retarded persons be afforded the opportunities to participate in physical activities that closely coincide with the Special Olympics, such as modified track and field, swimming, and wheelchair events. Sherrill recommends that this program be ongoing, rather than a special event.

EMOTIONAL AND BEHAVIOR DISORDERS

Tracy

Tracy, a third grader, is almost a year behind in academic skills. She is considered to be anxious and fearful, particularly in new situations and when asked to perform new and unfamiliar tasks. She often says that "she can't" when asked to do a new task. At times, when in group activities in physical education, her attention span is short and she will often exhibit hostility when she does not want to do a skill. She may hit other children or become verbally aggressive. Tracy requires a good deal of individualized attention from the teacher, and because of her behavior problems, she receives physical education in an adapted classroom with only seven other students. Plans for placing her in regular physical education are being considered as soon as her behavior improves and fears lessen.

Steve

Steve is a sophomore in high school and has a poor self-concept. He often tries to please his peers by doing things that get him into trouble. He is often creating disturbances in class because some of his pals think it is funny. He has failed several subjects and has little motivation to study. Steve does not like to have physical education. He is overweight and has difficulty performing many skills in team sports. Students tease him when he does go to class. Steve is placed in an adapted class to concentrate mainly on weight loss, increasing his self-concept, and improving his skills. Steve goes to regular physical education for some activities. The regular teacher is trying to develop more positive acceptance from regular students while Steve is in the adapted class. Hopefully, this combination will improve Steve's self-image.

Emotional and behavior disorders are difficult to identify since the perceivers of the behavior may view disturbed acts differently. What is disruptive or disturbed behavior to one teacher may not be to another. Haring (1978) classifies children as emotionally disturbed when someone with authority so labels them. Some handicapping conditions are quite visible, whereas behavior and emotional disorders are visible by behaviors that are observed. Behaviors can range from extreme withdrawal to extreme aggressive acts.

Definitions

Emotional disturbance is defined under P.L. 94–142 as:

a condition exhibiting one or more of the following characteristics:

- an inability to learn which cannot be explained by intellectual, sensory or health factors.
- an inability to build or maintain satisfactory relationships with peers and teachers.
- inappropriate feelings or actions under normal circumstances.
- general mood of unhappiness or depression.
- tendency to develop physical symptoms related with personal and school problems. (Federal Register, 1977, August)

This definition refers to the seriously emotionally disturbed and not to those who may be socially maladjusted.

According to Hallahan and Kauffman (1982), there is general agreement as to what emotional disturbance and the behaviors manifested by the condition may be. Their definition includes:

- behavior that goes to an extreme and not that which is slightly unusual
- behavior that is different and chronic which does not readily disappear
- behavior that is unacceptable because of social and cultural expectations

General Learning Characteristics of Disturbed Students

Peer relationships are a problem for disturbed students, since they are often rejected by their peers (Schultz & Turnbull, 1984). Many children who are disturbed try desperately to be accepted. Unfortunately, the harder they try the more they are rejected because of their disruptive or annoying behaviors.

Classroom problems occur from a variety of behaviors, such as acting out, clowning as a way of avoiding feelings and academic responsibilities, verbal aggression, physical aggression, withdrawal, daydreaming, etc. These forms of behavior, which indicate emotional disturbance, affect the student's academic ability.

Hallahan and Kauffman (1982) indicate that the myth that many emotionally disturbed children are intelligent is false. They report that intelligence measures of emotionally disturbed children fall into the dull normal range. Many more disturbed children fall within the slow learner category. Mildly retarded children may also demonstrate signs of behavior and emotional disorders. Such children are more likely to be underachievers in school.

Behavioral Characteristics

Geddes (1981) explains that behaviors exhibited by disturbed children may be outward expressions of their inner feelings. These may include:

- frustration
- fear
- anxiety
- insecurity
- poor self-concept
- feelings of worthlessness and inadequacy
- anger and hostility

These feelings may be demonstrated by moods of crying, depression, temper tantrums, emotional outbursts, and physical abuse of other children.

Behaviors can be placed into the two major categories of aggression or withdrawal.

Aggression

Aggressive acts are the ones teachers most often address in the classroom. Examples of aggressive behaviors often noticed in school settings include:

- hitting
- fighting
- teasing
- noncompliance
- destructive acts

Withdrawal

Withdrawn behavior is more noticeable when it reaches a severe stage. Mild forms of withdrawal are usually not addressed by teachers. Examples of withdrawn behaviors include:

- passivity
- daydreaming
- immature behaviors: baby talk, thumb sucking, etc.
- lack of social interaction
- playing by oneself
- feelings of sadness
- listlessness and fatigue

It is important to remember that all individuals do experience these feelings at one time or another. When in a child the feelings become chronic and interfere with the normal routine, the child can be considered emotionally disturbed or behavior disordered.

Characteristics of the Severely Emotionally Disturbed

Severely disturbed children exhibit behaviors that are extremely different from their normal peers. These may include severely depressed and withdrawn behaviors, self-injurious behaviors such as biting oneself or banging one's head. Severe behavior disorders and emotional disturbance may accompany other handicapping conditions such as mental retardation and multiple disabilities, although not in all cases. Severely disturbed students may be deficient in other areas of abilities. Other deficits in severely disturbed individuals reported by Hallahan and Kauffman (1982) include:

- language and speech deficits
- self-stimulating behaviors
- patting one's body or body parts
- hand clapping and arm flapping
- spinning the body or objects for extended time periods
- overaggression toward objects and other persons
- biting, scratching, kicking, or other self-injurious behaviors

Autism

Attempts have been made to define autism as early as 1943. However, Knoblock (1982) defines autism as a developmental disability that appears during the first three years of life. Autism is a complex psychological disorder that may result from brain disorders. Knoblock (1982) suggests that autistic children may have many characteristics, however, those that are generally common among this group include:

- Impairments in emotional relationships that result in abnormal responses to people and objects.
- Extremes in movement from hyperkinesis to catatonic statue-like postures.
- Speech and langauge may be absent or idosyncratic words may be spoken.
- Responses to visual, tactual, and auditory sensations can range from excessive to none.
- Intellectual ability may appear normal at times and as severe retardation at other times.
- Self-stimulating behaviors occur in the forms of rocking, rolling, gazing, and hand flapping.

Psychomotor Characteristics

Students with emotional disorders are a heterogeneous group in terms of psychomotor skill development. No definitive set of psychomotor deficits can be generalized to this group. Wiseman (1982) explains that the psychomotor performance of emotionally disturbed and behavior-disordered students may vary. In many cases some of the following difficulties in motor performance have been observed, as reviewed by Wiseman:

- poor eye-hand coordination due to distractability
- poor body control leading to poor spatial relationships
- poor development of refined movements
- low vitality as a result of inactivity and poor nutrition

LEARNING DISABILITIES

Learning disabilities are the most difficult of handicapping conditions for educators to understand since the handicaps are not as obvious as physical disabilities or mental retardation. Thus, teachers are not able to readily observe the handicap and, at times, do not understand why this handicap may cause the student to have learning problems. Learning disabilities were not clearly defined or presented as a separate category in special education until the mid 1960s. The term *learning disabilities* was coined by Samuel Kirk (1963).

P.L. 94–142 defines learning disabilities as:

a disorder in one or more of the basic psychological processes involved in understanding or in using language, which includes spoken or written. This may manifest itself in an imperfect ability to listen, think, speak, read, write, spell, or do mathematical calculations. Included in the term ''specific learning disability'' are conditions such as perceptual motor problems, dyslexia and developmental aphasia. Specific learning disabilities are not a result of visual, hearing, mental retardation, emotional disturbance, environmental, cultural and economic disadvantage. (*Federal Register*, Section 5(6)4, 1977, December)

Learning-disabled students are different from mentally retarded students in intelligence levels, in spite of having learning difficulties. In nearly all cases learning-disabled students exhibit a discrepancy between intelligence and achievement. They may show average or above average intelligence but have difficulty with learning and achievement. Many times these students are labeled as lazy and simply perceived as not trying in school by uninformed teachers.

Learning-disabled students may have difficulty in only one area such as language. However, several problems may be encountered that may include social and academic or motor and academic difficulties. Each learning-disabled student is unique. Generally, students with learning disabilities have their problems in the following categories: verbal disabilities, nonverbal difficulties, behavioral and social problems. Verbal disabilities may include the disorders of language, reading, writing, and so on, while nonverbal disabilities may include perceptual motor problems and difficulties with motor coordination. Behavioral difficulties may also occur. Not every learning-disabled student will have problems in all areas.

General Characteristics

The physical education teacher needs to be aware of the many characteristics that may be found among learning-disabled students. However, this chapter will concentrate on the characteristics that are most likely to affect performance in physical education.

Gearheart (1981) and Geddes (1981) have described characteristics of learning-disabled students. Geddes has concentrated heavily on the characteristics that affect performance in physical education.

Nonverbal Disabilities

Body coordination deficits may manifest themselves in different forms. Some specific problems observed in learning-disabled students are listed in Table 2–2.

Table 2–2 Body Coordination Deficits

Problem	Characteristics
Clumsiness	Sometimes learning-disabled children are awkward and clumsy. They may bump into objects, trip, or seem to fall over their own feet.
Balance	Problems with maintaining stationary balance may occur. When dynamic balance is a factor, such as walking a balance beam, the learning-disabled student may run across to avoid balance. Poor balance may be the result of a neurological problem. It may also be due to impulsivity.
Kinesthesis	Kinesthesis is the ability to determine the body's position in space. Winnick (1979) reports that kinesthesis aids in determining the correctiveness of movement. Learning-disabled students may have difficulty with self-correction of their movement skills because of poorly developed kinesthetic discrimination.
Motor Planning Deficits	Motor planning is the ability to place a sequence of movements in proper order or plan a series of movements. As a result of thought disorders and memory problems, some learning-disabled students find it difficult to plan a sequence of complex motor acts or responses.
Visual Motor Coordination	Accurate responses to visual cues result in coordinating the body to produce smooth motor responses. Poorly integrated responses may occur because of inaccurate perceptions of visual cues.

Perceptual Motor Problems

Perception occurs as a result of interpretation of stimuli, which may include vision, tactile, auditory, and kinesthetic sensations. Stimuli must be accurately received and interpreted before accurate responses can be made. Learning-disabled students with specific perceptual disorders and disorders in thinking will have difficulty making motor responses that use the perceptual system which is not intact. Motor responses may be affected at both the gross and fine motor levels.

Visual Perceptual Disorders

The main channel for receiving information is via the visual modality. Visual perception, therefore, would involve the interpretation of visual stimuli. It includes several areas.

Visual figure-ground skills include the ability to select the relevant visual stimulus from a background of other visual stimuli.

Visual constancy refers to the ability to see objects as the same even though they may be presented in different forms. Learning-disabled students may not recognize targets at which they are to throw if the target is presented in various ways or forms.

Visual memory requires the ability to recall visual presentations or cues. Learning-disabled students may not remember a sequence of movements presented by the teacher. Thus, it will be difficult to reproduce a series of connected movements or to remember skill demonstrations.

Visual tracking skills require that the eyes follow or pursue a moving target in a coordinated manner. Students with a problem in this area may have difficulty catching a fly ball.

Visual discrimination is the ability to distinguish between objects visually. Learning-disabled students may not be able to distinguish different-size balls, or may be selective in following movement patterns given by the teacher or another student.

Auditory Perceptual Disorders

Auditory perception is used frequently while the student is engaged in game-type activities, dance, and other rhythmic skills.

Auditory memory requires skill in recalling what is heard. The student may not be able to remember a sequence of rhythmic beats or directions given verbally.

Auditory figure-ground ability enables the student to select relevant auditory stimulus from background noise. Difficulties in this skill may prevent a student from hearing the physical education teacher's verbal instructions while a game is in progress.

Auditory discrimination allows the student to discriminate or differentiate between various sounds. Students with auditory discrimination problems will have difficulty in accurately perceiving rhythmic sounds and differentiating auditory cues in game activities.

Body Awareness

Body awareness refers to the child's ability to name and locate body parts and understand their relationship to one another. Spatial relationships may be inaccurate when children do not understand their body and its relationship to space. Learning-disabled students may have difficulty in perceiving their body parts and consequently have difficulty in moving about related to direction, such as left or right. Difficulty may be encountered when having to move in relationship to other children or objects in the environment.

Other concepts about the body may be confused by learning-disabled children. Concepts of laterality and directionality are often difficult for these children to comprehend.

Laterality refers to awareness of both sides of the body and identification of left and right. At times learning-disabled students may be confused about the left and right sides of objects and about identifying their own right and left sides. They may be confused in motor activities requiring much lateral movement when the right and left sides must be identified. For example, if children with this problem are asked to hop left then hop right, they become confused about which foot to use. Laterality problems may also interfere with participation in games of a complex nature that require precise use of the left and right sides of the body.

Directionality is often referred to as projecting laterality outside of the body (Kephart, 1971). However, directionality also includes differentiation of forward, backward, and sideways. Problems with directionality may be present in some learning-disabled children. They often are confused about which way to move and have difficulty with forms and shapes.

Behavior Problems Associated With Learning Disabilities

Learning-disabled students may actually not be able to control their own behavior in some instances as a result of minimal brain damage. The teacher should be aware of the behavioral difficulties some learning-disabled students exhibit. Some of the problems can be controlled with medications. However, learning-disabled students respond to sound behavior management techniques and structured environments. All three may be necessary to help some learning-disabled children to manage themselves in an appropriate manner.

There are four common behavior problems that learning-disabled students may exhibit.

Hyperactivity is a condition of being unable to sit or hold still. Hyperactive students are in constant motion or most of the time are moving some part of their bodies. They may

rock, finger tap, shake their leg, or simply move about. Many forms of hyperactive behavior can be controlled by medication. However, caution needs to be used concerning medications. Some students are either over- or undermedicated. Parents may forget to refill medications or forget to administer them properly. A change in nutritional practices is often strikingly beneficial.

Distractability refers to attention problems. Students may attend to almost any irrelevent stimulus. They may be distracted by a fly, a horn, a voice, or any other kind of stimulus other than the relevant one at the time. These students will have short attention spans and a poor ability to concentrate.

Impulsivity refers to acting without any forethought. Students who are impulsive may respond in a haphazard fashion without thinking about the behavior or its consequences. They will generally have difficulty separating cues from the teacher and respond in a selective manner. For example, the impulsive student may be on first base and suddenly dart to second base without even contemplating a "steal" at second.

Perseveration refers to problems in changing quickly from one movement to another or one activity to another. Students with this behavior problem seem to "get stuck." For example, when the student is asked to hop on the left foot then quickly change to the right, the student gets stuck and cannot change feet quickly. Also, if an activity is in progress and the teacher changes to something else, the student who perseverates may not be able to make the proper adjustment and will continue doing what he or she was doing. If the teacher does not understand this problem, there may be confusion and the behavior may be misinterpreted as a discipline problem.

NEUROLOGICAL AND ORTHOPEDIC DISABILITIES

Orthopedic disabilities and neurological impairments may often accompany each other. These are disorders referred to by Cratty (1980) as disabilities that cause interference with the normal use of muscles, bones, and joints. Some orthopedic problems are congenital and permanent, while others may be only temporary. In several cases physical problems are the only disability. However, many physically disabled children have other associated disabilities along with the orthopedic disability. Some children may be classified as multi-impaired.

Cerebral Palsy

Cerebral palsy is a nonprogressive disorder of movement that results from brain damage before or during birth. Cerebral palsy may range from mild to severe, depending on the extent of brain damage.

Associated disabilities may accompany cerebral palsy, depending largely on the location and extent of brain damage. Bleck and Negel (1975) report that mental retardation may accompany 75 percent of cerebral palsy cases. Not everyone who has cerebral palsy is mentally retarded. Other disabilities may be present.

Visual impairments may include nearsightedness, farsightedness, and crossed eyes.

Hearing impairments may range from mild to severe, but are not as frequently found as visual loss.

Seizure disorders accompany spastic forms of cerebral palsy more so than any other type. Seizures may range from mild to severe with low to high frequency. Medication is frequently used to control seizures.

Speech and language deficits occur in almost half of persons with cerebral palsy. These disorders may result from paralysis of muscles controlling speech. Language disorders may result from several problems, mainly due to mental retardation or minimal brain damage causing a specific language problem.

Perceptual disorders are found among students with cerebral palsy in the form of visual, auditory, kinesthetic, and tactile perception difficulties. Visual perceptual disorders are probably the most common.

Poor visual motor integration may be observed when the cerebral palsied student has difficulty integrating movements in response to what the eye sees. This may be observed while the student is cutting shapes, copying, or kicking a moving ball.

Types of Cerebral Palsy

Umbreit (1983) defines various types of cerebral palsy according to the movement problems associated with this disorder.

Spasticity refers to tight or hypertonic muscles that respond to stretching by contracting. The body movement that results is a jerky motion. Affected limbs are usually held in more flexed positions.

Athetoid types of cerebral palsy include involuntary motions rather than the hypertonic musculature that is found in spasticity. Many voluntary attempts at movement may be contorted.

Ataxic forms of cerebral palsy may be observed in those who have difficulty with balance and coordinated movements. As the student ambulates, a high stepping and weaving gait can be observed.

Rigidity is a result of very tight musculature. This lack of movement results in a great deal of resistance to passive movement. Moving the limbs of students with rigidity is similar to bending a stiff pipe.

Tremors may be observed as rhythmic forms of movement with oscillating characteristics. Generally, no other forms of neurological damage are present in tremor forms of cerebral

palsy. Most of the time the tremor may be observed only when movement occurs in the limb or limbs involved.

Psychomotor Characteristics

The type of cerebral palsy, severity, and accompanying disorders will determine the psychomotor characteristics observed in each student. Another factor will include the number of limbs involved. In some cases all four limbs may be involved. While cerebral palsied students are a heterogeneous group, the following general characteristics may be observed:

- reduced mechanical efficiency of movement
- lack of coordination between upper and lower extremities, particularly in jumping and hopping
- decreased balance using a narrow base of support
- slow reaction time
- reduced movement time
- presence of primitive reflexes
- inaccurate movement
- perceptual motor deficits if perceptual disorders are present
- clumsiness, with frequent tripping and falling

These characteristics may not be present in every student with cerebral palsy and they will also tend to vary according to the degree of involvement.

Muscular Dystrophy

The Muscular Dystrophy Association of America reports that several types of muscular dystrophy exist. The most common types in childhood are Duchenne's Dystrophy, progressive muscular dystrophy, and pseudo hypertrophic muscular dystrophy. Research is progressing on muscular dystrophy, but the exact cause is not known at this point. Duchenne's Dystrophy is the most common form encountered by teachers in public schools.

Duchenne's Dystrophy affects boys and is transmitted by the mother via the X chromosome. In Duchenne's Dystrophy, as in most dystrophies, a progressive degeneration of the voluntary muscles occurs. Duchenne's Dystrophy may be noticed by age 3 by parents or others who observe children.

The early signals of Duchenne's Dystrophy include:

- awkward movements when walking or running
- postural deviations—lordosis and protruding abdomen
- clumsiness and frequent falling
- hands used to push up from floor to assume a standing position

- legs pushed up to stand up from sitting (Gower's sign)
- slowness in climbing stairs

Later signs include:

- Weakening abdominal muscles with weakness progressing to shoulder region, hands, face, and neck areas
- Tendency to put on weight as activity decreases
- Skeletal deformities resulting from muscular weakness

Many with Duchenne's Dystropohy may be in wheelchairs by age 10 (Bleck & Negal, 1975).

Spina Bifida

Umbreit (1983) defines spina bifida as open defects in the spinal canal or vertebra. Spina bifida is the least severe of several spinal defects. Two other common forms are meningocele and myelomeningocele.

Meningocele involves the protrusion of the covering of the spinal cord through the spinal defect.

Myelomeningocele is the most severe form as a result of the protrusion of the spinal cord itself through the opening in the vertebra.

Those defects may occur anywhere in the spinal column. As Bigge (1982) reports, the most frequent location is in the lumbar or lower region of the vertebral column.

The defects are usually corrected surgically. However, depending on the amount and severity of damage to the spinal cord, other problems result. These include:

- loss of bowel and bladder control
- muscular weakness and possible paralysis of the lower extremities
- trunk weakness, depending on how far up the spinal column the defect is located
- deformity of bones and joints due to muscular imbalances that may result in dislocations
- loss of sensation in the skin, which may result in pressure sores if the student is not moved periodically and frequently from one position to another
- retardation
- hydrocephalus (more in myelomeningocele)

Hydrocephalus results when the flow of cerebral spinal fluid is blocked from the brain to the spinal cord. The procedure is to surgically insert a drainage tube called a shunt, which keeps the fluid circulating. The shunt is inserted into the brain and leads usually to the abdominal cavity, where the excess fluid is drained and eventually eliminated. If this procedure is completed soon enough, the head does not enlarge from excess fluid and mental retardation or other damage does not result.

Psychomotor Characteristics

- Some students will be ambulatory, using braces and crutches, while some need wheelchairs.
- Motor skills will vary with each student, depending on the severity of the condition.
- Motor skills may range from ambulation with crutches to the aid of a wheelchair for assistance.
- A variety of motor skills can be learned, from swimming to simple ball skills or activities that can be completed from a wheelchair.

SENSORY IMPAIRMENT

Sensory-impaired individuals include those with visual or hearing deficits. Both impairments may be found together in some individuals.

Visual Impairments

P.L. 94–142 defines the term *visually handicapped* as an impairment which, when corrected, will adversely affect the student's educational achievement. This term includes not only the blind but those who are partially sighted as well. Visual impairments may be viewed in two ways. The first involves measuring the disability in terms of visual acuity and the field of vision. The second is to view visual impairment in terms of how well the student can function in an educational setting.

Individuals are defined as legally blind when vision is corrected in the better eye to no greater than 20/200 or when the visual field is no more than 20 degrees. An acuity of 20/200 means that the visually impaired person can see at 20 feet what the person with normal vision is able to see at 200 feet.

Field of vision refers to the range in degrees that the person is able to see. Persons without impaired vision can see 180 degrees. Thus, a person with a field of vision of 20 degrees or less is seeing much like looking at the world through a tunnel (Heward & Orlansky, 1984).

A student may be legally blind but function fairly well in a physical education setting. Each student will need to be taught to use the amount of residual vision he or she has available.

General Learning Characteristics

Intelligence levels in blind students can vary from above average to below average. Even when intelligence is above average, achievement may be lower than that of students who are not visually impaired. This is because of slower reading speed. Blind students, however, have achieved as much as their sighted peers in the academic classroom.

Body image may be distorted with posture deficiencies resulting from the inability to have a sighted point of reference for good posture. Cratty (1971) studied the body image of blind children and, although deficiencies were found, improvement in body image was achieved after a period of instruction.

Abstract concepts are difficult for blind individuals to grasp, possibly as a result of difficulty in understanding spatial relationships (Jansma & French, 1982).

Psychomotor Characteristics

Blind and partially sighted students may progress through normal motor developmental sequences but at a slower rate than their nonimpaired peers. However, this may not always be the case. Blind students may be overprotected from their environment and consequently be deprived of motor experiences as young children. This may lead to delays and omissions of the normal motor developmental milestones. Because of deprivations in play experiences, social skills may be deficient in many blind children. They may be shy and withdrawn as a result.

The following psychomotor characteristics may be observed to some extent in blind and visually impaired students. Some or several of the problems may be exhibited.

- Complicated movements may be difficult and at a level below that of sighted peers.
- Physical fitness levels are generally lower than those of sighted peers, particularly on items that require locomotion (Buell, (1973).
- Stationary fitness skills do not differ significantly among blind and sighted peers, as reported by Buell (1973).
- Discrepancies in fitness skills tend to decrease as age increases. Current research by Winnick and Short (1984) suggests that the age of onset of blindness was not a significant factor on the performance of physical fitness test items that included running, throwing, jumping, and the shuttle run. These findings conflict with earlier research indicating that age of onset of visual impairments significantly affected performance among visually impaired children.
- Blind children who run unassisted have better running speeds than those who need some form of assistance.
- Balance abilities appear to be lower in blind and visually impaired students since visual orientation is used for balance.
- Stationary motor skills may be more highly developed than locomotor skills.

- Underweight and overweight among visually impaired students may be more prevalent than in the normal population due to under- or overeating and a lack of exercise (Jansma & French, 1982).
- Stereotyped movements, called blindisms, are more prevalent among severely visually impaired. Blindisms consist of rocking, swaying, eye poking, hand flapping, and lateral head movements.

Implications for Physical Education

The physical education program for the blind student needs to encompass a broad range of skill areas. To be definitely included are:

- body image and spatial orientation
- development of good locomotor skills for the future development of independent orientation and mobility
- a well-rounded sports program, particularly including individual and dual sports
- team sports with modifications.

Hearing Impairments

In P.L. 94–142 hearing-impaired students are discussed under two categories: deaf and hard of hearing.

Deaf is defined as having a hearing impairment that is so severe that the student is unable to process language through hearing, with or without the use of an amplification device. The loss must be severe enough to affect the student's educational performance adversely (*Federal Register*, 1977, August).

Hard of Hearing refers to having a hearing impairment that may be permanent or fluctuating and adversely affects the student's educational achievement or performance (*Federal Register*, 1977, August). Hearing losses may range from mild to severe and can be of two types, including conductive and sensorineural.

Conductive losses are defined by Heward and Orlansky (1984) as hearing losses that result from obstructions in the outer and middle ear. These also include any malformations that interfere with conduction of sound waves from the middle ear to the inner ear.

Several procedures may be used to correct or improve conductive hearing losses. Some forms may be corrected by surgical procedures or medication or a combination of both. In instances where total restoration is not possible, hearing aids may be beneficial.

Sensorineural losses include hearing losses that result from auditory nerve damage or damage to the inner ear. Sounds in this type of hearing loss are highly distorted. As surgical techniques advance, some forms of sensorineural losses may be corrected. However, at present this type of hearing loss is normally not corrected by surgery (Heward & Orlansky, 1984). In some cases, a hearing aid may be helpful. More severe forms of hearing losses are found in this category.

Measuring Sound

Sound is measured in several ways. Intensity is the primary means of measuring sound using the decibel (dB) scale. Levels of hearing impairment can range from slight to profound. Table 2–3 outlines the range of hearing losses and the resulting student abilities.

General Learning Characteristics

Intelligence may vary among hearing-impaired children from above to below average. When multiple disabilities are present, such as in Rubella children, intelligence may be moderately to severely retarded. Achievement in school may be affected because of the difficulty with communication. With advances in electronics, however, such as computers, language boards, and other devices, hearing-impaired students may not lag far behind their nonimpaired peers.

Social skills vary from one hearing-impaired student to another. There may be delays in social development as a result of reduced social interaction and isolation.

Psychomotor Characteristics

Moores (1978) and Cratty (1980) have reported the findings of some studies that attempted to define the psychomotor characteristics of hearing-impaired students. Those students with sensorineural losses are more apt to be deficient in psychomotor skills and to a more severe degree than those with conductive losses.

Table 2–3 Range of Hearing Losses

Hearing Level	Decibels	Student Ability
Normal Hearing	0–27 dB loss	Not affected.
Slight	28–40 dB loss	Functions well.
Mild	41–55 dB loss	Needs to face and be within 5 feet of the teacher's voice to hear conversation.
Marked	56–70 dB loss	Voices must be loud to be heard; some speech is defective.
Severe	71–90 dB loss	Primarily uses vision; speech and language are defective; hears only very loud noises.
Profound	91 dB or greater	Relies totally on vision; may feel only sound vibrations.

Balance

Those with sensorineural losses are more deficient in balance than hearing-impaired persons with other types of losses. Static balance is probably the most deficient skill area. Dynamic balance skills also seem to be a problem with children who have a sensorineural loss, particularly when the problem is in the semicircular canal of the inner ear. Since balance is a problem, the walking style of hearing-impaired children may be similar to that of blind children. In this case the feet are not lifted well, but shuffled instead. Sherrill (1981) reports that walking form can be improved with training.

Posture and Fitness

Postural deformities may result if the student tilts the head frequently or assumes other unusual postures in order to hear better. Fitness levels of hearing-impaired children are similar to levels of their nonimpaired peers. However, if hearing-impaired students are socially isolated and choose to participate in more sedentary activities, cardiovascular endurance may be less than that of students who are active in sports and games. The endurance, however, is not directly related to the hearing impairment itself.

Implications for Physical Education

Hearing-impaired students respond well to good physical education programs. Most students can be accommodated in the regular classroom provided that the teacher can communicate with the student with sign language, finger spelling, or some other means. Elementary level students need to be involved in developmental skill progressions and their utilization in games and lead-ups to sports. This approach would help develop social skills and prepare the student for secondary physical education activities.

COMMUNICATION DISORDERS

The ability to communicate depends on the skills of expressing oneself and receiving language, or the ability to communicate in other ways. Disorders of communication fall within the abilities of speech and language. (See Table 2–4.)

Language Disorders

Language disorders involve delays in the ability to express and/or understand ideas and extreme delays in language that would seriously affect communication. Table 2–4 lists the types of language disorders and their characteristics.

Table 2–4 Types of Language Disorders

Type	Characteristics
Aphasia	An acquired language disability resulting from brain damage. Person forgets words and/or symbols.
Language Delay	Individual cannot understand and express language that would be appropriate for his or her chronological age. May not understand how words are ordered in a sentence like "Shoe my tie." Makes many grammatical errors.
Language Difference	Language that is different from the dominant culture.

Types of Speech Disorders

Speech, according to Van Riper (1978), is considered defective when it (1) draws attention to itself instead of what the person is saying, (2) interferes with the ability to communicate effectively, and (3) causes social maladjustment in the person speaking. Speech disorders vary and in more severe cases an individual may have more than one type. Table 2–5 lists the types of speech disorders and their characteristics.

Learning Characteristics

The intelligence of persons with speech and language disorders may not differ significantly from the norm. Differences in intelligence, however, that do exist may result from the organic causes of speech and language disorders that are particularly related to brain damage or other associated handicapping conditions that might accompany the language problem.

Some secondary reactions can occur that may indirectly affect the student's social and emotional development. The student may be bothered by the speech defect and be reluctant to socialize and interact with peers. Some students with more severe problems may exhibit aggression and hostility from not being able to make their needs known.

Table 2–5 Types of Speech Disorders

Type	Characteristics
Articulation	Speech sounds are heard as being omitted, substituted, distorted, and added.
Speech Flow	Includes stuttering, abnormal repetitions and hesitations, cluttered speech, fast or poor articulation of words, and disorganization.
Voice Problems	Vocal quality may be related to the loudness and pitch (high or low).

Psychomotor Characteristics

Unless children have speech and language disorders associated with some other handicapping condition, there should be no physiological reason for poor psychomotor skill performance. Students who may have secondary problems from their speech or language deficits may have poor psychomotor responses as a result of reduced opportunity to participate with their peers in motor activities and games.

Implications for Physical Education

The physical education program should be designed to aid the enhancement of social interaction and the development of a good self-image. Physical education activities should be used to reinforce language concepts. Whenever possible, the physical educator should take the opportunity to incorporate language development into the motor skills being taught. For example, new words should be taught along with a new game.

Physical education activities can provide a means for fostering communication. Group activities can be particularly good for discussion. Physical education activities can provide interesting topics to talk about during class, relating, for example, to sports events seen or attended.

HEALTH IMPAIRMENTS

Students who do not fit into a particular category of handicapping condition such as mental retardation or physically impaired could possibly receive special education services under the category of health impaired. Health impairments may be permanent or temporary. They include a variety of disabilities that can adversely affect the students' educational achievement. The health impairments to be discussed in this chapter include juvenile rheumatoid arthritis, congenital heart problems, and juvenile diabetes mellitus.

Juvenile Rheumatoid Arthritis

Juvenile rheumatoid arthritis has its onset in early childhood. Bleck and Nagel (1975) report that this form of arthritis primarily manifests itself with inflammation in the joints. Bigge (1982) explains that the disease may begin as early as three years of age. If the disease is untreated, permanent damage may result from scarred and damaged tissue. Treatment of the inflammation with proper rest and exercise usually will alleviate any secondary complications.

Secondary Complications

Many students with this condition have to either remain in bed or use a wheelchair. When acute inflammation stages are present, weight bearing on the affected joints is not recommended. Umbreit (1983) explains that the objectives for treating a child with arthritis include the following procedures:

- Reduce inflammation in the joints generally through the use of medication.
- Prevent deformities and weakness using sound physical therapy programs and physical education.
- Provide knowledge to the family on how to manage the child's condition so that maximum use is made of the opportunities to move and reduce the problems associated with arthritis.

General Learning Characteristics

Students with juvenile forms of arthritis may function quite well in school. However, when inflammation is severe, they may fall behind in their school work. Achievement may fluctuate with the severity of the condition. Bigge (1982) reports that some students with arthritis may undergo personality or behavioral changes, including shyness, self-consciousness, and withdrawal from peers. Irritability can occur when inflammation is present, even though the condition is being treated with medication. It is important that teachers be understanding when their students are going through periods of inflammation and discomfort.

Psychomotor Characteristics

A major problem with arthritic students will be restricted movement in the joints affected. Other problems include:

- side effects from medications
- limping from irritated joints
- atrophy in the musculature as a result of restricted mobility
- muscular weakness
- restricted range of motion in affected joints

Implications for Physical Education

If the student is having pain and swelling, physical education will most likely be quite restricted, or the student may be on homebound instruction. The physical educator needs to work closely with the student's physician and physical therapist. Exercise is a very important part of the arthritic student's treatment. Exercises should be developed to provide range of motion, maintain strength, and prevent or reduce atrophy of the affected areas. Swimming in warm water of 82-85 degrees is recommended since movement can occur without the effect of gravity. This kind of activity will provide all the overall exercise for maintenance of flexibility and strength. Recreational games are particularly good for

arthritic children. Activities that involve body contact or where falling is more of a risk should be eliminated from the student's program.

Congenital Heart Problems

The rate of heart disorders in children is not as high as in adults, particularly for those disorders that are acquired. The rate of congenital heart defects in children is lower than acquired defects. Umbreit (1983) reports that out of every 1,000 children born, six will have some form of congenital heart defect. Some specific handicapping conditions such as Rubella and Down's Syndrome include congenital heart defects.

Many congenital heart disorders have no known causes. Several types of defects are related to defects in the internal tissue of the heart. A common type of defect consists of a hole in the septum, or the dividing wall between the two chambers of the heart. This condition can usually be repaired by surgery and the child generally recovers quite well. Another defect is called Tetralogy of Fallot. Four defects within the heart itself are involved. The defects result in return blood mixing with newly oxygenated blood from the lungs. This leaves the individual with poorly oxygenated blood, often resulting in a bluish color to the skin, lips, and nails. Tetralogy of Fallot can also be corrected by surgical techniques.

General Learning Characteristics

Unless the congenital heart defect is associated with some other handicapping condition, the intelligence of students with congenital heart defects will be very similar to the distribution found in the normal population. If the condition has not been totally corrected by surgery, achievement may vary somewhat as a result of the student's need to take longer to complete work and assignments.

Psychomotor Characteristics

No particular set of characteristics can be defined for students with congenital heart disease. Some characteristics, however, need to be considered while the disease is present.

Implications for Physical Education

The physical education instructor should not attempt any physical activities with the student until a medical consultation or some form of instruction from the medical personnel responsible for the care of the student has been obtained. The major problem that the student will encounter will be fatigue from physical activity. The student and teacher both need to be aware of those activities that are permitted and those that are to be avoided. Umbreit (1983) concludes that these students do not have to be exempt from physical education, only that certain types of activities should be avoided.

The physical educator and the student should both be aware of signs of undue physical stress in students with congenital heart disease. The signs include:

- cyanosis
- rapid pulse
- shortness of breath
- chest pains or neck and arm pains

Competitive sports should be avoided. The student should be involved whenever possible in the choice of activities. When the student feels fatigue, a rest period should be allowed.

Juvenile Diabetes Mellitus

Juvenile diabetes mellitus occurs in childhood within the first ten years of life. Insulin is needed to convert glucose into energy sources for the body. If glucose is used properly, it is burned and converted to carbon dioxide and excreted from the body. However, when glucose is not converted and utilized by the body as a result of little or no insulin in the body, it is excreted by the kidneys.

Some of the first signs of juvenile diabetes in children are:

- frequent thirst
- weight loss
- poor performance in school
- fatigue
- frequent skin infections (Umbreit, 1983).

General Learning Characteristics

Diabetic children can learn and achieve as well as any other student if coping with the disease is positive. If the student copes in a negative manner, achievement in school may be adversely affected. These students need understanding from the physical educator about the disease. Generally, the student's personality may change when coping skills become less than positive.

Many students undergo some difficulty and need appropriate counseling to aid them in managing their problem. During periods when the student is not coping well, academic and other school performance may fall behind.

Psychomotor Characteristics

If diabetes is kept well under control, normal growth will occur. Diabetic children show no significant deviations in psychomotor skill performance when compared with normal

peers. However, if the student adjusts poorly to the condition, then psychomotor performance may be affected. Poorly adjusted students may exhibit the following characteristics:

- fear of performance in physical education
- inconsistency in performing exercises
- no pacing while exercising and therefore becoming unduly fatigued
- underweight or overweight from an inconsistent diet

Insulin Reactions

It is important for the physical educator to recognize the symptoms of an insulin reaction. The signs of too much insulin are:

- low blood sugar level
- nausea
- blurred vision
- dizziness
- headaches

If the insulin reaction is not counteracted by giving a sweetened juice or a candy bar, the student may actually go into a diabetic coma.

Implications for Physical Education

Keeping weight under control is important for diabetic students because it may decrease the need for insulin. The amount of exercise must be regulated with the amount of insulin or vice versa. Fait and Dunn (1984) point out that care needs to be taken to avoid infection in diabetic students, since they are highly susceptible.

The teacher must be aware of the needs of the diabetic student and cooperate when the student feels the need for juice or candy to compensate for low glucose levels.

POINTS TO REMEMBER

1. Although the causes may be different for certain disabilities, in mild conditions, some of the behavioral and motor characteristics can be similar.

2. With other handicapping conditions such as with the health impaired and severely handicapped, the instructor should be familiar with any medical problems the student has and their implications for physical exercise.

3. The teacher should view the characteristics of handicapped students in terms of their implications for physical education. One cannot stereotype or overgeneralize, since each student must be considered as an individual.

4. The more severe the handicapping condition, the more gaps will exist between disabled students and their non-disabled peers.

5. Mildly retarded students have difficulty with more abstract and reasoning skills. Motor skills that are complex are difficult for retarded students because of the reasoning involved.

6. Retarded youngsters respond favorably to sound physical education programs.

7. Physical education programs for disabled students should focus on their individual needs, but for the group as a whole develop leisure, fitness, and social integration skills through physical activities.

8. Students with special health problems can participate in physical education if medical advice is followed and the program is highly individualized.

REFERENCES

Ayres, J.A. (1972). *Sensory integration and learning disorders*. Los Angeles: Western Psychological Services.

Bigge, J.L. (Ed.). (1982). *Teaching individuals with physical and multiple disabilities* (2nd ed.). Columbus, OH: Charles E. Merrill.

Bleck, E.E., & Nagel, D.A. (Eds.). (1975). *Physically handicapped children: A medical atlas for teachers*. New York: Grune & Stratton.

Buell, C.E. (1973). *Physical education and recreation for the visually handicapped*. Washington, DC: American Association for Health, Physical Education, and Recreation.

Chasey, W.C., & Wyrick, W. (1970). Effect of a gross motor developmental program on form perception skills of educable mentally retarded children. *Research Quarterly, 41*, 345–352.

Corder, W.O. (1969). *Effects of physical education on the psycho-physical development of educable mentally retarded girls*. Doctoral dissertation, University of Virginia.

Cratty, B.J. (1980). *Adapted physical education for handicapped children and youth*. Denver: Love.

Cratty, B.J. (1974). *Motor activity and the education of retardates*. (2nd ed.). Philadelphia: Lea & Febiger.

Cratty, B.J. (1971). *Movement and spatial awareness in blind children and youth*. Springfield, IL: Charles C. Thomas.

Crowe, W.C., Auxter, D., & Pyfer, J. (1981). *Principles and methods of adapted physical education and recreation*. St. Louis: C.V. Mosby.

Fait, H.F., & Dunn, J.M. (1984). *Special physical education* (5th ed.). Philadelphia: Saunders College Publishing.

Folio, M.R. (1975). *Validation of a developmental motor assessment instrument and programmed activities*. Doctoral dissertation, Peabody College of Vanderbilt University, Nashville, TN.

Folio, M.R. (1981). Trace mineral profiles of Down's Syndrome subjects compared to normal laboratory standards. Final Report of a Faculty Research Grant, Tennessee Technological University, Cookeville, TN.

Francis, R.J., & Rarick, G.L. (1959). Motor characteristics of the mentally retarded. *American Journal of Mental Deficiency, 63*, 792–811.

Gearheart, B.R. (1981). *Learning disabilities: Educational strategies* (3rd ed.). St. Louis: C.V. Mosby.

Geddes, D. (1981). *Psychomotor individualized educational programs for intellectual, learning and behavioral disabilities*. Boston: Allyn & Bacon.

Goodwin, L.A. (1970). *The effects of two selected physical education programs on trainable mentally retarded children*. Doctoral dissertation, University of Utah.

Grossman, H.J. (Ed.). (1983). *Manual on terminology and classification in mental retardation*. Washington, DC: American Association on Mental Deficiency.

Hallahan, D.P., & Kauffman, J.M. (1982). *Exceptional children: Introduction to special education*. (2nd ed.). Englewood Cliffs, NJ: Prentice Hall.

Haring, N.G. (Ed.). (1978). *Behavior of exceptional children* (2nd ed.). Columbus, OH: Charles E. Merrill.

Heward, W.L., & Orlansky, M.D. (1984). *Exceptional children* (2nd ed.). Columbus, OH: Charles E. Merrill.

Jansma, P., & French, R. (1982). *Special physical education*. Columbus, OH: Charles E. Merrill.

Kanner, L. (1964). *A history of the care and study of the mentally retarded*. Springfield, IL: Charles C. Thomas.

Kephart, N.C. (1971). *The slow learner in the classroom*. Columbus, OH: Charles E. Merrill.

Kirk, S.A. (1963). Behavioral diagnosis and remediation of learning disabilities. Proceedings of the conference on exploration into the problems of the perceptually handicapped child. Chicago.

Knight, R.M., Hyman, J., and Wozny, M.A. (1965). Psychomotor abilities of familial brain damaged and mongoloid retarded children. *American Journal of Mental Deficiency, 70*, 457.

Knoblock, P. (1962). Teaching and mainstreaming autistic children. Denver: Love Publishing Co.

MacMillan, D.L. (1982). *Mental retardation in school and society*. Boston: Little, Brown.

Moores, D.F. (1978). *Educating the deaf: Psychology, principles and practices*. Boston: Houghton Mifflin.

Morrison, D. (1972). Two different remedial motor training programs and the development of mentally retarded preschoolers. *American Journal on Mental Deficiency, 77*, 251–258.

Neisworth, J.T., & Smith, R.M. (Eds.). (1978). *Retardation: Issues, assessment and intervention*. New York: McGraw-Hill.

Rarick, G.L., Dobbins, A., & Broadhead, J. (1976). *The motor domain and its correlates in educationally handicapped children*. Englewood Cliffs, NJ: Prentice-Hall.

Rarick, G.L., & McQuillan, J.P. (1977). The factor structure of motor abilities of trainable mentally retarded children: Implications for curriculum development. Final Report for the Office of Education, Project No. H23–2544, Berkeley, California: University of California.

Rarick, G., Widdop, J.H., & Broadhead, G.D. (1970). The physical fitness and motor performance of educable mentally retarded children. *Exceptional Child, 36*, 509–519.

Schultz, J.B., & Turnbull, A.P. (1984). *Mainstreaming handicapped students: A guide for classroom teachers* (2nd ed.). Boston: Allyn & Bacon.

Sengstock, W.L. (1966). Physical fitness of mentally retarded boys. *Research Quarterly, 37*, 113–120.

Sharpe, G.D. (1968). Effectiveness of specified physical education programs and establishment of selected motor performance norms for the trainable mentally retarded. Doctoral dissertation, University of Wisconsin, 1968.

Sherrill, C. (1981). *Adapted physical education and recreation* (2nd ed.). Dubuque, IA: William C. Brown.

Smith, R.M. (1971). *An introduction to mental retardation*. New York: McGraw-Hill.

Taylor, G.R. (1969). The relationship between varying amounts of physical education upon the development of certain motor skills in trainable mentally retarded children. Doctoral dissertation, The Catholic University.

Umbreit, J. (Ed.). (1983). *Physical disabilities and health impairments: An introduction.* Columbus, OH: Charles E. Merrill.

Van Riper, C. (1978). *Speech correction: Principles and methods* (6th ed.). Englewood Cliffs, NJ: Prentice-Hall.

Webb, R.C. (1969). Sensory motor training of the profoundly retarded. *American Journal on Mental Deficiency, 74,* 283–295.

Winnick, J.P. (1979). *Early movement experiences and development: Habilitation and remediation.* Philadelphia: W.B. Saunders.

Winnick, J.P., & Short, F.K. (1984). *The physical fitness of sensory and orthopedically impaired youth.* Brockport, NY: State University of New York at Brockport. (ERIC Document ED 240 764)

Wiseman, D.C. (1982). *A practical approach to adapted physical education.* Reading, MA: Addison-Wesley.

RECOMMENDED READINGS

Mental Retardation

Education and Training of the Mentally Retarded. Publishes four issues per year on educational studies and articles relating to the education of the mentally retarded.

Kolstoe, O.P. (1972). *Mental retardation: An educational viewpoint.* New York: Holt, Rinehart & Winston.

MacMillan, D.L. (1982). *Mental retardation in school and society* (2nd ed.). Boston: Little, Brown.

Mental Retardation (American Association on Mental Deficiency). Publishes bimonthly studies on teaching approaches, methodology, and general research related to mental retardation.

Learning Disabilities

Arnheim, D., & Sinclair, W. (1979). *The clumsy child* (2nd ed.). St. Louis: C.V. Mosby.

Learning Disability Quarterly (Council for Learning Disabilities). Contains articles with applied research on the learning disabled. Published four times annually.

Lerner, J.W. (1981). *Learning disabilities: Theories, diagnosis and teaching strategies* (3rd ed.). Boston: Houghton Mifflin.

Myers, P.I., & Hammill, D.D. (1982). *Learning disabilities: Basic concepts, assessment practices and instructional strategies.* Austin, TX: PRO ED.

Smith, D.D. (1981). *Teaching the learning disabled.* Englewood Cliffs, NJ: Prentice-Hall.

Wallace, G., & McLoughlin, J. (1979). *Learning disabilities: Concepts and characteristics* (2nd ed.). Columbus, OH: Charles E. Merrill.

Emotionally Disturbed/Behavior Disordered

Hewett, F.M., & Taylor, F.D. (1980). *The emotionally disturbed child in the classroom: The orchestration of success.* Boston: Allyn & Bacon.

Kauffman, J.M. (1981). *Characteristics of children's behavior disorders* (2nd ed.). Columbus, OH: Charles E. Merrill.

Visually Impaired

Journal of Visual Impairment and Blindness (American Foundation for the Blind). Publishes articles on education and rehabilitation of visually impaired children and adults. Published ten times annually.

Mangold, S. (Ed.). (1982). *A teacher's guide to the special educational needs of blind and visually handicapped children.* New York: American Foundation for the Blind.

Willoughby, D.M. (1980). *A resource guide for parents and educators of blind children.* Baltimore: National Federation of the Blind.

Hearing Impaired

Moores, D.F. (1978). *Educating the deaf: Psychological principles and practices.* Boston: Houghton Mifflin.

O'Rourke, T.J. (1973). *A basic course in manual communication.* Silver Spring, MD: National Association of the Deaf.

Shames, G.H., & Wiig, E.H. (Eds.). (1982). *Human communication disorders.* Columbus, OH: Charles E. Merrill.

Physically Disabled

Umbreit, J. (Ed.). (1983). *Physical disabilities and health impairments: An introduction.* Columbus, OH: Charles E. Merrill.

Part II

The Psychomotor Domain and Motor Skill Acquisition

Chapter 3

Psychomotor Development and Motor Learning

Focus

- Defines the psychomotor domain and its use in designing motor programs
- Discusses factors that affect motor learning
- Explains motor learning principles and teaching implications

Most educators are familiar with the cognitive and affective domains of learning. The psychomotor domain refers to observable voluntary human motion (Harrow, 1972). The domains of learning provide a framework for classifying skills into a meaningful hierarchical sequence. This method of classifying movement aids in developing meaningful motor development curricula. The psychomotor domain also assists in formulating sequential instructional objectives.

Several taxonomies have been developed for classifying motor skills in a logical sequence. Harrow's (1972) taxonomy follows a developmental model of motor skills. It is organized into six major categories that include:

- reflexive movements
- basic fundamental movements
- perceptual abilities
- physical abilities
- skilled movements
- movement communication

Reflexive movements are movements that are involuntary responses to stimuli. They occur automatically and are present at birth. Reflexes are precursors of voluntary movement and aid in positioning the body for movement. They assist with righting the body and maintaining its position. Harrow states that reflexes do not need programming, but there are some instances where they do, such as in the case of students with neurological damage and in severe disabilities.

Basic fundamental movements are general movement patterns that form the basis for more complex specialized movements. Examples include locomotor, nonlocomotor, and manipulative skills. Many of these skills are developed by age 6.

Perceptual abilities are made up of interpreted sensory information from the sensory modalities, such as vision, hearing, touch, and kinesthesis. These are essential in interpretation through the brain and for the making of correct motor responses.

Physical abilities refer to the efficient functioning of the body's organic vigor. These include endurance, strength, flexibility, and agility.

Skilled movements refer to efficient movements when performing a skill. These include adaptations of basic fundamental movements that are involved in games, sports, skills requiring the use of implements, such as rackets, bats, etc., and movements requiring the use of advanced body mechanics, such as tumbling, diving, and other advanced skills.

Movement communication refers to creative, expressive movements often used in rhythms and creative dance.

The framework of the psychomotor domain provides the instructor with a developmental approach to the teaching of motor skills. This approach assists with focusing on learner strengths and deficits, individual needs, and the designing of a program of motor activities that allows for maximum development.

Other chapters in this text address the levels within the psychomotor domain. The intent at this point is to discuss principles of motor skill acquisition within the framework of the domain. The aim is to provide a basic foundation of how motor skills are learned and the implications for teaching them.

FACTORS AFFECTING MOTOR SKILL ACQUISITION

Learning is often defined as a relatively permanent change in behavior that results from experience. Motor learning, as explained by Drowatsky (1971) refers to the modification of motor behavior that occurs from specific training procedures and the surrounding environmental conditions that act upon the individual. Learning is a relatively complex task and many factors play a part in the acquisition of motor behavior. By examining variables that affect motor skill learning in general, the variables that affect learning for the handicapped student may be more clearly understood.

Many factors affect the motor learning process. These include individual characteristics and teacher characteristics.

Individual Characteristics

Relative factors that influence motor learning include:

- intelligence
- maturation and growth
- environmental experience
- motivation
- personality
- perception
- physical development
- sensory ability

Intelligence

Intelligence affects the rate at which an individual can acquire and process information. Studies that have researched the relationship between intelligence and motor proficiency have reported positive but low correlations between these two factors. Black and Davis (1966) reported significant correlations between the ability to localize movements, speed, and dexterity. Moran and Kalakian (1974) reported that very little relationship exists between intelligence and motor performance.

While no conclusive research data point to a direct relationship between intelligence and motor performance, the physical educator working with students with intellectual impairment will need to gear teaching strategies to the intellectual level of the student. The more complex the motor task and the greater the number of component parts of the task, the more difficulty will be seen with students who have lowered intelligence. Generally, as students approach the lower end of the intellectual scale, more motor and physical problems may be observed.

Maturation and Growth

Crowe, Auxter, and Pyfer (1981) explain that physical growth may occur without the development of high-level motor skills. Heredity has a significant effect on growth in terms of size, body structure, and growth rates. However, environment, disease, and nutritional practices can also affect growth patterns.

Extreme deviations in weight may affect motor skill performance. Extremely underweight children may lack the necessary strength and vitality to perform specific motor tasks. On the other hand, extremely overweight children may not be able to perform specific types of motor skills efficiently. Malnourished children may have a variety of physical problems that interfere with the performance of physical and motor skills.

Environmental Experience

The early acquisition of basic fundamental motor skills depends on maturation. McClenaghan and Gallahue (1978) emphasize that refinement and further skill development are highly related to practice and experience.

Environmental conditions refers to the type of motor development experiences young children receive. This applies to both handicapped and nonhandicapped children. Nonstimulating environments may produce children who acquire basic motor patterns and skills as a result of maturation but who may have a low level of refined specific skills. McClenaghan and Gallahue (1978) recommend that young children and those in the early elementary grades have ample opportunity to explore, experience, and practice basic fundamental motor patterns and skills. Particularly important is the fact that refinement of skills occurs through exploration and a variety of environmental experiences. Young children who experience a wide variety of movement activity generally are better coordinated than children who are placid and do not move adequately.

Motivation

Motivation plays an important role in the development and refinement of motor skills. Usually, young children do not have to be externally motivated to develop motor skills or use them in play. Motor skills are a natural part of young children's methods for interacting with peers and the

environment. Educators and parents should be careful not to "unmotivate" children to explore and utilize their motor patterns. Unfortunately, parents may sometimes become overly concerned with children's academic skill development and restrict the opportunities for their children to participate in motor activities during preschool and early elementary years. Similarly, in grades K-3, children do not receive adequate structured time to refine and further develop motor skills. Many schools simply offer a free-play approach to physical education. This type of situation leaves the unmotivated student with less opportunity to practice motor skills.

Motivation may be reduced because of previous experiences with motor skills where injury has resulted. For example, a student who is unsuccessful in catching a softball and has been injured as a result will need some type of motivation to catch. A NeRF® ball with a lead-up activity to catching might motivate the student to participate in such activities.

Personality

Children's personalities may have significant effects on their willingness to engage in a variety of motor and physical activities. Drowatsky (1971) reported deficiencies in personality characteristics between children highly skilled in motor development and those with low levels of motor skill development.

Motor skill achievement plays an important role in the social actions of children and adolescents. Usually, those who have well-developed motor skills will experience more social and psychological gratification than peers with lower-level motor skills. Children with low motor ability may experience failure and some frustration in trying to participate with peers in game activities requiring motor skills. Although this does not apply to all children, the rejection and ridicule that may result can be detrimental to the child's self-concept.

Children who are shy and withdrawn tend to have lower motor skill development than their peers who are more outgoing and enjoy group-type games and motor activities. This may simply be a result, however, of more opportunity to engage in such activities by the outgoing child. Shy and withdrawn children may enjoy more sedentary activities or prefer adult company.

Family and cultural practices may also affect motor development, more so in the elementary and upper grades than at the preschool age. Some families have lifestyles oriented toward physical and motor activities. Consequently, their children are exposed to a variety of motor or physical activities. If the child's maturation is developed, rather sophisticated motor skills can be achieved.

Folio and Fewell (1983) found evidence during the standardization procedure with the *Peabody Developmental*

Motor Scale that some five- and six-year-olds far exceeded the performance of the other subjects included within their age group. Interviews with the parents revealed that the more advanced children had been receiving gymnastics instruction since age 3.

Non-nurturing families who do not supply the basic needs of children may seriously affect their growth and personality development. Abusing parents can affect motor development as a result of structural damage to their children. The psychological damage may leave the child unmotivated and fearful.

Seaman and DePauw (1982) explain that culturally determined forms of movement are made up of refined complex motor skills. These skills are often employed in games and sports that are practiced in various cultures.

Perception

The ability to interpret stimuli properly will affect the rate at which students can learn and retain motor skills. Perception requires that the student be able to discriminate and interpret a stimulus in order to make the correct motor response. Deficits in perception will reduce the rate at which students can learn motor skills. Specific perceptual abilities are discussed in Chapter 5. Visual perception is very important in the learning of motor skills. Children with perceptual disorders will have difficulty selecting and interpreting stimuli in order to make a decision about the correct motor act.

Physical Development

Motor performance depends on physical ability. Those students who lack strength and endurance, in particular, will have difficulty learning motor skills. Other components of physical fitness affect the learning of motor skills. These are discussed in more detail in Chapter 6.

Sensory Development

The degree to which the major sensory modalities are intact will affect the rate at which students will acquire and retain motor skills. Blind students may have more difficulty learning a motor task because of not being able to see the sequence of movements and body positioning that are necessary to perform the skill. The learning rate will be slower in these instances. Once the skill is learned, however, it is retained generally to the same extent as found in sighted persons.

Teacher Characteristics

The personal qualities of the teacher can have some effect on the learning of motor skills. Several factors determine how effectively handicapped students learn skills in this area. These include the teacher's personal qualities, teaching style, and knowledge of subject matter.

Personal Qualities

The personal qualities of enthusiasm and empathy are important for enhancing the motor learning environment for handicapped students. These qualities would enable the teacher to motivate the student. They also give the student the impression that the teacher wants the student to achieve and be successful. For example, an empathetic teacher will convey to the student that the student's problems are recognized. The teacher can say to a student who is withdrawn "I know you are afraid to play on a team. Let me help you. I'll be your buddy in the field during the softball game." This acknowledges the fact that the student is having difficulty, but the teacher does not demonstrate an attitude of "Oh, you poor thing." The teacher recognizes the student's problem, acknowledges it in an objective manner, and offers a solution.

Teaching Style

Teaching style should be flexible so that different methods may be available for the handicapped student during a motor learning lesson. Students have their own learning styles. Unless the teacher is able to match teaching style to the student's best learning style, the rate of learning may be negatively affected. For instance, if a learning-disabled student has difficulty with auditory processing and requires a considerable amount of visual input and cues to learn a skill, the flexible teacher will take this into account and add more visual aids and cues in the teaching process. If a teacher is working with a group of mentally retarded students in a difficult activity, the teacher should be willing to modify or completely change to some other activity for a change of pace.

Knowledge of Subject Matter

Knowledge of subject matter reflects the extent to which the teacher is able to break down the motor skill into small components. This is important in teaching handicapped students with poor learning ability. If the teacher is unable to task analyze the motor skills involved, handicapped students may have a difficult time grasping the skills to be learned.

Those providing physical education services to handicapped students need a broad knowledge base, since these teachers are working with the entire child. In addition, many other professionals may be involved with the adapted physical educator in working with the exceptional student. Open and effective lines of communication among professionals greatly enhance the programs offered to special education students.

An example of the need for a broad knowledge base might be the physical educators who are asked to assist in implementing a strict behavior management program with a student. When working with the school psychologist, the special education teacher, and the educational diagnostician, physical educators need to know the principles of sound behavior management in order to carry out their portion of the management techniques.

MOTOR LEARNING PRINCIPLES

The adapted physical education instructor needs to understand factors that affect motor learning. Basic motor learning principles should start with knowledge of the students, particularly related to the factors included in the preceding section of this chapter. The principles and strategies discussed below should generally be employed while teaching motor skills.

Corbin (1973) suggests that the following principles be applied in the initial learning of motor skills.

1. The maturational readiness of the student should be assessed. Developmental and physical tests can be applied to determine the student's maturational status.

2. The teaching progression should occur from what is already known by the student, based on assessment data, to what is related and unknown.

Implication: It is important to establish what skills the student has mastered, those that are emerging and those that are unknown.

3. Positive successful experiences must be provided early in the learning sequence.

Implication: Even if the equipment or teaching method needs to be altered, the success the student experiences in the beginning will serve as a motivator to continue.

4. The aspect of too much fear should be eliminated or reduced during the initial learning phases.

Implication: Students need to approach a task with the notion that it is achievable. If students are overly fearful, the task may be perceived as too difficult and unattainable.

5. Expectations in initial learning stages should be flexible, allowing for exploration and experimentation.

Implication: Students should be allowed to explore movements and variations of the skill until they learn the more precise aspects of the skill.

6. Practice strategies should generally be short with high concentration levels maintained.

Implication: Practice time needs to be varied in accordance with the age of the learner, the attention span, and the difficulty of the skill. The teacher should make it a point to know the learner's characteristics, particularly related to these aspects.

Practice sessions should be shorter and more frequent if the following conditions occur:

- The skill is very tiring.
- Movements are simple and boring.
- Intense concentration is required.
- Learners have short attention spans and are unable to concentrate for long periods.

7. Practice sessions can be longer, but with less frequency if the skill

- requires many complex movements.
- contains several components.
- is new, novel, or maintains the attention of the learner.

8. Drowatsky (1971) reported that fatigue, boredom, and decreased motivation were factors that entered into massed practice (practice over long periods of time). School schedules are better set up to have distributed practice, or more practice over shorter periods of time. Practice that is distributed over short periods appears to help in the long-term remembering of the skill.

9. Mental and verbal rehearsal of a skill can aid in understanding cognitively what is to be learned.

Implication: A good method, according to Sage (1984), is to describe to oneself the movements involved in the skill. According to Sage, this approach helps one develop a greater memory for the movements involved. Students who have poor memory should be allowed time to rehearse a skill before actually physically practicing the skill.

10. Learning can be enhanced if students are able to selectively attend to relevant stimuli in the task.

Implications: Students with learning problems may not be able to attend to relevant stimuli in an instructional setting. Consequently, attention is given to irrelevant stimuli and not those that are significant to the task. Shea (1984) reports that stimuli have characteristics that help to focus attention. These include:

- size, intensity of color, noise, and speed
- novelty of the task
- expectation of a stimulus, i.e., calling the student's attention to the stimulus

Figure 3–1 helps to illustrate this point. In the scene the teacher is trying to have two students catch a ball. While the teacher is asking the student to catch, other stimuli are occurring, other than the teacher's voice. One student is running by, shouting "Hi." Another is bouncing a ball nearby. Students must focus on the teacher's verbal cue and the ball being thrown to them. Some students will have difficulty attending to the relevant stimuli, i.e., the ball being thrown and the teacher's verbal instructions.

Figure 3–1 Relevant Stimuli Selection

11. Learning will occur more quickly if the student is motivated to learn the skill.

Implication: Motivation is closely related to satisfying needs. The need to achieve, learn, and become more proficient at performing motor skills will motivate the student to participate in motor skills. Those who provide motor development instruction should not automatically assume that students will be motivated to learn these kinds of activities. Sage (1984) notes that teachers will need to employ many types of motivational techniques that will excite the learner's attention and willingness to participate. Examples of motivators include rewards, recognition, competition, and establishing levels of achievement.

12. Students will learn better if the teaching is geared to their best learning style.

Implication: Students have their own unique styles of learning. Some need many concrete experiences and much visual input in order to understand a skill. Auditory learners will require verbal instruction and verbal rehearsal of the task, while students who are more tactile oriented may need manipulative experience with the task. Fortunately, the learning of motor skills involves most of the learning channels. The key is to find the channel that best aids the student and utilize it in teaching.

13. Flexibility of the skill helps the student to generalize it and use it in different situations.

Implications: Rothstein, Catelli, Dodds, and Manahan (1981) suggest that skills be practiced in different settings, particularly if they are open skills, where the elements change from one effort to the next. For example, catching a ball is an open skill since the speed and direction change from one effort to the next. Many games and team sports are made up of open skills. The individual must be able to perceive the changes in order to make the correct motor response. Closed skills do not require as much diversity because the elements

do not change as much. An example is shooting a foul shot. Basically, the elements stay the same from one situation to another. These skills do not require as much information processing as open skills. Practice should offer diversity in performing the skill.

Students with learning problems will need to practice skills in different settings in order to generalize the skill and make more decisions as the skill changes.

14. The initial learning of a skill can be enhanced by first eliminating the locomotor aspects associated with it.

Implications: When teaching a student to dribble a basketball, no movement should be required. Thus, dribbling in a stationary position at first allows the student time to focus on the elements involved. This also helps to reduce the complexity of the skill. The teacher should build a skill sequence that begins with little transport and progresses to the actual transport involved. The following example illustrates a sequence that might be followed while learning to pass a soccer ball.

- Remain still and kick the ball to a stationary player.
- Run forward and kick the ball to a stationary player.
- Dribble the ball with the feet, then pass it to a stationary student.
- Dribble the ball and pass it to a moving player.
- Dribble the ball and pass it to a moving player being guarded.

15. The complexity of a task can be reduced if the information that has to be processed can be reduced until the skill is learned.

Implication: The more factors there are, thus creating more decision making, the more complex the task. The early stages of learning a complex task can be enhanced by reducing the number of decisions to be made (Rothstein et al., 1981). For example, if the main skill involves dribbling and passing a basketball to another player, the skill can be simplified by reducing the number of decisions to be made. Environmental stimuli can be decreased, such as reducing the number of players involved and reducing the speed of movement. As students become more skilled at dribbling and passing, more decision-making factors can be used in the motor task.

16. Feedback is critical in improving and/or correcting motor skills. Feedback should immediately follow the learner's trials so that adjustments and errors can be eliminated.

Implication: Feedback is information received by the learner after performing a task (Sage, 1984). However, feedback can occur at any stage during motor responses. *Concurrent* feedback refers to information given while the learner is still performing. *Terminal* feedback occurs after performance is completed. *Instrinsic* feedback is that supplied by the performers themselves. It is the feeling, seeing, and hearing of how one is responding. *Augmented* feedback is external and is usually provided by the instructor. The instructor generally presents feedback in terms of knowledge about the end result, or knowledge about performance aspects, i.e., why an error occurred or how to improve performance. Feedback from the instructor will eventually help the student to correct errors independently.

POINTS TO REMEMBER

1. The psychomotor domain provides a sequential developmental model for classifying motor skills and developing behavioral objectives.

2. The psychomotor domain can be used for developing sequential and meaningful instruction of motor skills.

3. By classifying movement and application of sound learning principles, instruction can be more easily accomplished.

4. The application of motor learning principles aids in designing teaching methods that will motivate students and enhance the instructional process.

5. The initial learning of motor skills can be enhanced by simplifying the task, distributing practice, and providing knowledge of results and performance.

6. The teacher should develop a flexible teaching style that can be readily adapted to the student's best learning style.

REFERENCES

Black, A.H., & Davis, L.J. (1966). The relationship between intelligence and sensorimotor proficiency in retardates. *American Journal of Mental Deficiency* 71, 55–59.

Corbin, C.B. (1973). *A textbook of motor development*. Dubuque, IA: William C. Brown.

Crowe, W.C., Auxter, D., & Pyfer, J. (1981). *Principles and methods of adapted physical education and recreation* (4th ed.). St. Louis: C.V. Mosby.

Drowatzky, J.N. (1971). *Physical education for the mentally retarded*. Philadelphia: Lea & Febiger.

Folio, M.R., & Fewell, R. (1983). *Peabody developmental motor scales and activity cards*. Allen, TX: DLM-Teaching Resources Corporation.

Harrow, A.J. (1972). *A taxonomy of the psychomotor domain: A guide for developing behavioral objectives*. New York: David McKay.

McClenaghan, B.A., & Gallahue, D.L. (1978). *Fundamental movement: A developmental and remedial approach*. Philadelphia: W.B. Saunders.

Moran, J., & Kalakian, L. (1974). *Movement experiences for the mentally retarded or emotionally disturbed child*. Minneapolis: Burgess.

Rothstein, A., Catelli, L., Dodds, P., & Manahan, J. (1981). *Motor learning: Basic stuff series I*. Reston, VA: American Alliance for Health, Physical Education, Recreation and Dance.

Sage, G.H. (1984). *Motor learning and control: A neuropsychological approach*. Dubuque, IA: William C. Brown.

Seaman, J.A., & DePauw, K.P. (1982). *The new adapted physical education: A developmental approach*. Palo Alto, CA: Mayfield.

Chapter 4

Fundamental Motor Patterns and Skills

Focus

- Discusses and describes the basic milestones of normal motor development.
- Defines and discusses fundamental movements, their development, problems encountered by handicapped students, and teaching activities.
- Explains common problems encountered when trying to learn skills of nonlocomotion and locomotion and projectile management skills.

Adapted physical educators need to clearly understand the normal sequence of motor development in order to evaluate and implement motor programs for handicapped youngsters. The developmental model of motor skill acquisition is the reference point from which disabled students may be assessed and the extent of any deviations determined. This model is particularly useful with handicapped students during the first six years of life since most of the basic fundamental motor patterns and skills have been developed within the normal child. The model can actually be applied with any level student.

This chapter will provide an overview of normal motor development and how basic fundamental patterns of locomotion and nonlocomotor skills develop. This will serve as a reference point in understanding the motor deviations and problems that might be encountered by students with disabilities. Projectile management skills will also be discussed similarly. While these skills may develop simultaneously, presentation in this format facilitates the organization of the material and information.

NORMAL MOTOR DEVELOPMENT

Corbin (1977) emphasizes that the most important and significant task of children during the first two years of life is to master sensory motor control over their environment. Much of what a young child does in the first three years of life is tightly interwoven in the development of motor skills. Basic fundamental patterns allow the child to move and explore the environment.

The majority of the literature on the development of basic fundamental motor patterns and skills has resulted from the study and work of several researchers, such as Shirley (1931), Bayley (1935), McGraw (1943), Gesell and Amatruda (1947), Wickstrom (1977), and Rarick (1973). The following are some basic concepts regarding motor development:

- Motor development occurs in a predictable, orderly sequence.
- Motor development proceeds from the head toward the feet and from the midline of the body outward.
- The motor development process is cumulative, such that higher-level skills generally are built on the development of lower-level skills.
- Generally, gross motor skills are more refined than fine motor skills. However, some fine motor skills can develop simultaneously with gross motor skills. For example, sitting, reaching, and grasping may develop during the same developmental time frame.

- Growth, maturation, environmental opportunity, and cultural practices affect the rate at which motor skills are developed.
- The rates at which children develop the normal motor milestones may vary widely, based on the factors mentioned above.
- Children will rely more on a lower-level skill until the newly acquired skills are learned and integrated.
- Children develop from a relatively reflexive state to one of voluntary motor acts. Many of the basic skills, such as walking, normally develop as characteristics of the human species, whereas other skills must be learned.

Handicapped children may not progress through the normal basic motor patterns and skills as normal children do because of the particular effects of their disability, the lack of motivation to learn, or impaired learning ability. The more severe the handicapping condition, the more evident the motor impairments.

The basic motor patterns and skills discussed in this chapter include:

- major motor milestones
- reflexes
- locomotor skills
- nonlocomotor skills

MOTOR BEHAVIOR STAGES

The postnatal motor behavior change can be divided into three basic stages: the neonate from birth to one month; babyhood, one month to two years; and early childhood, two years to six years. These stages are not necessarily clearly demarcated, but the developmental process is a continuation of what has occurred in previous stages.

The Neonate

The infant is primarily in a reflexive state with little or no voluntary motor responses present. Most of the movements observed in the first month or two of life are basic primitive reflexes. Fiorentino (1972) describes reflexes as involuntary responses to stimuli.

Babyhood

The development that occurs in babyhood provides a basis for some of the most significant accomplishments that will take place in a child's lifetime. One of the most important achievements is the development of upright locomotion. Achievement of upright locomotion is the culmination of a long complex sequence of progressive and interrelated skills.

This pattern, as studied by Shirley (1931), follows a predictable sequence. First, the infant must gain control of the muscles of the head and neck. For a short period during the first month, infants are able to hold up their heads. Later, by four months, infants are able to turn their heads from side to side and hold up their heads in a prone position. Considerable control of the head and trunk are developed by six months. During this time some forward progress is attempted while in a prone position. More strength has developed in the lower trunk, enabling the infant to sit with support at four months and independently at seven months.

Creeping (movement on the hands and knees) is generally developed by seven to nine months and greatly expands the baby's environment. The trunk and legs have further developed by seven to ten months, which allows the baby to stand with support and pull erect while holding on to stable objects. This leads to independent walking, which usually develops into a preferred method of locomotion by thirteen to fourteen months. Arnheim and Pestolozzi (1973) emphasize that walking is a tremendous milestone in the child's lifetime, as it increases the environment immensely and the possibilities for exploration.

The initial walking form is uneven and the steps are short. Frequent falling occurs as the baby is still trying to perfect balance skill. A wide base of support is assumed with the arms abducted to compensate for balance. However, as muscular strength increases, balance improves and the walking pattern becomes more mature. By twenty-four to thirty months, the child usually walks fairly well with little or no falling or bumping.

Early Childhood

Early childhood is also a time of rapid changes in motor skills. From the period of two to six years, most of the fundamental movement patterns develop to a fairly high level, provided the environment furnishes ample opportunity. Many of the motor skills that will be further developed actually have their beginnings before the age of 2. For example, walking is basic to the development of other movement patterns such as running, jumping, hopping, galloping, and skipping.

MAJOR MOTOR MILESTONES

Major motor milestones are the motor skills that constitute the important achievements for a given age period. These serve as a guide for measuring whether or not a child may be developing normally or on target. One of the most recent comprehensive motor development standardized tests is the *Peabody Developmental Motor Scales* (Folio and Fewell, 1983), which serves as a measure for children's motor development from birth through six years of age. While the

Peabody Developmental Motor Scales is primarily a standardized instrument, it may also serve as a means for viewing the developmental motor milestones of normal children. The test goes beyond the milestones, providing a comprehensive selection of motor skills that may be observed at particular age segments. Table 4–1 lists some of the major motor skills that develop at particular age sequences. The descriptions provided in this table do not include the exact criteria as presented in the *Peabody Scales*. The purpose here is to offer a basic picture of the unfolding and development of motor skills.

REFLEXES

Reflexive behavior is present at birth and continues to develop at higher levels as the brain matures in the course of normal development. The first reflexes present are referred to as primitive reflexes (Bobath & Bobath, 1975). These usually disappear or are integrated into higher levels of movements or postures. If higher-level reflexes do not appear, such as protective reactions and righting reactions, motor development can be delayed (Fiorentino, 1972). The primitive reflexes that occur during the first four months of life are controlled by the brain stem. These include the

- asymetrical tonic neck reflex
- symmetrical tonic neck reflex
- Moro reflex
- grasp reflex
- tonic labyrinthine reflex

The physical therapist usually tests for reflexes and provides therapy to inhibit or integrate them. The adapted physical educator needs to be aware of some of the basic reflexes in order to understand how motor skill acquisition might be affected. In some cases the adapted specialist may assist with the program designed by the physical therapist.

The Asymmetrical Tonic Neck Reflex

The asymmetrical tonic neck reflex may be observed when the infant is placed on the back. As the infant's head turns to the right or left, the body on the side to which the face is turned extends and the side of the body next to the back of the head flexes. In some instances, the body position is curved. Also, the arm on the face side may extend while the arm on the skull side may flex slightly.

This reflex is present at birth and will disappear around 4-6 months of age. If this reflex persists beyond 6 months, it may well interfere with using the hands at the midline of the body, or coordinated movements of the hands and knees may be

Table 4–1 Major Motor Skill Attainment of Specific Age Segments

Age Category	Motor Behaviors	Age Category	Motor Behaviors
0–1 month	• Demonstrates basic reflexive postures. • Arms thrust. • Legs flex.		• Begins throwing with intended directionality. • Stands with one foot on a line.
2–3 months	• Begins to hold head in body's midline. • Begins weight bearing, but legs sag. • Walking reflex present. • Bears weight on forearms while on stomach.	18–23 months	• Throws a ball three feet within 45 degrees of a straight line. • Runs flat footed at least 10 feet without falling. • Walks on 4-inch-wide beam at least 10 feet, one foot on and one foot off. • Jumps down from 10-inch height with one foot leading. • Jumps forward at least 4 inches without falling.
4–5 months	• Brings arms to midline of body. • Rolls from back to side. • Raises chest from prone position, supporting body with arms. • Sits supported for three seconds. • Pulls self to sitting while holding adult's fingers.	24–29 months	• Walks up steps one foot per step with support (alternating feet). • Throws a tennis ball at least 7 feet without deviating more than 20 degrees. • Balances on one foot at least 3 seconds. • Takes at least three steps on a 4-inch-wide beam without falling off. • Walks on a circular line 1 inch wide without stepping off more than five times.
6–7 months	• Protecting reactions emerge by extending arms. • Rolls from back to stomach. • Moves forward on stomach. • Sits and manipulates a toy at least 30 seconds.	30–35 months	• Balances on one foot for 5 seconds. • Jumps forward at least 24 inches. • Hops at least three times without losing balance.
8–9 months	• Assumes position on hands and knees—may or may not move forward. • Scoots in sitting position. • Recovers lost balance in sitting position.	36–41 months	• Climbs stairs unsupported alternating feet. • Descends stairs without support alternating feet. • Jumps down from 30-inch height using two-foot takeoff and landing. • Catches a ball with elbows bent in front of body. • Begins skipping—may forget to keep the same lead foot.
10–11 months	• Stands and moves while holding on to furniture. • Lowers self to sitting position from standing position while holding on to furniture or an adult. • Takes three or four steps foward while holding on to an adult's hand.	42–47 months	• Throws ball at targets 2 feet square hitting the target from 5 feet away. • Bounce passes a ball at least 5 feet. • Jumps forward on one foot at least 6 inches. • Balances on one foot for 10 seconds. • Walks backward on a 1-inch-wide line without stepping off more than once.
12–14 months	• Assumes kneeling position without losing balance. • Climbs stairs on hands and knees. • Stands and pivots. • Picks up a toy from a standing position. • Walks four or five steps unsupported. • Flings a ball while standing.	48–53 months	• Runs using arms in good reciprocal movement. • Walks four steps forward on a 4-inch-wide beam unassisted. • Begins to do somersaults.
15–17 months	• Walks using a narrow base of support with reciprocal arm movements. • Walks up stairs with both feet on each step (marking time). • Walks backward. • Walks down steps holding rail with both feet on each step (marking time). • Attempts to kick a ball.		

Table 4–1 continued

Age Category	Motor Behaviors
54–59 months	• Jumps and turns 180 degrees. • Walks backward with heel-to-toe pattern at least five steps on a 4-inch-wide beam. • Skips well eight to ten skips integrating arm and leg movements. • Catches a ball with elbows placed at sides. • Throws at a 2-foot square target from 12 feet hitting the target two of three trials. • Jumps forward 36 inches.
60–71 months	• Walks on tip toes 15 feet without losing balance. • Jumps over a hurdle 10 inches high. • Bounces and catches own ball. • Hops 20 feet in 6 seconds. • Gallops in a smooth rhythmical pattern. • Kicks a ball in the air at least 12 feet forward.
72–83 months	• Kicks a rolling ball straight ahead with no more than a 20 degree deviation. • Moves toward a ball and kicks with a continuous coordinated motion. • Shuttle runs a 12-foot distance in 12 seconds.

Source: DLM-Teaching Resources

impaired. In severe cases, hip dislocation and curvature of the spine may result.

The Symmetrical Tonic Neck Reflex

The symmetrical tonic neck reflex can be observed by holding the child across an adult's lap. When the head is bent or flexed, the arms will also flex and the legs will extend. When the head is extended, the arms extend and the legs flex.

This reflex is present at birth and will usually disappear by 5 months of age. If the reflex persists, it interferes with hand and knee positioning in creeping.

The Moro Reflex

The Moro reflex, sometimes referred to as the startle reflex, may be observed by holding the child in a semisitting position while holding the trunk and head. As support is released momentarily from the head, the child's arms will fan away from the body with the fingers spread. This reflex disappears at about 5 months of age. If it persists, balance may be hampered.

The Grasp Reflex

The grasp reflex is fairly simple to elicit. By placing the child on the back and touching the palm of the hand with an object, an instinctive grasp will occur. No vision is needed to find the object. Later, this reflex helps to coordinate movements for grasping objects and ultimately to a mature grasp and voluntary release of objects. If the reflex is not integrated, voluntary release of objects becomes difficult.

Tonic Labyrinthine Reflexes

Montgomery and Richter (1977) report that the tonic labyrinthine reflexes may be observed both in prone and supine positions. While in a prone position, if the reflex persists, the child cannot achieve arm and head extension. While in a supine position, the child will be unable to lift the head off the floor. The reflex may be observed as the child is pulled to a sitting position. If the reflex is present, the trunk will remain stiff without bending in the direction of the pull. Or if the child is on a stomach position and the reflex is present, resistance will be noticed as the head is lifted by an adult. This reflex generally disappears by the fifth month.

The Landau Reflex

Beginnings of the Landau reaction may be seen around 5 months. The reaction becomes stronger between 6 and 8 months. By at least two years of age the reflex disappears. Montgomery and Richter (1977) explain that this reflex can be observed when holding a child across an adult's lap. While the child is on the stomach and the head is lifted by an adult, the trunk and legs will also extend.

The Landau reflex is important because it begins the development of extensor tone, which serves to strengthen the extensor muscles of the body. When the reflex disappears, the trunk and legs are not extended when the head is extended. The Landau reflex interferes with coordinated creeping on all fours if it persists.

Body-Righting Reaction

The body-righting reaction can be observed with the child in a back-lying position. As one knee and hip are bent to the right or left, the trunk should rotate sequentially beginning with the hips, trunk and shoulders moving toward the direction of the bent leg. This reflex may be seen around 6 months of age and allows for the breakup of the total patterns of extension and flexion. Consequently, both flexion and extension patterns can occur simultaneously, allowing the child to sit or do other motor activities where both patterns are necessary (Fraser, Galka, & Hensinger, 1980).

Protective Extension and Equilibrium Reactions

Protective extension and equilibrium reactions generally appear at about 6 months of age and persist throughout life. These reactions are important in trying to block a fall and maintain balance.

One of the first protective reactions to develop is called the parachute reaction. It can be observed as the child is lowered slowly toward the floor. If it is present, the arms will extend toward the floor in an attempt to protect the body. This reflex can be first observed around 6 months of age and remains throughout life. It helps to protect the body as it falls and aids in maintaining balance in a number of positions.

Righting Reactions

Fraser, Galke, and Hensinger (1980) refer to righting reactions as movements from the head when the body is tilted from the midline. These can be observed by tilting the body from a suspended position. When this occurs, the head will try to maintain alignment with the trunk.

Righting Reactions While Sitting

Righting reactions occur while sitting. If the child is tipped sideward, the head will return to the vertical position. This reaction may be seen as early as 6 months and remains throughout life. Later, the reaction develops as balance is lost sideward while sitting and then backward.

Equilibrium Reactions

Equilibrium reactions develop in standing within a 12-18-month range. As the child loses balance in any direction the body adjusts by moving in the opposite direction, using the head, shoulders, trunk, and extension of the leg in the direction of the fall. These reactions are obviously needed for standing, locomotor activities, landing, and prevention of falls.

LOCOMOTOR SKILLS

Locomotor skills provide transport to the body. In fact, any motor skill that moves the body from one base of support to another is referred to as a locomotor skill. The adapted physical educator should be able to analyze a motor skill to determine problems that handicapped students may encounter while performing motor activities that transport the body. The following section provides an overview of basic fundamental locomotor skills, problems encountered by handicapped students, and activities for teaching each skill.

Rolling

Rolling is an early childhood skill used for locomotion. In addition, rolling can be a higher form of movement when used in a somersault. Infants use rolling to move in different directions before age 1. Some handicapped children may use rolling well beyond the time higher levels of locomotor skills should have developed.

Rolling should be taught to young children with developmental delays in order to provide a foundation for higher-level skills to develop. Another important need for rolling skill is to absorb the force of a fall.

First attempts at rolling may be initiated by an arm or leg movement in the infant. This form of rolling by the infant is different from basic forms of rolling used in beginning stunt activities. The most commonly used roll is the sideward roll.

Sideward Roll (Right or Left)

Evans (1980) explains that a true sideward roll should be initiated with the hips as the body is held straight with arms over the head. The body segments should move together evenly.

Problems Observed in Handicapped Children

- Roll is initiated with an arm or leg rather than the hip.
- Legs and arms may not remain positioned together.
- Rhythm may not be maintained while rolling.
- Body is bent rather than kept straight.

Teaching Activities

1. Wrap student in a blanket and unroll the student so the feel of rolling is achieved.

2. Let students roll down an incline board; this aids in initiating the roll in the beginning stages.

3. Once students learn to roll using proper techniques, let them roll using different speeds and in different directions.

4. For students having difficulty keeping their legs together, tie the legs together loosely with wide sewing elastic. This will keep the legs together without binding them (Evans, 1980).

Walking

Walking occurs after the child has developed sufficient strength in the back, hip, and leg muscles. Generally, walking is preceded by crawling, creeping, and walking around furniture or large obstacles while holding on for support. By the time the child is ready to begin walking, many of the postural reactions to the loss of balance are intact. These are noticed in nonlocomotor skills and then transferred to walking and other locomotor skills.

Careful observation and evaluation of walking in young children is essential. Sometimes poor walking gaits may be indicative of delays or specific disabilities. For example, some children with cerebral palsy may have deficiencies or deviations in their walking gait if the limbs are affected. They may scissor the legs when walking, walk with heels elevated, or use a high-stepping gait. Some children may fall frequently; others may have poor postural alignment. Extraneous movements or wasted movements may be present and produce inefficient movement. Some of the errors can be modified and some corrected.

Correct Walking Pattern

Several key points should be observed when evaluating the child's walking pattern:

1. The body should be aligned correctly. The head should be over the shoulders, the shoulders in line with the hips, and knees should be over the ankles. The head should also face forward.

2. The heel of the forward foot should come in contact with the supporting surface first and the body weight should be shifted to the ball of the foot and then the toes. The back leg should swing forward, with the heel contacting the ground first. The feet should point fairly straight ahead. The arms should swing freely in opposition to the moving foot. This cross pattern is first seen in crawling and creeping.

Problems Observed in Handicapped Students

- Head is held out of alignment, too far back, forward, or to the side.
- Shoulders are tilted forward or uneven.
- Feet are turned too far outward or inward.
- Feet shuffle.
- There is more lateral movement than anterior posterior movement.
- Arms are not coordinated with leg movement.
- Body posture is too rigid.

Teaching Activities

1. Blind students can be taught to improve their walking gait. Some problems observed are a shuffling gait, head tilt, and lateral movement in the body.

2. Cratty (1980) suggests that students with coordination problems be placed in a kneeling position to practice the cross-extension pattern of the arms with the legs.

3. Marching activities where the arms are exaggerated help students get the feel of the arm and leg movements.

4. Students should be allowed to walk on a variety of surfaces to practice balance.

5. If foot placement is a problem, footprints can be set down in a straight path and the student can practice proper foot placement.

6. Students who must use assistive devices should be taught the most efficient method for using them. This is generally done by the physical therapist, but the teacher should evaluate the student periodically to be sure that the equipment is used properly. Also, the teacher should examine the equipment for wear, tear, and loose screws or other methods of joining the pieces together.

7. Devices such as sticks, push toys, and ropes provide the student with support other than always holding hands. These should be used for students who cannot yet walk independently to make them feel secure.

8. For young handicapped children, it may be necessary to motivate the child to walk. A favorite toy, for example, can be placed just ahead of the child.

9. Having children observe themselves in the mirror as they are being led while walking gives them encouragement as well as a model to strive for.

10. Videotaping or filming older students as they walk can provide feedback where errors need to be corrected.

11. Varying the base of support from wide to narrow provides a progression in small increments.

Walking Up and Down Stairs

Most children can negotiate a flight of standard stairs and climb objects rather well by 3 to 4 years of age (Folio & Fewell, 1983). Stair climbing may actually be observed first as the child tries to climb two or three steps on the hands and knees around the first year of life. Caretakers often may deny early opportunities to learn this skill. Children are carried up and down steps when adults are in a hurry or are fearful of children falling even though assistance is provided. Climbing ladders or gym equipment often parallels the patterns developed in stair climbing. Children will normally pass through several sequential stages when ascending and descending stairs.

The following sequence may normally be observed for ascending stairs:

- Creeps up stairs on hands and knees, or hands and feet.
- Walks up steps with adult help, placing two feet at one time on each tread (marking time).
- Walks up steps with assistance, alternating feet (one foot per step).
- Walks up steps unassisted, marking time.
- Walks up steps unassisted, alternating feet.

The following is the sequence for descending stairs:

- Descends stairs by scooting down.

- Descends stairs with adult assistance with a marking time pattern.
- Descends with assistance, alternating feet.
- Descends stairs without assistance, marking time.
- Descends without assistance, alternating feet.

Ladder Climbing

Ladder climbing and climbing gym equipment follow the same pattern as seen in negotiating stairs.

Teaching Activities

1. Begin with lead-in activities such as having students walk up and down inclines working on balance.
2. Have students march in place as if climbing stairs.
3. Have students step over low objects, rope tied between two chairs, or between the rungs of a ladder placed flat on the floor.
4. Visually impaired students should be allowed to try the activities barefooted to stimulate tactile awareness.
5. Begin stair climbing first, since it appears to be the easiest developmentally. A motivating toy can be placed three steps from the bottom step so that it aids the child in climbing two steps to retrieve it.
6. Begin with steps low in height. If steps are not readily available, secure wooden boxes or cement blocks can be used.
7. Place footprints on steps to show the child where to step.
8. Students who have to use assistive devices should be taught to negotiate stairs for safety, if they are able to do so.
9. Similar strategies should be used to teach the student to descend stairs. However, students who are fearful should begin on the bottom step, then step down. Gradually increase the number of stairs to walk down.

Running

Burton (1977) explains that running differs from walking primarily in the speed of locomotion. Also, while running, there is no base of support temporarily, making the skill more difficult and less stable than walking.

The body position and mechanics of running are similar to those of walking. Wickstrom (1977) reports that early forms of running are characterized by body rotation. The legs seem to have more lateral and rotational movements than anterior-posterior movements. The arms are held rather stiff and abducted during the beginning phases of running.

McClenaghan and Gallahue (1978) describe more mature phases of running. The middle stage is characterized as follows:

- There is more leg stride and less rotation about the vertical axis of the body.
- More pushoff occurs with the weight-bearing leg.
- The arm movements are more coordinated with the leg movements.
- Less falling occurs than in earlier stages and more speed is acquired.

More advanced stages of running have some significant changes. McClenaghan and Gallahue (1978) point out the following:

- More extension and height in the running stride occurs.
- Well-coordinated cross-extension movements are observed in the arms and legs.
- The elbows are bent at near right angles.
- More agility is developed as the child is able to negotiate obstacles and start and stop quickly.

Problems Observed in Handicapped Students

Similar kinds of faults noted in walking can also be observed while the student is running since the movement patterns are similar. In addition, children who are uncoordinated may stumble and fall frequently.

Teaching Activities

Burton (1977) recommends that beginners be allowed to practice running in an open space. Before teaching running, be sure that the student has a mature or somewhat stable walking pattern. Frequent falling may occur during the initial stages of running, so it is important to arrange for a safe environment.

Evans (1980) suggests that the movements for the different body segments and parts involved in running be taught separately and then combined. The arm movements should be practiced in front of a mirror and the instructor can help manipulate the student's arms.

1. Have student practice raising the knees or march using arm and leg movements.
2. Let student walk quickly over objects placed on a course.
3. Have student march using exaggerated arm and leg movements.
4. Hold student's hand and run slowly.
5. Have students run with a partner.
6. Have students run a race with a partner.
7. Have students run to designated points and return.
8. Have students play simplified games that involve running, tag, relays, etc.
9. Have students run short distances for time.

Jumping

Moran and Kalakian (1974) define jumping as the ability to take off on either one or two feet and land on two feet. Jumping can occur in any direction. Most often, jumping occurs straight ahead. However, jumping may be used to dismount or jump down from objects. Vertical jumping can also occur and is used in many different sports.

McClenaghan and Gallahue (1978) provide a good description of the different stages of jumping. The beginning stages are characterized by little movement of the arms during first attempts. The body is used very little to give direction to the jump. Actual first attempts at jumping are more like elongated steps. Landing may not first occur simultaneously on both feet. Instead, one foot may land before the other until sufficient coordination in jumping is achieved.

In the second or intermediate phases of jumping there is more integration of the upper and lower extremities of the body. During this phase, children may be seen using the arms more to initiate the beginning phase of jumping. McClenaghan and Gallahue (1978) report that the arms are also used more in flight to maintain balance. More body crouch can be observed during the takeoff than in the previous stage. Also, the legs begin to extend more after takeoff.

The mature phase of jumping is characterized by more precision and coordination of all the body segments. The trunk is used more extensively to propel the body in the desired direction. In the horizontal jump, the trunk is usually angled at 45 degrees. The arms are used extensively to initiate the jump and reach forward to carry momentum. The legs are straightened after takeoff and then bent for landing in a crouched position. The trunk leans forward as weight is absorbed on landing.

Other Forms of Jumping

Jumping down from objects can be observed as early as 2 years of age. However, prior attempts may resemble an elongated step downward from the obstacle. Young children and handicapped children are usually fearful of jumping down from heights. The same movement patterns used in forward jumping should also be used in jumping downward. By age 5 or 6 children can jump down from 2-2½-foot heights in a fairly sophisticated manner (Folio & Fewell, 1983).

Vertical Jumping

Jumping upward or vertical jumping begins around age 4 among normally developing children. Initial attempts may resemble the immature stages of other forms of jumping. The motivating factor for jumping vertically for young children is to try to obtain something out of reach.

Problems Observed in Handicapped Students

- Retarded children may exhibit immature patterns of jumping observed in normal children.
- The upper portion of the body is not well integrated into the total movement cycle while jumping.
- The arms may not be used for takeoff, may not be held in position while in flight, or may not be used to balance while landing.
- The upper portion of the body may be held at the wrong angle for takeoff, too far forward or backward.
- The legs may not be extended sufficiently to produce maximum takeoff.
- Handicapped students in Project PERMIT exhibited other jumping deviations as reported by Folio (1983). These included using one side of the body more than the other, landing flat footed, or stepping forward instead of jumping. These characteristics were observed more in children with Down's Syndrome, neurological impairments, and sensory impairments.
- Similar difficulties have been observed as handicapped students attempt to jump down from objects.

Teaching Activities

These strategies may be employed across most handicapping conditions.

1. Be sure the student is ready for jumping; muscular strength is important. The student may practice climbing, tricycle riding, and walking to strengthen the leg muscles.

2. Let the student practice bouncing, using the arms for balance. Basic trampoline activities or other bouncing devices are helpful to teach the idea of bouncing and becoming airborne.

3. When holding the student's hands for support, try to hold them in the natural position they will be in while performing the jump, away from the side and not straight overhead.

4. Hold the student's hands and bounce in place.

5. Allow time for exploration of jumping skills. Ask students to jump in or out of taped shapes, hoops, ropes, or other designated spaces.

6. Challenge the students to jump over ropes placed in a "V" shape, pretending to jump across a river or other imaginary object.

7. For students who have difficulty with balance, use mats or a soft landing spot.

8. Ask students to use their imagination and jump like a kangaroo, frog, jack-in-the-box, or popcorn popping.

9. Ask students to jump in different directions, or jump through an obstacle course.

10. Students who become somewhat skilled may begin combining other movements with jumping, such as jumping and bouncing a ball or running and jumping.

Hopping

The differences between jumping and hopping is that hopping is a takeoff and landing on one foot. Hopping requires more skill refinement of balance and coordination than jumping. Hopping is generally considered a locomotor movement, but it can be accomplished in a stationary position. More often than not, hopping is used as a locomotor movement.

When hopping, the body's center of gravity must be kept over the supporting foot while the arms and opposite leg are used for balance. The takeoff and landing are completed on the ball of the foot. During takeoff, the hip and leg should be bent slightly to initiate the force to drive the body upward. The arms should be bent at the elbow and raised to aid in the lift of the body. This will help increase the height and lift of the hop.

Landing properly is important. The ball of the foot should absorb the force, with the leg and hip bending also to absorb force. This procedure prepares the body to begin another hop.

Hopping can vary in form from simple hopping on one foot to rhythmical hopping where more timing and skill are required. The activity can be made more complicated by hopping in designated patterns.

Actual hopping begins to appear in normal children around age 4. By the sixth year, hopping can become more refined and precise. Speed also increases by age 6. Children can hop from one point to another at age 6 at a fairly fast rate and still maintain balance. Hopping is also used in some perceptual motor tests to evaluate neurological development and body coordination.

Problems Observed in Handicapped Students

Handicapped students exhibit problems when hopping which may be similar to those in jumping. These include:

- poor balance
- improper positioning of the nonsupporting leg
- lack of strength in the support leg for pushoff and landing
- arms not integrated into the liftoff
- legs stiff on flat-footed landing
- center of gravity not over the supporting foot
- bounces instead of leaving the floor

Teaching Activities

The physical educator should first conduct an informal assessment of each student's motor skills prior to teaching hopping. Some students will lack the prerequisite skills. The teacher should look primarily for the readiness skills described below:

- The student should have the ability to balance on one foot.
- Jumping skill should already be developed on two feet.
- The support leg should be strong enough to support the student's weight, particularly on landing.
- There should be adequate coordination of the upper and lower extremities.

A good teaching progression should be developed, particularly if the students demonstrate a variety of hopping skills.

1. Begin by reviewing jumping in place on two feet.
2. Let students stand next to a wall for support. While holding the wall for support, students can bounce on one foot. Other stable support devices should be available, such as parallel bars.
3. Repeat the procedure in activity 2 but have students jump rather than bounce.
4. Have students bounce in place on one foot holding hands with a partner, then hop in place.
5. Ask students to hop forward three or four steps, then change the hopping foot. Students having difficulty may still use a wall for support.
6. Have students hop using different speeds.
7. Have students hop into designated spaces on the floor.
8. Have students hop into bicycle tires, taped shapes, or other objects arranged in a circuit.
9. Use rhythms and have students hop on one foot for so many counts, then switch the hopping foot. For creativity allow students to explore their own rhythms and make up their own patterns.
10. Introduce combining other locomotor skills with hopping, such as walk and hop, run and hop, etc.

Leaping

Schurr (1980) describes the leap as being very similar to a run, except that the time in the air is longer and more height is achieved. Usually, a leap is preceded by a run of several steps. Since the body is elevated more than in the run, more absorption of force is necessary on landing. During the suspension phase when the body is airborne, the stride is elongated. More force is exerted with the pushoff leg and more lift comes from the arms than in the run. In the leap, the takeoff is on one foot and landing occurs on the opposite foot. The leap is used to navigate over objects while running and is basic in many dance routines.

Landing is an important component in the leap and should be carefully taught. The idea of landing softly and absorbing force needs to be stressed.

Problems Observed in Handicapped Students

Leaping requires balance and coordination since it is usually combined with running steps. Handicapped students may exhibit some of the following difficulties while trying to leap:

- They may not gain sufficient height.
- The arms are not used enough to gain height.
- The arms may be used unevenly during takeoff.
- Landing may be on both feet or with the leg stiff.
- The legs may not be stretched out enough during the takeoff and airborne phases.
- Perseveration may occur during the running phase, resulting in an inability to push off; instead, the student continues to run.

Teaching Activities

1. Have students practice taking long giant steps forward.
2. Tape lines on the floor 6 to 12 inches apart in a parallel pattern and have students leap over the lines.
3. Have students take several running steps before leaping and practice trying to gain height.
4. Tie ropes between cones or chairs at heights ranging from 3-12 inches and have students leap over them.
5. Use imagery and have students imagine they are leaping like a deer over a log.
6. After they have developed some skill, allow students to leap to different rhythms. A drum may be used or other forms of sound.
7. Not all students with disabilities will be able to leap with perfect form, but they should be allowed to try to develop the skill, if that is possible.

Sliding

Sliding is a sideward movement with the same foot leading throughout the movement. In sliding to the left the left foot leads; in sliding to the right, the right foot leads.

Dauer and Pangrazzi (1979) suggest that bouncing while sliding should be kept to a minimum and the movement should be smooth. Some students may try to move forward instead of sideways. This movement would be a gallop rather than a true slide.

Sliding is an important fundamental skill because it is used in many games and sports, such as moving sideways to guard an opponent or dodge an object. When used in games and sports, sliding requires some agility in order to quickly change directions.

Problems Observed in Handicapped Students

- change of the lead foot.
- sliding flat footed rather than on the ball of the foot.
- taking short steps and bouncing while sliding.
- moving forward instead of sideways.
- body weight not shifted smoothly.

Teaching Activities

1. Teach the slide by standing in front of the student and facing away. This will help the student see the correct movement pattern.
2. Place a piece of tape on the lead foot so the student can be reminded to keep the same foot in the lead.
3. Slide at a slow pace until the student can maintain a correct pattern.
4. To develop rhythm in the slide, face the student and hold hands while sliding together. Verbal cues can be used, such as "Step, step, step," at the beginning of each movement of the lead foot.
5. Practice sliding to the right, then to the left.
6. Play follow-the-leader and have students imitate each other while sliding.
7. Add music and slide at different tempos.

Galloping

After students have learned to slide, galloping can be easily taught since it is very similar to sliding. The difference is that in galloping, the movement is in a forward direction rather than sideward. The basic techniques involved in sliding are also applicable to galloping.

Problems Observed in Handicapped Students

Problems observed while galloping will be similar to those of sliding.

- Steps may be unrhythmical.
- The lead foot is changed by moving the back foot too far forward.
- The arms may be held too stiffly at the sides.
- Changing directions may be difficult or confusing.

Teaching Activities

1. Review sliding to familiarize student with the movements. Describe or demonstrate moving forward instead of sideward.
2. Let student use a broomstick to pretend he or she is riding a horse.

3. Tie a rope around another student's waist and have the handicapped student hold the rope while imitating the front student galloping.

4. In the beginning, have students stop before changing and practice with the opposite foot as the lead foot.

5. Use tape or a different-colored sock for the lead foot if students get confused.

6. Have students gallop to music or a drum beat.

7. Let students gallop with a partner, holding hands side by side.

8. Ask students to combine other movements with galloping.

Skipping

Skipping may be more difficult to teach handicapped students because it combines several movements. The walk and the hop are combined to form a skip. Many times when handicapped students try to skip, they will actually gallop. The hop part of the skip is usually omitted.

The actual skip is a step forward on one foot and then a hop on the same foot, with the cycle being repeated on the opposite foot. Since hopping is involved in skipping, it requires some degree of dynamic balance. Skipping is used in many simple dance routines, games, and relays. Also a step hop is used in landing in some cases, such as dismounting from an apparatus or maintaining balance after jumping. The hop portion of the skip gives propulsion to the body in an upward direction. The arms, when used properly, add height and momentum to the skip.

Problems Observed in Handicapped Students

- Steps forward on one foot, but hops on the other.
- Fails to change the lead foot for the next step.
- Has difficulty maintaining balance while skipping.
- Arms are not well integrated with leg movements.
- May perseverate and take too many hops.
- Uses one side of the body more than the other.
- Rhythm may be difficult to achieve or maintain.

Teaching Activities

1. Review balance skills and hopping skills as lead-in activities.

2. Let peer tutors demonstrate skipping. A small rhythmic routine can be performed, or a relay using skipping.

3. For students who have difficulty, let the peer tutor work separately with them on skipping.

4. Give cues such as "Step, now hop." Colored tape can be placed on one foot to remind the student to complete both the step and the hop on the same foot before changing the lead foot.

5. Hold student's hand and skip.

6. Once some understanding and ability have been developed, let students explore the movement by asking them to skip at different speeds, in different directions, and to different locations.

7. Play records or tapes of different rhythms and ask students to skip in time to the music.

8. Play a simple game using the skip, or develop a relay race.

9. Combine other movements with skipping.

NONLOCOMOTOR SKILLS

Nonlocomotor movements consist of movements around the different axes of the body and do not transport the body as do locomotor movements. More often, nonlocomotor movements are used in everyday routines or are combined with locomotor movements. These skills are important for handicapped students to learn in order to function in a daily routine. Some of these movements may be important actions in particular vocational skills. Nonlocomotor skills are also used as warm-up activities before exercising and executing locomotor skills.

Bending

Bending involves movement around a joint—the location where two bones join—in which the angle of the joint is decreased. *Flexion* is a term used to mean bending. The amount that one can bend a joint depends on the amount of flexibility and the structure of the joint itself. Flexion in a joint is also accompanied by stretching or extension. These two movements are combined to bend and straighten a body part at a particular joint.

Most of the time more than one body part is combined while bending. For example, bending of body parts at several joints occurs when a person squats down to pick up an object. Another important aspect of bending or flexing is the fact that the amount of flexion in certain body parts, such as the legs, will affect the amount of force exerted when executing a skill, for example, jumping (Schurr, 1980).

Problems Observed in Handicapped Students

Normally, young children remain quite flexible, but as age increases, flexibility usually declines unless activities are continued to maintain flexibility. Bending ability may vary widely among handicapped students, depending on the nature of the disability and the opportunity to exercise and develop physically.

Orthopedically Handicapped

Children with cerebral palsy may develop orthopedic problems resulting in limited range of motion and rigidity in the musculature structures. Range of motion activities are often recommended as part of everyday routines for students with specific types of cerebral palsy. Keeping the range of motion in joints is of primary importance.

On the other hand, certain forms of cerebral palsy may leave the musculature totally flaccid with too much flexibility. This is particularly evident in infants, and later may develop into spasticity leading to reduced flexibility in the movements around particular joints.

Mentally Retarded

In cases of mild mental retardation with unknown causes, flexibility may not be seriously affected. Flexibility and bending that is less than optimal may be due to improper body mechanics. Some mentally retarded students may lack the ability to bend as a result of inactivity.

Down's Syndrome students, on the other hand, may possess extreme ranges of motion in particular joints as a result of too much flexibility. This is particularly true when Down's children have not had the opportunity to benefit from good physical education programs.

Teaching Activities

Unless there are particular problems that would interfere with bending activities, handicapped students should be taught to bend properly and integrate the skill in a variety of activities.

1. When describing flexion actions, language that the student understands should be used. Concrete examples must also be provided. Blind students may be allowed to feel the movement as another person or a manikin performs it.

2. Begin with small bends such as the small parts of the body, including the finger, wrist, ankles, neck, etc.

3. Ask students to bend their arms, then a leg. Provide a demonstration or model. Then ask students to think of body parts to bend.

4. Have students bend larger portions of the body. Bend at the waist, hips, and so forth.

5. Use bending in an activity, like touching your toes, picking up an object, sitting down. Ask students to think of other activities that use bending.

6. Have students bend several body parts at one time.

7. Have students bend different body parts from different postures, lying down, sitting, standing, and so forth.

8. Have students move around the room and bend different body parts.

Stretching

Stretching is commonly referred to as extension or increasing the angle of a joint. Any extension beyond 180 degrees is referred to as hyperextension at a joint. Some individuals may normally have hyperextension in some joints, the elbow and knees being the most common joints. Burton (1977) defines extension as the return of a body part to a straightened position after it has been flexed or bent. Bending and stretching, as mentioned previously, act together to alter or change the characteristics of movements or body positions.

Stretching is recommended before performing more vigorous movements with the body. Muscles need to be warm and stretched before performance to prevent injury. Stretching muscle groups also helps the body to remain flexible. Stretching aids in achieving maximum extension while performing. Many motor acts would not reach maximum performance if stretching was not included in the movement.

Stretching should be done carefully in order not to injure muscles. Bouncing excessively to stretch muscle groups is not recommended. This is true of all levels of students, particularly those who have orthopedic problems.

Teaching Activities

1. Stretching should begin by mild reaching and extending the body. Hints such as "Reach for the sky," if standing, or "Make your body long," are helpful. For students who cannot stand and stretch, lying positions are effective. Stretching of particular body parts may also be done from a wheelchair or sitting position.

2. Total body stretching can be accomplished or specific body parts can be emphasized. Students should begin slowly and not bounce.

3. Stretching can be active, where the student moves independently, or passive, where the teacher moves the body part. If the teacher has any concern about whether or not a student should participate in stretching activities, a physician or physical therapist should be consulted.

4. Hanging from a horizontal ladder or stall bar can also be a method for stretching.

5. Partner activities are motivating for students.

6. Partners can sit and face each other pulling a rope back and forth. This can help stretch the leg muscles. Stress that this should be done slowly. If ropes are not available students can hold hands.

7. Partners can sit side by side, hold hands, and rock to each side.

8. Have different bases of support and combine bending and stretching of several body parts.

Twisting

Twisting, or rotation around the vertical axis of the body, is also used in many motor activities. Twisting movements most often occur at the hip, neck, and shoulder joints. Twisting is used in the daily routine and in gymnastics, dance, and diving skills.

Many levels of handicapped students can learn to twist the body properly. If neurological problems are present, the movements may be uncoordinated or possibly restricted. When twisting to a particular rhythm, the rhythm may be uneven.

Teaching Activities

While students are standing ask them to turn the trunk without moving the feet. Tell them to pretend to look for someone behind them.

2. Have students stand and look from side to side.

3. Have students twist or turn the hips from side to side.

4. Play a record, tape, or the radio, even if students have difficulty maintaining rhythm.

5. Have students twist smaller body parts, such as the wrists and fingers.

6. Do dance activities that use twisting movements. For students who cannot stand, let them twist another body part in time to the beat.

PROJECTILE MANAGEMENT COMPONENTS

Many sports and recreational activities in which handicapped students might engage require the abilities of throwing, catching, or other forms of imparting force or stopping an object. These skills may be slightly delayed, immature, or not present at all in handicapped students. They should be developed with locomotor and nonlocomotor skills and used together.

Projectile management may indirectly affect other areas of development. For example, as a child moves through space while imparting force to an object, spatial relationships may be formed. These activities may also be used to teach and refine skills in depth perception and other visual motor coordination skills. A child who possesses skills such as throwing, kicking, striking, etc., will be able to enhance social interaction among peers. This will allow the child to participate in many leisure and recreational activities.

The following sections will explain the stages of development of skills that children use to impart and receive force to and from objects. Also, activities for teaching these skills to handicapped children will be suggested with modifications provided when necessary for some children with specific handicapping conditions.

Throwing

Throwing is a very noticeable skill as it normally develops. Parents are usually very much aware of their child's first few attempts at imparting force to objects in the form of throwing. A sequence of throwing skills generally follows. The patterns vary from random flinging of objects to more precise movements related to form, speed, and accuracy.

McClenaghan and Gallahue (1978) reported studies of the patterns of throwing. Their summary indicated that children pass through specific stages of development in acquiring a mature throwing pattern. The stages include several features, as seen in Table 4–2.

Overarm Throw

Several throwing patterns occur, including the sidearm, underarm, and overhand throw. The most frequently used form is the overarm or overhand throw.

Overarm throwing requires that the ball be held in the right hand for a right-handed person and the opposite for a left-handed person. Vannier and Gallahue (1978) outline the overarm throw as including the following sequence:

1. The ball is held in the right hand with the first two fingers on top of the ball, while the third and fourth fingers are spread along the side.

2. The thumb is held underneath the ball with the palm not touching it.

3. Body weight is distributed equally on both feet. The left side faces the target with the left foot forward.

4. The right arm is brought back to a position slightly behind the ear and the body's weight is shifted to the right foot. The elbow is held away from the body and the wrist is cocked backward.

5. As the release is begun, the left foot moves toward the target, and the body begins to rotate, with the hips and

---

Table 4–2 Stages of Development: Throwing

Stage	Task Component
Stage 1	Forearm imparts force forward in a fairly high short path. Little body movement is involved and the feet remain stationary.
Stage 2	Some trunk and foot action enters into the throwing pattern on the same side of the body as the throwing hand.
Stage 3	More shift in body weight is observed. The arms and feet move in opposition to each other. Followthrough begins to appear, with evidence of hand and wrist control.
Stage 4	A definite shift of weight, trunk rotation, and overarm extension are noted. Hand control and wrist followthrough are more precise. All of the throwing dynamics of movement and form are observed in the final mature stages.

arm brought forward. As the arm straightens, the wrist is snapped and the ball moves forward off the fingers.

6. The force of the arm motion will carry the arm downward and across the body. The body continues to rotate so that the right side of the body is facing the target.

This integrated pattern is seen emerging in six- and seven-year-olds. However, if proper opportunities have not been made available for throwing in the earlier years, the more immature patterns may be observed even in older students and those who are handicapped. Students with disabilities may be taught mature throwing patterns provided the neurological basis for throwing is intact. Even severely retarded subjects have been taught fairly mature throwing patterns. This can be observed in the softball throw included in the Special Olympics.

Problems While Throwing Overarm

Handicapped and nonhandicapped students may encounter similar problems in trying to develop a mature throwing pattern. Some common problems include:

- positioning the body improperly such as facing the target, rather than turning the shoulder toward the target
- gripping the ball with the palm rather than the fingers
- keeping the wrong foot forward such as extending the right foot forward when throwing with the right hand
- failing to shift the body weight from one leg to the other
- keeping the wrist stiff
- releasing the ball too soon or too late
- using little or no followthrough

General Adaptations

In general, the following modifications may be used with several types of handicapped students. Specific modifications and adaptations will be given for particular handicapping conditions, where necessary, following this section.

1. Determine if throwing equipment fits the student's skill level and grip size.
2. Use modeling and demonstrations with peers or videotapes.
3. Manually guide the student's body when necessary.
4. Stand close enough to the student to give immediate feedback.
5. Provide ample opportunity to practice the skill.
6. Begin in an orderly progression from simple to complex skills.

Modifications for Blind Students

1. Provide an auditory cue in the direction of the target.
2. Use a ball with a beeper.

3. Give verbal feedback regarding the results of the throw, particularly the proximity to the target.

Modifications for Physically Impaired Students

1. Tie a string to a wiffle ball so that students with limited mobility can retrieve the ball themselves while practicing.
2. Pair a physically disabled student with one who is nondisabled.
3. Allow students to practice throwing against a backstop.

Teaching Activities

These suggested activities will be presented from the least difficult to the most difficult. Many activities may be used to teach the overarm throw. However, only a few will be suggested.

1. Begin activities at the level of the student.
2. Use two hands or one hand, relying on the preference of the student.
3. Have the student throw in the general direction of another person.
4. Throw the ball over objects, i.e., a rope tied between two poles.
5. Suspend large hula hoops for students to throw objects through.
6. Allow students to throw a variety of objects.
7. Gradually set up different types of targets and increase the distance as skill is gained.
8. Let the student experiment with different throwing patterns.

Catching

Like throwing, catching is also used in many games that children play, ranging from individual and dual to team play. Children tend to be fearful of catching a ball, particularly when they have experienced difficulty or have been injured while catching. Injuries may occur in the early stages of catching as a result of poor skills or inappropriate objects used for catching.

The sequence of catching skills has been noted by McClenaghan and Gallahue (1978). (See Table 4–3.)

Problems While Catching

- failure to align the body when the object is approaching
- not positioning the hands properly
- failure to give with the object to receive force
- eyes not following the ball
- stance too narrow
- arms held improperly, too stiff, etc.

Table 4–3 Stages of Development: Catching

Stage	Task Component
Stage 1	Initially, the head may be turned away from the ball. The arms are usually held stiffly in front of the body. Timing is usually delayed, and the response is not made until the ball touches the arms and hands. The child attempts to scoop the ball toward the chest rather than using the hands to catch it.
Stage 2	The head remains steady, but the eyes may close when contact is made with the ball. The arms remain in front of the body, but there is bending at the elbow. Timing is generally still poor at this stage of catching. Some attempt is made to catch with the hands, but the object is still corralled at the chest or abdomen.
Stage 3	A mature catching pattern may be observed in the third stage of catching. The eyes begin to follow the ball closely and avoidance reactions have been eliminated. The hands are held in the proper position, either with the thumbs next to each other or the little fingers next to each other in the case of an underhand catch. The hands are used to make the catch in a well-timed action. The arms are positioned at the sides with the elbows flexed. More give in the arms and hands may be noticed upon contact with the object. A good stance, permitting balance, is assumed.

General Adaptations

1. Alleviate fears about catching.
2. Use lightweight objects so that injury while catching can be minimized or avoided until the student is able to develop some degree of skill.
3. Use objects that move slower.
4. Begin with a sitting position, then progress from kneeling to standing, or at whatever level the student needs to begin.

Modifications for Blind Students

1. Allow the student to catch a rolled ball.
2. Use a ball with a beeper.
3. Work from behind the student moving arms and hands until the feel of catching the ball on the ground is developed.
4. Provide verbal cues.

Modifications for Physically Handicapped Students

1. Use lightweight objects when necessary and ones that move slowly.
2. Begin catching in an enclosed space so the balls or other objects do not go very far if missed.

Modifications for Learning-Disabled Students

1. Use a suspended object for those who have very poor timing.
2. Arrange for practice to be in an uncluttered area and a nondistracting environment.
3. Use slow-moving objects such as balloons or NeRF® balls.

Modifications for Hearing-Impaired Students

1. Make sure student is aware that the object is going to be thrown.
2. Provide a visual signal that indicates the object is about to be thrown.

Teaching Activities

1. Begin with catching rolled objects in a sitting position.
2. Have student move to other positions, kneeling, then standing.
3. Let student toss the object up and catch it independently.
4. Have student bounce and catch a large ball.
5. Toss balloons in the air and catch them.
6. Catch objects that are suspended, such as a tether ball, yarn ball, or other types.
7. Have students catch objects thrown from different heights and angles.
8. Let student throw the ball against a wall and catch it on the first bounce.
9. Have student catch different shaped balls.
10. Play lead-up games that involve the skill of catching.

Kicking

Kicking is another projectile management skill used in many games that children play. Kicking requires some degree of eye-hand coordination just as catching and throwing do. Kicking is the motor act of imparting force to an object with the feet. Various forms of kicking are implemented in games ranging from simple kicking of a stationary ball to more sophisticated forms. Dauer and Pangrazi (1979) describe the stages of kicking through which children normally progress. (See Table 4–4.)

Problems While Kicking

- Eyes do not remain on the ball.
- Too short a backswing and little or no followthrough may be used.
- Body is improperly aligned with the ball.
- Upper and lower extremities are not integrated.

Table 4–4 Stages of Development: Kicking

Stage	*Task Component*
Stage 1	A stationary ball is generally involved in the first stages of kicking. Most of the kicking action is done with little movement in the arms or trunk. Contact is not well coordinated and no followthrough is used in this stage. The backswing is done only by bending the leg at the knee, rather than moving the entire leg backward. First attempts at kicking may be characterized by the child stepping on the ball.
Stage 2	In this stage, some action in the arms is observed as the upper extremity is somewhat integrated with the lower extremity. The leg is still bent at the knee on the backswing. However, some followthrough can be observed in this stage.
Stage 3	The child begins to coordinate the arm and upper body movements when kicking. The arm on the opposite side of the kicking foot will swing forward and the body balances smoothly with increase in followthrough. At this point the child may walk or run toward the ball before kicking it.
Stage 4	Less knee bend and more movement from the hip are observed in the mature stage of kicking. The backswing and followthrough create a longer range of motion. The arms are well integrated with the leg movements. The support leg is raised by toe elevation and bending at the waist occurs as the leg follows through after contact with the ball. A small hopping step may be used to maintain balance.

General Adaptations

1. Use a ball that will travel short distances at first.
2. All students kicking the ball should be kicking in the same direction.
3. Provide a model for students to follow.
4. Use lightweight equipment for less-skilled students.

Modifications for Blind Students

1. Allow the blind student to feel where the ball is placed before kicking it.
2. Have the student take a step back from the ball to measure the distance before kicking.
3. Use an auditory ball.
4. Have a partner for the student or provide an auditory signal in the direction the ball is to be kicked.
5. Give verbal feedback regarding the accuracy and distance of the kick.

Modifications for Physically Impaired Students

1. Let the student use whatever form of support is necessary to stand and kick the ball: a crutch, partner, wall, or whatever is comfortable to the student.

2. Allow a crutch to substitute for the kicking leg if applicable.
3. If students have shunts or are prone to seizures, protective headgear should be worn.

Modifications for Students with Learning Disabilities

1. Arrange for practice to be in an uncluttered area.
2. Have only one ball at a time available for each student.
3. Allow the student who is easily distracted to kick with a buddy or in a more secluded area.

Modifications for Hearing-Impaired Students

1. Be sure the student sees all signals to begin and stop.
2. If balance is a problem, allow the student to hold on to a stable object.

Teaching Activities

1. Let students begin from a sitting position, if balance is difficult.
2. Have students begin kicking from a stationary position with a lightweight ball.
3. Experiment with several sized balls until the right size for each student is determined.
4. Let student take a short step back, then kick the ball.
5. Have student kick a slowly rolled ball.
6. Have student take a step and kick a moving ball.
7. Increase the speed of the rolling ball and have student take two or three steps before kicking the ball.
8. Have student approach a rolling ball with which the body must be aligned before kicking.

Striking

Arnheim and Sinclair (1979) explain a variety of striking skills that are used in various sports. However, they point out that the sidearm pattern or movement in the horizontal plane is the beginning striking action to be learned first. Adaptations of this basic movement skill are applied to sports, such as the overhead and underhand strike.

Most striking skills are first learned with an implement such as a bat or racket, though the bare hand is also sometimes used. When striking, however, the body position and movement in the sidearm form are very similar. Striking in this chapter will be explained in terms of imparting force with a bat.

Unlike throwing, catching, and kicking, striking does not appear to follow well-defined stages in its development. To understand the development of striking, the proper form should be studied.

Striking Form

The body is positioned for the right-handed student so that the left side is facing in the direction of the approaching object to be hit. The feet are spread about shoulder width apart, with the weight evenly distributed on both feet. The right-handed person should grasp the bat with the right hand above the left and hold the bat slightly elevated over the right shoulder.

The swing begins with a step forward and the bat is brought around parallel at the height of the ball or object to be struck. The eyes should be kept on the ball and the arms brought on around the body for followthrough.

Learning to swing appears to take place in three stages. (See Table 4–5.)

Problems While Striking

Handicapped students will exhibit some of the same problems as their nonhandicapped peers while striking. Some common problems include:

- bending forward or backward
- not extending the arms fully during the contact and followthrough
- failing to step forward as the swing is begun
- swinging too early or too late
- gripping the bat improperly or holding it in the wrong position

General Adaptations

1. Give practice in striking a stationary object first.
2. Give practice in striking using a larger piece of equipment.
3. Simplify the procedure and work on a few components at a time.

Table 4–5 Stages of Development: Baseball Swing

Stage	Task Component
Stage 1	The arms are used only to initiate the swing and impart force. The eyes may close as contact is made. The bat is brought around more in an arc or "golf" swing.
Stage 2	The weight begins to shift toward the front foot. The bat is brought around more in the horizontal plane.
Stage 3	The set position is more definite and the feet are distributed properly. A step initiates the swing and a well-timed swing occurs.

4. Use a lightweight object to strike and one that is large enough for the student to make contact.

Modifications for Blind Students

1. Manipulate body parts until the blind student gains the concept of striking.
2. Use an auditory ball.
3. Use a white or yellow ball.
4. Let the student bat from a batting tee.

Modifications for Physically Impaired Students

1. Allow the racket to be taped to the student's hand or use a special grip on a bat if grip strength is weak.
2. Allow the student to bat with one hand.

Modifications for Students with Learning Disabilities and Mental Retardation

1. Fit the size of the striking implement to the ability and size of the student.
2. Keep the background uncluttered in the direction the student is facing.
3. Give cues concerning important points, i.e., "Eyes on the ball," "Step forward," "Grip," and so forth.
4. Use a batting tee.
5. Moving objects should move slowly at first, or until some skill is achieved.
6. Be sure the student understands the instructions.

Teaching Activities

1. Begin with prestriking activities such as batting a balloon with either hand or using modified paddles or other lightweight forms of equipment.
2. Let student hit suspended objects with different striking implements.
3. Have student hit a ball from a batting tee.
4. Have student hit a rolled ball on the ground.
5. Have student hit a bounced playground ball.
6. Have student hit a lightweight pitched ball.
7. Have student toss the ball up to himself or herself and hit it.

POINTS TO REMEMBER

1. Basic motor skills follow a natural progression in both handicapped and nonhandicapped children, with the exception that handicapped students are delayed in proportion to the severity of their handicapping conditions.
2. The period from two to six years of age is a time of rapid growth and change in motor skills.
3. The majority of fundamental motor skills develop to a fairly high level by age 6.

4. Major motor milestones can be used as predictors of how well the child is progressing motorically.

5. The developmental sequence of motor skills can serve as a model for planning a program of motor activities for disabled students.

6. The sequence that motor skills follow is more significant in developing programs than the actual timelines at which they occur.

7. Mildly handicapped students may exhibit the same problems seen in normal children during the initial stages of learning a motor skill.

8. The instructor needs to find a logical skill sequence of activities so that the disabled student can be allowed to develop a level of fundamental skills.

9. Not all handicapped students will be able to reach the same level of skill development. The teacher should concentrate on mastery of the skill level at which the student can perform most efficiently.

REFERENCES

Arnheim, D.D., & Sinclair, W.A. (1979). *The clumsy child: A program of motor therapy* (2nd ed.). St. Louis: C.V. Mosby.

Bayley, N.A. (1935). The development of motor abilities during the first three years. Monograph, *Society for Research in Child Development, 1,* 1–26.

Bobath, B., & Bobath, K. (1975). *Motor development in the different types of cerebral palsy.* London: International Press.

Burton, E.C. (1977). *The new physical education for elementary school children.* Palo Alto, CA: Houghton Mifflin.

Corbin, C.B. (1977). *A textbook of motor development* (2nd ed.). Dubuque, IA: William C. Brown.

Cratty, B.J. (1980). *Adapted physical education for handicapped children and youth.* Denver: Love.

Dauer, V.P., & Pangrazzi, R.P. (1979). *Dynamic physical education for elementary school children* (6th ed.). Minneapolis: Burgess.

Evans, J.R. (1980). *They have to be carefully taught: A handbook for parents and teachers of young children with handicapping conditions.* Reston, VA: American Alliance for Health, Physical Education, Recreation and Dance.

Fiorentino, M.R. (1972). *Normal and abnormal development.* Springfield, IL: Charles C. Thomas.

Folio, M.R., & Fewell, R. (1983). *Peabody Developmental Motor scales and activity cards.* Hingham, MA: Teaching Resources Corporation.

Fraser, B.A., Galka, G., & Hensinger, R.N. (1980). *Gross motor management of severely multiply impaired students.* Baltimore: University Park Press.

Gesell, A., & Amatruda, C.S. (1947). *Developmental diagnosis.* New York: P.B. Hoeber.

McClenaghan, B.A., & Gallahue, D.L. (1978). *Fundamental movement: A developmental and remedial approach.* Philadelphia: W.B. Saunders.

McGraw, M.B. (1943). *The neuromuscular motivation of the human infant.* New York: Columbia University Press.

Montgomery, P., & Richter, E. (1977). *Sensori motor integration for developmentally disabled children: A handbook.* Los Angeles: Western Psychological Services.

Moran, J.M., & Kalakian, L.H. (1974). *Movement experiences for the mentally retarded or emotionally disturbed child.* Minneapolis: Burgess.

Rarick, G.L. (Ed.). (1973). *Physical activity: Human growth and development.* New York: Academic Press.

Shirley, M.M. (1931). *The first two years: A study of twenty-five babies, 1, Postural and locomotor development.* Minneapolis: University of Minnesota Press.

Schurr, E.L. (1980). *Movement experiences for children: A humanistic approach to elementary school physical education* (3rd ed.). Englewood Cliffs, NJ: Prentice-Hall.

Vannier, M., & Gallahue, D.L. (1978). *Teaching physical education in elementary schools* (6th ed.). Philadelphia: W.B. Saunders.

Wickstrom, R. (1977). *Fundamental motor skills.* Philadelphia: Lea & Febiger.

Chapter 5

Perceptual Aspects of Motor Responses

Focus

- Explains how perception and the process of sensory interpretation affects motor performance.
- Develops a working process or model for analyzing and teaching the integration of information processing as it relates to making a motor response.
- Defines perceptual abilities within the psychomotor domain.
- Suggests training activities to integrate perceptual skills and motor skills.

Motor responses require the processing of information received through the senses. When the individual is able to put these two aspects together, perceptual motor integration occurs and correct motor responses are made. The individual combines sensory skills and movement to enhance the integration of these two processes. As perception is enhanced, the decision about how to respond is made more accurate. These two aspects need to be trained together. Isolated instruction does not foster the integration of perception and movement. Nor does training in one aspect necessarily enhance the other.

There are many theoretical models for how perceptual data and motor data are integrated. The intent is not to provide a rationale or review the theories. This notion is fairly well documented in the literature. Suggested readings at the end of the chapter list publications that explain perceptual motor theory in detail.

This chapter will focus on a model of perceptual motor integration that can be used for understanding how motor responses are made. It is based on information processing and explores how problems occur with handicapped students. Suggestions are provided for programming.

PERCEPTUAL MOTOR SKILL COMPONENTS

Just about every skill performed in a physical education classroom requires the integration of perception and motor acts. Thus, it is very difficult to separate the terms *perceptual* and *motor*. First, view the term *perception*. Actual perception occurs in the brain and involves the interpretation of sensory data transmitted from the sensory organs, i.e., eyes, ears, etc. The instructor should view any motor response that is voluntary as a process, a perceptual motor process.

There are several stages in the process that can be simplified or quite complex. Kephart (1971) describes four stages:

- input
- processing
- output
- feedback

If one thinks of the brain as a computer, it may be helpful to understand the perceptual motor process in these terms:

Input is the first stage, where sensory information is received through the primary sensory channels of vision, hearing, kinesthesis, and touch. These four sensory channels are the primary ones used to receive sensory data in physical education classrooms. One rarely uses smell to shoot a basketball!

Once the information is received, it is sent to the brain via nerve pathways. Interpretation of the sensory information

Figure 5–1 Perceptual Motor Process

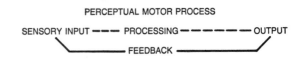

occurs in the brain. However, prior to actual interpretation, the sorting of information must occur.

In *processing,* the information received is sorted by various means such as prior experience, memory, perceptual skills, and coding of information.

Output involves the actual response made on the basis of the interpretation or processing of actual information. These first three stages actually occur very rapidly and often throughout the day in each individual.

Feedback is another important component or stage in the perceptual motor process. Feedback serves as a self-correcting mechanism during the process. It can also serve as an indicator of the response accuracy itself. In this situation, feedback is internal. However, feedback can also be external, from the teacher or others present. External feedback, while not a part of the perceptual motor process itself, is important for the learner to increase skill levels and to continue to be motivated. Methods of providing external feedback should vary and be of a positive nature. Figure 5–1 will aid in understanding the perceptual motor process.

The following illustration is an example of how the perceptual motor process might work. The instructor tells the student, "John, practice shooting at least 20 foul shots." In viewing the perceptual motor process, several events might occur. At this point, input includes auditory information as the teacher speaks to John. What the instructor said must be heard and processed correctly using auditory perceptual skills, language, memory, etc. The correct motor response would be for John to get a basketball, go to the foul line, and begin shooting. However, in order to shoot foul shots, other processing must occur. First, John needs to be familiar with the task. Visual information must be processed in terms of the height of the basket, the distance, and so forth. Also, kinesthetic memory will aid John in positioning his body to prepare himself for the shot. After the shot is made, feedback will come into play as to whether the shot was correct and accurate. If John missed the basket, feedback should help him to make corrections if the information during feedback is interpreted correctly. The teacher can also provide external feedback with suggestions on how to improve performance.

Perceptual-Motor Errors

According to Rothstein, Catelli, Dodds, and Manahan (1981), handicapped students may make errors at all levels of the perceptual motor process. By focusing on the segment where the student is having errors, better instruction can be provided. The summary of errors at each level, according to Rothstein et al. (1981), includes the following:

Input Errors

- Student focuses at the wrong part of the playing area.
- Student may focus on the wrong cues.

Interpretation Errors

- Student may misinterpret the speed, direction, or path of an object or another player.
- Student may incorrectly judge distances, heights, and weights of objects, targets, etc.
- Student may select the wrong movement, force, or timing of a response.

Output Errors

At this level the student does not execute the movements as planned, i.e., the child with cerebral palsy moves to kick a ball but misses because of spasticity in the legs.

Feedback Errors

- Student does not remember movements used to execute the task.
- Student does not determine the errors.
- Student does not determine what caused the error, i.e., does not know that the improper grip may have led to poor release or control while throwing.

The perceptual motor process must be kept in mind when working with handicapped students. Most handicapped students will have difficulty with primarily one stage of the perceptual motor process. However, Kephart (1960) mentions that a breakdown in one stage will ultimately affect the entire process.

Mentally retarded students will have the major difficulty at the processing or interpretation stage in the perceptual motor process. Generally, the mentally retarded student will adequately receive the information provided that sensory receptors are intact and functioning properly. The difficulty arises when the information must be correctly interpreted. Obviously, the correct motor response will depend on how accurately the incoming sensory information is interpreted.

Learning-disabled students will also have difficulty at the processing level, depending on the particular kind of disability. For example, if the learning-disabled student has a visual perceptual disorder, processing and interpretation of visual information will be difficult and possibly inaccurate. This will ultimately result in making an inaccurate motor response.

Sensory-impaired students, on the other hand, will have the most difficulty at the input level. If information is not accurately received, it cannot be accurately interpreted and, again, the motor response is affected.

Physically handicapped students will have the most difficulty at the motor output level of the perceptual motor process. They may be able to receive information, interpret it, but make an incorrect response because of a motor disability.

Students with neurological impairments may have difficulty at several levels of the perceptual motor process, depending on the location and extent of the brain damage. A similar problem exists with students who have multiple disabilities.

The physical educator needs to keep in mind the process and be aware of how each handicapping condition affects performance. This will aid the teacher in being more effective in presenting information to the student during the instructional process.

PERCEPTUAL SKILLS

Perceptual skills are important for interpreting stimuli sent to the brain via the sensory channels. Harrow (1972) describes a hierarchy of perceptual skills in the psychomotor domain. These include:

- kinesthetic discrimination
- body awareness
- balance
- body image
- body and spatial relationships
- visual perception
- auditory discrimination
- tactile discrimination
- eye-hand coordination
- eye-foot coordination

Kinesthetic Discrimination

Kinesthetic discrimination allows students to determine the body's position in space. Kinesthesis is often referred to as "muscle sense" (Lerch, Becker, Ward, & Nelson, 1974). Sensations from sensory receptors in the muscles, tendons, and joints send messages to the brain about position. These then must be interpreted. Knowledge about body parts and space is needed to interpret the sensations. Kinesthesis is complex, but interpretations occur very quickly and are continuous during motor performance. Kinesthesis is highly developed in well-trained athletes.

Some handicapped children have difficulty with kinesthetic discrimination because of various problems related to their handicapping conditions. For example, if a student has a poor level of body awareness, it will be difficult for the student to make accurate interpretations about position in space. In addition, if improper nerve impulses are sent to the brain, the student may receive inaccurate feelings or sensations related to movement and body positions.

Body Awareness

Body awareness involves a cognitive understanding of body parts and their functions. Recognizing their relationship to one another and their functioning enables the student to interact accurately and make motor responses, provided that other systems in the body are intact. Understanding the body is important because it serves as a reference point for making judgments about spatial relationships (Kephart, 1971). Movement experiences reinforce the notion of spatial dynamics observed by the child. Movement is important in the beginning stages of making spatial judgments but becomes less of a factor once spatial concepts are learned.

Corbin (1977) lists the stages that children generally pass through in becoming aware of their bodies. Actually, children are quite aware of their bodies from early infancy. Corbin states that after the child becomes visually aware of the body, verbal identification of body parts occurs as language is developed. Left and right concepts are then learned and finally dimensions of external space are related to the body.

Balance

Flinchum (1975) defines balance as the ability to maintain control of the body when stationary or moving. Movements can be simultaneous, individual, or alternating. Harrow (1972) states that balance involves reflexes, body awareness, and body mechanics. Other factors are also involved in trying to maintain balance. According to Arnheim and Sinclair (1979), the other mechanisms include tactile sensations, vestibular sensations, and vision. Handicapped students having deficits in any of the balancing mechanisms will have difficulty maintaining equilibrium.

There are two types of balance: static and dynamic. Static balance refers to holding a stationary position over a period of time, such as standing still, sitting up, and other postures where no locomotion is involved. Dynamic balance is the ability to maintain body support while moving through space.

Balance is maintained by keeping the center of gravity over the base of support while stationary. If movement is involved, the center of gravity will move out of the base of support, so balance must be lost and regained temporarily as in walking or running.

Body Image

Harrow (1972) distinguishes between body awareness and body image. Body awareness is more of a cognitive understanding of the body and its movement capabilities. Body image, on the other hand, refers to the emotional or affective responses and visions about the body. The two may be closely related. Corbin (1977) indicated that as body awareness develops in young children, they acquire feelings and opinions about themselves related to their physical capacities. Body image, then, is in a state of constant change. Eventually, children's self-concepts and basic personality structures will evolve out of body-image perceptions. Also, the way children feel about themselves as physical beings may greatly influence their performance of perceptual motor skills.

Visual Perception

Visual skills, particularly visual perception, are important in performing perceptual motor skills. Improving visual acuity is generally not in the realm of the physical education teacher. However, other visual skills play a significant role in motor performance.

Visual tracking is important in following moving objects. It involves the ability to follow objects with the eyes. In physical education it is necessary, for example, to follow a moving ball or other players in a game. Students who cannot follow a moving ball or other moving objects in a physical education classroom will have difficulty making accurate motor responses.

Visual memory involves recall of what has been seen, either on a short- or long-term basis. Obviously, visual memory is very important in learning motor skills, since demonstrations and modeling are frequently used to teach motor skills. Students with visual memory problems may remember only the last part of what was demonstrated and have difficulty learning motor skills if only visual cues are used in teaching. The instructor needs to provide information about a particular skill by using the learner's best channel for receiving information. Auditory cues may need to be used more frequently, or shorter segments of information may be advisable.

Visual figure-ground discrimination is also involved in performing many motor skills. This visual skill includes the ability to select the relevant stimulus from a background. Tennis might be a good example. Suppose an optic yellow tennis ball is being used. The opponent hits a lob shot and in the background are large groups of trees with green leaves. As the ball reaches the height of the lob, it may be temporarily lost in the green background. Students with visual figure-ground problems may not be able to follow the ball in the cluttered background. Also, they may lose sight of their teammates in a game involving many players.

Auditory Discrimination

When auditory discrimination skills are properly integrated into motor acts students are able to react to sounds and make appropriate motor responses. Auditory discrimination has components similar to those of visual discrimination. Frostig and Maslow (1970) refer to the combining of auditory stimuli and motor responses as hearing and doing or auditory motor association and transfer. An example of this would be a verbal instruction or signal from the teacher followed by an appropriate motor response from the child.

Auditory memory is actual recall of what was heard. Physical educators will give a sequence of verbal instructions while teaching motor skills. Although visual demonstrations of skills are frequently used in physical education, auditory directions are also common practice. Students who have difficulty remembering what was heard may not be able to recall in what order the movement components of a particular motor task are to be carried out. Thus, it is important for the physical educator to know which modality is best for presenting information to students with discrimination difficulties.

Auditory figure-ground discrimination is the ability to select the relevant auditory stimulus from a background of other noise. Students who have this difficulty may be attracted to a passing car or other students who may be playing a game or discussing an activity nearby. The student is really unable to concentrate on what the teacher is saying. Some teachers mistake this problem for not listening or paying attention. Some students may even be punished for what is actually a learning problem.

Auditory tracking refers to the ability to follow a sound and localize it. This becomes important if the physical educator gives directions or signals from various locations around the gymnasium or from different positions outdoors. Auditory tracking is also involved in team games where players may be giving auditory signals to their teammates.

Tactile Discrimination

Discrimination through touch may be used in the physical education setting. Exploration, such as feeling the different shapes and textures of equipment, is often accomplished with tactile and visual discrimination combined. However, in the case of visually limited students, tactile discrimination becomes even more important. Tactile discrimination is done with the entire body and not necessarily the hands. Tactile experiences are important for all children, since they aid in confirming what the eyes see. It is through the combination of touch and vision that visual perceptual skills are sharpened.

Eye-Hand Coordination

Eye-hand coordination requires the matching of the hands with what the eye sees or the coordination of the body with visual stimuli. Winnick (1979) explains that adequate eye-hand coordination requires the combined skills of visual perception with coordinated movements of the hands, arms, and shoulders. Eye-hand coordination problems become evident when the child begins to reach and grasp, manipulate objects, and engage in various play activities.

Eye-Foot Coordination

Eye-foot coordination involves principles similar to those of eye-hand coordination. In this instance, however, the foot must react to the visual stimulus seen by the student. Eye-foot coordination is involved in many physical education activities, including agility in running, kicking, and other forms of movement requiring the feet to react to visual stimuli. Students may have poor eye-foot coordination as a result of poor balance, poor reaction time, or general coordination problems.

Other Perceptual Skills

Laterality is a perceptual skill that develops in several stages. Kephart (1971) refers to laterality as first an awareness that two sides of the body exist. Later, the child is able to identify right and left. Laterality is used in making interpretations about movements alternating from either side of the body and the left and right of objects.

Directionality develops after body awareness and laterality become integrated. Directionality can be viewed as the organization that the child gives to relationships in external space. This may involve interpretations of movements such as up, down, forward, backward, etc. These two perceptual skills aid the child in organizing external space.

PROBLEM INDICATORS

Perceptual abilities have been defined and discussed according to Harrow's taxonomy of the psychomotor domain. It is important that the physical educator have the ability to spot problem indicators for each skill. If deficiencies are caught early enough, improvements may be made by programmed activities designed to enhance each skill. Table 5–1 presents a summary of problem indicators.

Whenever a problem indicator is observed for any of the mentioned perceptual skills, the teacher should conduct more in-depth evaluation or look for other signs of the problem. Sometimes it is wise to confer with the classroom teacher since the problems may also show up in academic work, particularly in the elementary grades, K–6. If the problems are severe enough, the student may need to be referred for a full battery of tests. After testing is conducted, training activities can be designed and integrated into the student's physical education program.

Table 5–1 Perceptual Skills Deficits

Skill	Problem Indicators	Skill	Problem Indicators
Kinesthetic discrimination	• Is unable to identify body positions. • Has difficulty remembering body positions. • Has difficulty in planning a series of movements.	Auditory Memory	• Remembers only the last two or three things the teacher says. • May appear inattentive when verbal directions are being given. • Cannot repeat what is heard.
Body Awareness	• Cannot identify body parts and planes. • Has difficulty in identifying body parts of another person.	Auditory Figure-Ground Discrimination	• Cannot select what the teacher says in a noisy environment. • May not pay attention if other noises are present. • May hear only part of what was said.
Balance (Static)	• Has difficulty in maintaining specific postures. • Feet may be kept wide apart while standing. • Cannot maintain a heel-toe position. • Cannot sit in a tucked position.	Auditory Tracking	• Cannot follow a sound or signal. • Has difficulty finding where a sound is coming from. • May be inattentive if the teacher moves around the gym while talking.
Balance (Dynamic)	• Has difficulty moving while using a narrow base of support. • Avoids balance on a beam by moving across quickly. • May turn feet sideways or inward while walking on a beam. • Falls frequently in running games.	Tactile Discrimination	• Cannot identify objects via touch alone. • Has poor manipulative skills. • Exhibits rigidity and an inflexible grasp. • Has difficulty in interpreting sensations in various parts of the body.
Body Image	• Makes negative statements about self. • Makes statements like "I can't." • May be shy and withdrawn. Does not socialize well.	Eye-Hand Coordination	• Has difficulty in catching, striking, or other activities requiring the hands to react to visual stimuli. • May avoid activitites requiring catching, batting, etc.
Visual Memory	• Cannot remember all of what the teacher demonstrates. • Cannot remember what was in a film. • Often asks for demonstrations to be repeated.	Eye-Foot Coordination	• May have poor kicking skills. • Has difficulty completing an agility run. • May trip or fall frequently. • May avoid activities that require eye-hand coordination.
Visual Figure-Ground Discrimination	• Loses sight of objects in a cluttered background. • Cannot locate team members in a game. • Has difficulty catching or batting a ball if the background is cluttered.	Laterality	• May not be able to locate the sides of the body. • Cannot identify left and right. • May use one side of the body too much. • Has difficulty performing or integrating both sides of the body.
Visual Tracking	• Cannot follow a moving target well. • Moves head while following an object. • Eyes may move back and forth while following an object. • May exhibit poor eye-hand coordination.	Directionality	• Gets confused when asked to move in a specific direction. • Cannot identify sides of objects. • Has difficulty with prepositions such as *on, over, under, through,* etc.

TEACHING ACTIVITIES

Numerous training activities have been developed for perceptual skills. Many, however, are geared toward the academic classroom and involve paper and pencil tasks. A better method of training is to combine perceptual and motor skills. The following section suggests ideas and activities for developing perceptual motor skills.

Kinesthetic Discrimination

1. Have students walk on surfaces that require body reaction and vestibular stimulation such as a trampoline bed or an old mattress.

2. Have students engage in movement at different levels—high, low, rolling, creeping, crawling—to experience different sensations.

3. Have students imitate motor movements with the entire body or specific body parts to experience different body positions.

4. Have students move through an obstacle course where several body positions have to be changed to heighten kinesthetic awareness.

Body Awareness

1. Ask students to touch body parts while looking into a mirror, or touch body parts on a manikin or another person.

2. Have students place themselves in relation to an object, such as back to a chair, side to the wall, front to a ball, etc.

3. Provide a life-size tracing of students' bodies and let them identify parts and color them.

4. Play games where students have to identify body parts, such as "The Hokey Pokey," "Twister," or others.

Balance (Static)

1. Ask students to keep balance while assuming stationary positions, beginning with simple and less complex positions such as lying on the side, kneeling, two hands and one foot on the floor, and others.

2. Have students sit on a balance board and shift weight; repeat while standing.

3. Have students stand on a mattress or pillow with eyes open, then eyes closed.

4. Have students stand on a narrow line with heel in front of toes, eyes open, then eyes closed.

5. Have students stand on one foot or tip toes with eyes open, then eyes closed.

Balance (Dynamic)

1. Ask students to move close to the floor, on hands and knees, on hands and feet.

2. Ask students to walk on knees.

3. Ask students to walk on a trampoline bed, on a rope on the floor, taped lines, footprints, boards 6 inches wide and then on narrower ones.

4. Ask students to walk in a heel-to-toe pattern.

5. Ask students to walk around the room balancing objects on the head.

Body Image

1. Begin activities where students can be successful.

2. Have students practice movements in front of a mirror.

3. Ask students to keep a record of their successful accomplishments in physical education.

4. Send notes home to parents telling them how well students performed in physical education.

5. Have students repeat statements such as "I did well today," "I can do a lot of things."

Body and Spatial Relationships

1. Allow students to move about and in relation to objects, going over, under, around, and through objects.

2. Let students move in relation to one another, playing games such as dodge ball, "Follow-the-Leader," and others.

3. Have students move and tell where they are in relationship to an object.

4. Ask students to place an object in relation to their body parts or planes.

5. Other games can include tag games, steal-the-bacon, or activities that require movement through an obstacle course.

6. Ask students to form shapes using their bodies.

7. Ask students to find different objects in the gymnasium or outdoors and place them in other locations.

Visual Tracking

1. Hold hands with student or have students hold hands and follow movements with their eyes.

2. Let students roll a ball back and forth and follow the movements with their eyes.

3. Let students bat balloons with hands and follow movements with their eyes.

4. Have students visually follow a swinging ball from sitting or standing positions.

5. Have students play games like tether ball, "Follow-the-Leader," tag, and so forth.

Visual Memory

1. Do two movements, then have students repeat them. Gradually increase the number of movements.

2. Move or do a motor activity, then have students describe the movements in sequence.

3. Show a sport film or loop film and ask students to tell what happened.

4. Ask students to watch any sports event on television and tell what happened.

Visual Figure-Ground Discrimination

1. Allow students to imitiate each other's movements.

2. Let students select particular pieces of equipment from a box of equipment.

3. Have students engage in team games or relays where they have to sort and match objects in the relay.

4. Have students follow directions through an obstacle course.

5. Let students throw objects at several targets taped to a wall.

Auditory Tracking

1. Ask students to move toward or away from auditory signals, such as a bell, whistle, or the teacher's voice.

2. Let a student locate where another student is by listening to a sound being made.

3. Have students throw at a target blindfolded using a sound as a cue. A metronome can be placed behind the target or a student can ring a bell.

Auditory Memory

1. Give students three movements to do and have them do the movements in order.

2. Have students play "Simon Says."

3. Ask a student to tell another student how to demonstrate a skill.

4. With a rhythm instrument or just hand clapping, present a beat and have students repeat what was heard.

5. Let students listen to a record, tape, or the radio and try to repeat the beat by moving, clapping, or marching.

Auditory Figure-Ground Discrimination

1. Use auditory signals in game activities.

2. Let students count while jumping rope or singing chants.

3. Let students move, walk, or run. Then give signals for stopping and starting.

4. Have students repeat the instructions for an exercise while performing it.

5. Call simple dance steps or directions while students are moving to music, or try simple folk and square dances.

6. Have students march and sing the words to songs.

7. Have students assume a position, but change the position when they hear the change signal from several signals given.

Tactile Discrimination

1. Have students walk barefoot on a rug, mat, floor, or other textures to experience different sensations.

2. Have students touch body parts with different objects: yarn balls, bean bags, sandpaper, NeRF® balls, etc.

3. Let students roll on different surfaces: blankets, mats, grass, carpets, trampoline beds, or others.

4. Let students play catch with different textured objects.

5. Have one student lead another student who is blindfolded through an uncluttered area. Students should try to identify where they are or objects in the space.

Eye-Hand Coordination

1. Begin eye-hand activities at the level of each student. Use objects that are easily managed by each student.

2. Let students practice batting a balloon with both hands, then one hand.

3. Have students practice catching rolled objects of various sizes.

4. Have students bat from a batting tee.

5. Have students hit a suspended ball with a paddle.

6. Have students play catch with lightweight objects such as a bean bag, NeRF® ball, yarn ball, beach ball, etc.

7. Have students play relays where objects have to be passed or caught.

8. Have students move wands with streamers in various directions.

Eye-Foot Coordination

1. Have students kick stationary objects such as balls, balloons, bean bags.

2. Have students pass a ball with the foot to one student or to one another in a circle formation.

3. Have students dribble a ball with the feet, such as in a soccer drill.

4. Have students kick a ball between two objects using two flags, cones, or chairs as markers or a goal.

5. Have students complete an obstacle course where a ball must be moved around and between objects with just the feet.

6. Have students complete short dance routines with simple steps.

7. Have students walk through tires, hoops, over objects, and between objects.

Laterality

1. Let students practice moving body parts on one side of their body, then switch to the other side. This can be done with wands or other objects, or with no objects.

2. Let students walk on a balance beam while carrying objects in both hands.

3. Have students climb on outdoor jungle gym equipment to increase laterality awareness.

4. Have students bounce a ball with one hand, then the other, toss and catch with one hand, then the other, etc.

5. Have students ride a stationary bicycle or engage in swimming to develop laterality.

6. Ask students to move the left side or body part, then the right. Place a red ribbon on the right hand or wrist. Let students wear a red sock on the right foot and step on red footprints with the right foot.

Directionality

1. Ask students to move in different directions, saying the direction while moving.

2. Ask students to find the left and right sides of objects, or the front and back.

3. Have students hop on one foot then change to the other foot and change directions.

4. Have students follow arrows or taped trails on the floor.

POINTS TO REMEMBER

1. Perceptual motor training deserves a place in the physical education curriculum because of the necessity of integrating the two aspects in making accurate motor responses.

2. Perceptual motor development should be viewed as a continual process that improves as motor responses are made to interpreted stimuli.

3. The perceptual motor process model will aid the teacher in assessing where errors occur, providing feedback to students having problems, and selecting appropriate training activities to foster development and remediation of perceptual motor integration.

4. Harrow's taxonomy of the psychomotor domain provides a hierarchy of perceptual motor development that can be used as a point of reference regarding how these skills develop.

5. The two components, perception and motor action, cannot be separated. Consequently, programming for the integration of the two should occur together. Training in one area does not necessarily improve the integration of the two.

REFERENCES

Arnheim, D.D., & Sinclair, W.A. (1979). *The clumsy child: A program of motor therapy* (2nd ed.). St. Louis: C.V. Mosby.

Corbin, C.B. (1977). *A textbook of motor development* (2nd ed.). Dubuque, IA: William C. Brown.

Flinchum, B.M. (1975). *Motor development in early childhood: A guide for movement education with ages 2 through 6*. St. Louis: C.V. Mosby.

Frostig, M., & Maslow, P. (1970). *Movement education: Theory and practice*. Chicago: Follett.

Harrow, A.J. (1972). *A taxonomy of the psychomotor domain: A guide for developing behavioral objectives*. New York: David McKay.

Kephart, N.C. (1971). *The slow learner in the classroom*. Columbus, OH: Charles E. Merrill.

Lerch, H.A., Becker, J.E., Ward, B.M., & Nelson, J.A. (1974). *Perceptual motor learning—Theory and practice*. Palo Alto, CA: Peek Publications.

Rothstein, A., Catelli, L., Dodds, P., & Manahan, J. (1981). *Basic stuff series I: Motor learning*. Reston, VA: American Alliance of Health, Physical Education, Recreation and Dance.

Winnick, J.P. (1979). *Early movement experiences and development: Habilitation and remediation*. Philadelphia: W.B. Saunders.

RECOMMENDED READINGS

Ayres, A.J. (1964). *Manual of the Southern California motor accuracy test*. Los Angeles: Western Psychological Services.

Ayres, A.J. (1966). *Manual of the Southern California kinesthesia and tactile perception test*. Los Angeles: Western Psychological Services.

Ayres, A.J. (1973). *Sensory integration and learning disorders*. Los Angeles: Western Psychological Services.

Arnheim, D.D., & Sinclair, W.A. (1979). *The clumsy child: A program of motor therapy* (2nd ed.). St. Louis: C.V. Mosby.

Barsch, R.H. (1965). *A movigenic curriculum*. Madison, WI: State Department of Public Instruction.

Cratty, B.J. (1972). *Physical expressions of intelligence*. Englewood Cliffs, NJ: Prentice-Hall.

Flinchum, B.M. (1975). *Motor development in early childhood: A guide for movement education with ages 2 through 6*. St. Louis: C.V. Mosby.

Frostig, M., & Maslow, P. (1970). *Movement education: Theory and practice*. Chicago: Follett.

Rothstein, A., Catelli, L., Dodds, P., & Manahan, J. (1981). *Basic stuff series I: Motor learning*. Reston, VA: American Alliance for Health, Physical Education, Recreation and Dance.

Chapter 6

Health and Fitness for Exceptional Students

Focus

- Defines components of health-related, physical, and motor fitness.
- Discusses methods of posture screening.
- Provides guidelines for fitness training with disabled youngsters.
- Discusses nutritional problems of handicapped students and possible effects.
- Lists strategies for weight management and nutritional improvement.

Handicapped persons need physical, motor, and health-related fitness as much as nonhandicapped individuals. The everyday mobility of the handicapped person may require more strength than the average individual needs since ambulating with crutches and lifting oneself from a wheelchair will require considerable strength in the arms, shoulders, and grip.

All forms of fitness will aid in developing self-reliance and confidence among handicapped groups. When persons have achieved the optimum amount of fitness possible, they tend to feel good about themselves.

Often handicapped individuals are denied opportunities to engage in fitness activities. This is so for several reasons: overprotective parents, disinterested teachers, inaccessible facilities, and lack of interest in such activities by handicapped persons themselves.

Falls (1980) discusses modern concepts of physical fitness. Health-related fitness includes those aspects of fitness that have to do with prevention against modern degenerative diseases such as coronary heart disease and obesity. Falls also refers to traditional concepts of physical fitness and motor fitness. Traditionally, the components have included strength, endurance, agility, power, etc.

If fitness activities are taught to handicapped persons and the benefits explained, their interest and motivation to participate in such activities will increase. Too often handicapped persons become unfit and overweight as a result of little exercise. This affects many other areas of fitness and motor proficiency.

This chapter will provide information regarding the basic components of physical fitness, methods for assessment, modification of activities for special populations, and specific activities for developing each component. Weight and nutritional management for specific populations will be addressed.

FITNESS DEFINED

Physical fitness is related to the state of general health and well-being. It may be viewed in several ways. Generally, it is thought of as having enough capacity for daily work and recreation and sufficient energy stores for managing an emergency situation. This idea individualizes physical fitness to some extent since work and recreation vary from person to person. Fait (1978) defines physical fitness from a physiological viewpoint as the ability to perform and then recover from strenuous exercise.

Physical fitness is sometimes differentiated from motor proficiency. However, to have motor proficiency one needs an optimal amount of physical fitness ability. Kalakian and Eichstaedt (1982) refer to motor fitness as related to proficiency in performing motor skills. Part of motor proficiency

requires agility, speed, and other components of physical fitness. These authors also differentiate between general physical fitness, motor fitness, and fitness for a particular task. From this point of view, one may have a general level of fitness but lack task-specific fitness. For example, a student may be generally fit to participate in several sports and general physical education activities but may not possess the specific fitness levels for working on the rings or vaulting in gymnastics. The physical educator needs to be aware of both dimensions when planning a fitness and activity program for each handicapped student.

HEALTH-RELATED AND MOTOR FITNESS COMPONENTS

Physical and motor fitness include several components and each plays a part in the development of total fitness. Each requires specific training techniques and maintenance activities on a regular schedule. The components of fitness to be discussed in this chapter are those defined by Dauer and Pangrazzi (1979). These include:

- muscular strength
- muscular endurance
- cardiovascular endurance
- flexibility
- agility
- speed
- power

Reaction time and coordination are included under component of motor fitness. Certain qualities contribute to the performance of motor skills, such as reaction time and coordination, which can lead to motor proficiency. Some individuals include speed and agility as qualities contributing to motor proficiency. However, both physical and motor fitness are needed to execute motor skills.

Muscular Strength

Muscular strength is the ability to exert maximum or near-maximum force using a muscle or group of muscles. Exerting maximum effort in this instance is more important than duration. Handicapped students need large muscle activity on a regular basis with enough intensity and near-maximum effort to develop and maintain strength.

Muscular Endurance

Muscular endurance requires a submaximal effort extended over a long period of time. Duration or repetition is more a feature of muscular endurance while submaximal effort is being exerted. Strength of muscle groups is necessary for muscular endurance. A person with endurance is able to continue muscular effort long after the individual without endurance.

Cardiovascular Endurance

Cardiovascular endurance enables the heart and circulatory systems to respond to total body physical effort over prolonged time periods. Total body workload is important for handicapped persons. Too often educators expect too little from handicapped students. Dauer and Pangrazzi (1979) report that heart disease can start as early as childhood. Handicapped students are not exempt from heart disease. In fact, not allowing handicapped students to participate in physical fitness activities ignores their total well-being.

Flexibility

Flexibility is the range of motion in the joints. Flexibility gives the individual more freedom of movement. Because of the very nature of some handicapping conditions, such as cerebral palsy, it is important to work on flexibility in the specific limbs involved. Otherwise, the joints will become stiff and the range of motion will decrease.

It is also the case that because of decreased muscle tone some handicapped students have too much flexibility. Down's Syndrome pupils tend to be quite flexible at the joints. This is sometimes a result of weak musculature and supporting tissue such as ligaments and tendons.

Almost all motor skills require a specific amount of flexibility. Musculature that is not stretched and warmed up before a vigorous activity could be strained or torn. Flexibility should always be maintained for movement comfort and agility.

Agility

Agility is the ability to quickly and effectively change positions in space. Many activities encountered in games and sports require the participant to move and change directions quickly. Agility is also used in everyday activities, particularly to move quickly out of the path of an approaching object such as a car, or an airborne object that could cause injury. Handicapped students have below-average agility for several reasons. The student with brain damage may not have the total body coordination to change directions quickly, or some students may not be able to react to a stimulus quickly enough. Some students may have faulty body structure that interferes with agility movements.

Speed

Speed may be defined as rapid, successive movements of the same kind or quick movement from one point to another. Speed is based to some extent on muscular strength. Mentally retarded students tend to be below their normal peers in running speed, particularly as age increases (Rarick, Dobbins, & Broadhead, 1976).

Power

Power is the amount of strength that can be exerted by a muscle or group of muscles over a short period of time. Sometimes power is referred to as explosive strength and can be seen in motor skills like the broad jump or high jump, throwing, and quick starts. Both speed and strength are needed in explosive movements.

Reaction Time

The time elapsed between the presentation of stimulus and the individual's response is referred to as reaction time. Several factors may influence reaction time. While it is true that neurological effects cannot be changed to a great extent in handicapped students, if reaction time is slow because of inattention or failure to discriminate a stimulus, some training should improve reaction time among slow-learning and learning-disabled students.

Coordination

Kalakian and Eichstaedt (1982) recommend that coordination be considered as a component of motor fitness. They define coordination as the ability of muscles to contract together at the appropriate moment to create skilled motor responses. If one uses this definition of coordination, then almost all movements or motor acts that are well executed require coordination. Many factors can affect coordination, such as difficulty with kinesthesis, proprioception, motor planning, body awareness, discrimination, and physical abilities. The physical education provider should be aware of the handicapped student's problems in order to interpret deficits that are observed in coordination.

MEASURING FITNESS

Since fitness is part of the definition of physical education under P.L. 94–142, the handicapped student's IEP may need to include objectives and long-term goals related to fitness. There are several different kinds of physical fitness and motor proficiency tests available for the physical educator to use. Some handicapped students may be able to take standardized fitness tests, while others may need modifications of tests that have been standardized on handicapped populations. Some handicapped populations, however, are difficult to standardize fitness tests on since the populations may be so diverse. Chapter 7 provides a review of physical fitness tests.

There may be a need to use only portions of tests or teacher-made items can be designed or further modified to measure specific aspects of fitness. This approach is not diagnostic but may be used to measure progress or for additional programming guidelines. This procedure can also be used to obtain additional class norms or to establish a baseline from which to measure improvement.

Fitness Components

The following areas will be covered in an assessment and ensuing fitness program:

Muscular Strength

Abdomen	• sit-ups (modified versions)
Shoulder Girdle	• push-ups, pull-ups, crab and seal walk, other adaptations by teacher
Arms	• pushing objects, lifting, gripping
Legs	• jumping, hopping, bouncing, climbing

Muscular Endurance

Any of the above activities can be used to develop endurance by repeating more than the number used to develop strength. Generally, physical education providers will accept repetitions beyond ten as endurance development. The number of repetitions, however, will depend on the condition of the student.

Cardiovascular Endurance

- walking
- jogging
- aerobic dance or other forms of aerobics
- swimming
- bicycling
- rope jumping

Flexibility

- slow continued forms of bending and stretching (avoid bouncing)
- large circular movements
- twisting (trunk and waist)

Agility

- running in place with quick steps
- squat thrusts
- stepping over obstacles, tires, taped lines, etc. (Movement should be quick and lively.)
- shuttle run, modified forms (Place objects on a chair for those who cannot bend down easily.)
- running zigzag patterns
- shadowing someone, as in guarding in basketball

Speed

- engaging in an activity or movement in which student tries to reduce the time needed to complete it
- running short distances, 20–30 yards for time
- counting the number of seconds needed for a quantity of finger tapping, hand clapping, foot tapping, etc.
- counting the number of seconds needed for winding up objects or sorting objects into containers

Power

- vertical jump
- high jump
- throwing, kicking, and striking (Distance object travels is measured.)

Reaction Time

Reaction time may be improved only to a point and in some cases not at all. Some teacher-made activities can include:

- ringing a bell and having student clap hands as soon as bell is heard
- making a movement and having student try to quickly imitate it
- playing dodge ball

Coordination

Activities that combine movements for accuracy can be used to measure or develop coordination such as:

- throwing for accuracy
- hopping and clapping hands five times without missing
- counting the number of any combined movements correct in a 15–20-second range

FITNESS CHARACTERISTICS OF DISABLED STUDENTS

Winnick and Short (1982) completed an extensive investigation of the physical fitness characteristics of sensory-impaired and orthopedically-impaired students. The results of the findings of their study, called Project UNIQUE, have provided a new standardized fitness test for the populations covered and more current information on the fitness status of these subjects.

The findings have many implications for physical fitness development of sensory- and orthopedically impaired individuals. The factor studies indicate that the factor structure for physical fitness of sensory- and orthopedically impaired students does not differ significantly from that of normal peers. The rate of development of the factors, however, does differ. Major areas that need attention include body composition, muscular strength and endurance, cardiorespiratory endurance, and flexibility.

Of the populations studied by Winnick and Short, visually and orthopedically impaired students were found more often to need specially designed programs to meet their individual needs. The fitness levels of visually impaired students were not as much affected by age of onset of the disability as once previously thought. For partially sighted subjects, fitness scores were higher than those with less vision. In both cases, fitness levels of visually impaired students were lower than normal peers using group comparisons. This was particularly true for fitness items requiring movement through space. Another interesting fact was that subjects who participated in running events independently performed better than visually impaired students using a guide wire. Using a partner did not seem to affect the visually impaired students as much as the guide wire did. This was particularly true for the shuttle run.

Areas of fitness where visually impaired subjects were more like their nonimpaired peers were in skinfold measures, grip strength, and sit and reach. Other areas included sit-ups, leg raises, and arm hang. The greatest differences between sighted and nonsighted persons were seen in the softball throw, the 50-yard dash, and the shuttle run.

Hearing-impaired subjects in Winnick and Short's (1982) study in many cases had scores above the median scores found for normal subjects used for comparison. Measures included grip strength, pull-ups, the broad jump, and softball throw for males. Females were similar to normal subjects for grip strength and softball throw. Another finding was that deaf students who were in residential programs scored higher than deaf students in public school settings. Deaf students will not need as individualized a program of physical education as other sensory-impaired youngsters or those with orthopedic problems.

Orthopedic students in the study less often scored above the normal group than others with handicapping conditions. The one measure on which individuals with orthopedic impairments compared closest to normal subjects was for skinfold. The more severe the handicapping condition, the greater the difference in performance when compared with normal subjects and those with milder conditions. The researchers recommend that individuals with orthopedic conditions, such as cerebral palsy, and spinal neuromuscular disorders need individualized fitness programs to prevent atrophy and bone deformities and enhance mobility and overall health.

The fact that a commonality of factor structures exists between impaired and nonimpaired students suggests that the general fitness curriculum and its components can be similar for impaired and nonimpaired students.

Because lower levels of fitness were found among disabled populations when compared with normals, fitness programs will need to begin at different levels. The more severe the handicapping condition, the more basic the fitness program has to be. In all cases where disabled students are involved, fitness programs should be individualized.

Winnick and Short also suggest that age is a factor in fitness development. As age increases, fitness levels tend to improve in most handicapped populations, except for those with orthopedic impairments. Females tend to reach their peak in fitness between ages 12–14 years, whereas males reach their plateau between 10–17 years. In addition, sex differences were also found among disabled students. The implications are that fitness programs should vary in length, type of activity, intensity, and frequency.

ADAPTING ACTIVITIES

Many handicapped students can participate in almost all of the physical activities that are designed for regular students. Modifications may be made where necessary so that those who cannot participate in the regular activity may successfully participate at their own pace and level. There is a wide range of fitness levels among regular students and handicapped students as well. Some handicapped students may even have higher fitness levels than their nonhandicapped peers. Often, mildly retarded students who have participated in the Special Olympics for an extensive period are more physically fit than some of their nonretarded peers.

General Adaptations

Some modifications of physical fitness activities may be used with several kinds of handicapping conditions. The following are guidelines:

- Decrease the distance to be covered in walking, jogging, or running activities.
- Decrease the number of repetitions in an activity.
- Use lighter weights for strength training.

- Make activities interesting and appealing.
- Use stations so that students can progress more on an individual basis.

Adaptations for Particular Disorders

Physically Handicapped

- Allow students to use a wheelchair in mobility activities.
- Substitute an activity if the student cannot participate.
- Provide extra mats for exercising to provide protection from falls.
- Modify an activity to meet the particular needs of the student.

Blind and Visually Impaired

- Use sighted guides in mobility activities.
- Use guide ropes for short running activities.
- Have student use a buddy for jogging.
- Provide an auditory signal in throwing activities.
- Provide an exploration period for learning to use exercise equipment.
- Provide arm support, if needed, on jumping activities.
- Use touch to demonstrate body movements.
- Provide a board or other object with tactual input to indicate a throwing or jumping line.
- If a sighted partner is used on distance running, the visually impaired student's time and endurance should be measured.

GENERAL PRINCIPLES OF FITNESS TRAINING

1. Fitness activities must be done on a regular basis to be effective. Some individuals may need motivation and encouragement to keep on schedule.

2. To increase strength musculature must be overloaded. Overloading means providing a greater workload than the person normally experiences. For example, if a student is used to completing only 10 repetitions of an exercise, the number can be increased to 20 to create an overload, or more work output. Other means of providing an overload include using more weight, requiring that more distance be covered, increasing speed, or allowing less time for an exercise to be completed, i.e., more sit-ups in less time. The increase should be gradual and tailored to the individual. Overloading should not be generalized to groups of students since individuals have different fitness levels.

3. The total body needs to be considered in fitness training. As much of the handicapped student's body as possible should be involved in a total fitness program.

4. Progression in cardiovascular fitness should be carefully planned and slowly implemented. Children with special health problems such as cardiac disorders should have a medical exam and a physician's statement of approval prior to beginning any cardiovascular exercises.

5. Secondary students in particular should be asked to keep at least a weekly record of their fitness activities after they have been prescribed.

6. A warm-up activity must be included prior to any exercise routine.

7. Students must be allowed time to rest if they become overly fatigued during exercise, showing such signs as excessive sweating, pallor, heavy breathing, dizziness, or pain.

8. The physical fitness program should be individualized to meet the physical and mental ability of each student.

9. Rewards and incentives should be provided to keep motivation high.

FITNESS CIRCUITS

Stations that group exercises in an overall fitness course are an excellent means of providing total fitness training. This type of arrangement has an advantage over drill type exercises in a single large group. The major advantage of a fitness circuit is that students can progress at their own individual rates. Mildly handicapped students will have very little difficulty using this approach in a mainstreamed class. Moderately handicapped students can also participate in a mainstreamed setting if peer teachers or aides are available. This same format can be used with severely handicapped students. However, one-on-one instruction is necessary.

The number of stations to be used depends on the room available, the goals of the fitness program, and the number of students in the class. Usually, six to eight stations can be easily managed. Figure 6–1 illustrates how a circuit may be created indoors. The circuit can be set up for work on overall conditioning or on specific fitness components. Once students learn the circuit, the instructor can have more of a resource role for students experiencing difficulty.

Stations can be changed or variations added to each activity. Individual cards can be made for each student and progress recorded individually or by peer teachers. Stations should be geared to the students' ability to move. In some cases, levels may be very basic. For instance, beginning levels for some might consist of simple movements and stretching to increase the range of motion. Where severely disabled students are involved, these movements may be passive, with the teacher moving the student through the activity. Stations can be arranged from passive circuits to

Figure 6–1 Indoor Fitness Circuit

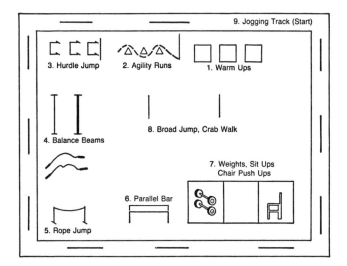

student-initiated movements. Combinations can also be set up where the instructor may work one-on-one for those needing passive movements at a level in a circuit and others can be initiating movements at other levels with supervision. Stations can be arranged from the least amount of movement to the most amount of movement. The instructor should keep in mind the flexibility of stations in programming.

POSTURAL FITNESS

Good posture adds an esthetic aspect to individuals. Moreover, the way in which persons carry themselves often reflects their psychological and emotional state. Poor posture may eventually interfere with normal functioning and the result is impaired circulation, breathing, and self-concept. Postural deviations can also affect movement efficiency by reducing the range of motion at a joint or reducing equal balance on both sides of the body.

Wiseman (1982) reports that postural fitness is one of the major anomalies found among school-aged populations. Handicapped students are not excluded from those found to be deficient. One of the major reasons students have poorly developed posture is the fact that insufficient screening occurs within the public schools. Also, postural fitness is not a major concern among handicapped populations.

Cratty (1980) found that, generally, healthy children had less postural deviations when compared with groups of children with a variety of health problems. Postural deviations occur in handicapped students much for the same reasons that they occur in nonhandicapped populations. They result largely from improper body alignment and combinations of other contributing factors. Fait and Dunn (1984) describe the causes of poor posture as being medical, emotional, or due to faulty body mechanics. In many cases combinations of these

conditions exist. Other factors include malnourishment, illness and infection, injury, and weak musculature.

Handicapped students may have particular kinds of postural problems.

Postural Problems

Blind Students

- poor walking gait (Feet may shuffle and more lateral movements may be observed.)
- head held to the side to see better

Hearing Impaired

- head tilted to hear better

Physically Impaired

- body imbalance because of missing limbs or differing limb lengths

Neuromuscular Disorders

- structural deviations and functional disorders
- poor body alignment due to muscular imbalances

Obese Students

- increased curve in lower spine from overweight
- flat feet

Types of Postural Problems

Functional Disorders

Functional disorders result from muscular and connective tissue being weak and unbalanced. This may be caused by overweight, lack of flexibility, or one group of muscles being overexercised and the opposing group being weakened. Such disorders respond fairly well to therapeutic exercise programs designed to get the musculature and connective tissue involved back into proper balance.

Structural Disorders

Structural deviations result from a deformity of the bony structures. These deformities need to be medically corrected either by surgery, bracing, or both. Exercises may be recommended later to maintain proper alignment.

Screening for Postural Deviations

Both handicapped and nonhandicapped students need to be screened for posture deviations and deformities. Functional deviations can eventually become structural deviations if not corrected.

Various forms of screening for postural deviations have been developed ranging from observations to the use of screening devices. Most posture screening is completed by having students assume a standing position. However, Schurr (1980) notes that students assume a variety of postures during the day including sitting, standing, and moving. After a general screening, students should be evaluated in several positions if deviations are suspected.

Sophisticated equipment is not always necessary to conduct a posture screening. Posture is evaluated from a standing position, viewing the student from the side, back, and front. Side views enable the evaluator to observe anterior-posterior deviations. Deviations such as forward head, lordosis, kyphosis, and hyperextended knees can be observed. Posterior views enable observation of lateral deviations such as scoliosis, head tilt, improper leg or foot alignment, and other deviations. Table 6–1 lists suggestions for observing proper alignment while the student is standing in a posterior stance. Table 6–2 covers the stance, with subject standing with right side to examiner.

Screening with a Plumbline

A quick check for body alignment can be achieved using a plumbline. This can be easily constructed by hanging a weight from a string. The string should be long enough to hang from the ceiling or a high place and it should rest about a ½ inch from the floor so the weight does not drag. The student should stand so the plumbline falls between the viewer and the student. Views should be observed from the side and rear.

Table 6–1 Clues for Posterior View

Observe	Proper Alignment
Feet	• should point straight ahead or with toes pointed slightly outward • toes fairly straight
Head	• should be held erect and balanced in the middle of the shoulders • should be fairly straight with no twisting right or left
Spine	• should be straight with no curve right or left in any segment
Shoulders	• even height between left and right shoulders, one shoulder not higher than the other
Hips	• should be very close to level

Table 6–2 Clues for Side View

Observe	Proper Alignment
Head	• should be held straight with ear in line with shoulder
Shoulders	• should be in line with head, chest slightly elevated • should not be rotating forward causing shoulder blade to protrude
Thoracic (Upper Spine)	• slight rounded look with trunk erect • buttocks not protruding • buttocks in good alignment with upper back
Abdomen	• stomach flat and not overly protruding or sagging
Lumbar Spine (Lower Back)	• should have only a slight rounded curve • lower back not hollow with buttocks protruding
Knees	• should be slightly flexed • should align with ankle

Side View Using the Plumbline

Crowe, Auxter, and Pyfer (1981) describe the points to look for related to proper posture alignment using the plumbline as a reference. If posture is properly aligned, the plumbline should fall at the following points on the body:

- about 1 inch in front of the ankle bone or external malleolus
- slightly in front of the knee
- through the center of the hips
- through the center of the shoulder
- through the center or midpoint of the earlobe

Anterior View Using the Plumbline

The student should stand so the plumbline falls between the student and the examiner. The line should divide the body into two equal halves. If posture is correct, the plumbline should fall at the following points on the anterior portion of the body:

- at the midpoint between the two ankle bones (internal malleoli)
- midway between the kneecaps
- middle of the hips
- center of the navel
- center of the breastbone
- center of the chin, nose, and forehead

Scoliosis Screening

Scoliosis, or curvature of the spine, is, according to Sherrill (1981), more serious than any of the other common posture deviations. If left uncorrected, it can eventually become an orthopedic handicap.

Scoliosis screening may be accomplished by having students assume certain positions in which the curvature may be observed. Two common screening procedures include the following techniques:

1. Adam's position is one method where the student is asked to bend forward at the waist while in a standing position. This relaxed, bent position should be held for several seconds. The student should be reminded to hold the knees straight. This allows observation of the curve. If the curve does not temporarily disappear or lessen, the curve is approaching a structural condition. The student in this stage should receive medical intervention and a referral should be made to a physician.

2. The vertical hang is a procedure where the student is required to hang from a horizontal bar using both arms. Again, as in the Adam's test, a referral should be made if the curvature does not temporarily disappear.

Implications

Posture development needs to be a part of every good physical education program. Screening, in particular, is essential. Developmental activities and exercises should be included and integrated into activities. The teacher should strive to have students use correct posture in performing motor skills, as this will add to mechanical efficiency.

Students with lowered intellectual ability, emotional difficulties, or other disabilities may not be able to see the necessity for developing good posture. The long-term benefits may not be meaningful to the student. In such cases the teacher will need to promote posture screening in addition to fitness development.

Activities associated with both programs need to be motivating and attractive to such students. Screening and developmental activities can be more easily facilitated if students are attracted to the notion of good posture. Students who are found not to have moderate to severe problems can participate in the regular program.

Functional disorders can be corrected or improved by exercises. However, the adapted physical educator should consult with a physician when a student is found with a postural deviation. School nurses may also be available to provide input. The adapted specialist can implement the prescribed exercise program to correct the postural problem.

A close working relationship should be developed among the adapted physical educator, physician, health specialist, and physical therapist to provide a sound program for students needing corrective measures. Kalakian and Eichstaedt

(1982) suggest that corrective programs should be conducted at least three days a week for students to receive maximum benefits from the program.

NUTRITION AND WEIGHT MANAGEMENT

One of the goals of a health and fitness program should be to provide motivation and education about good nutritional practices and weight management. Both are essential to good health and fitness. Thus, it is difficult to separate health, nutrition, fitness, and weight control. Often many different populations of handicapped students have nutritional problems, are overweight or underweight, and have low levels of physical fitness. The special physical educator should incorporate the health concerns of handicapped students within the physical education curriculum.

With the increase of teenage pregnancies, physical education programs can play an important role in the prevention of the birth of handicapped children by providing information regarding health, fitness, and proper nutritional practices.

With the passing of P.L. 94–142 and the implementation of the least restrictive environment, handicapped students, to the maximum extent possible, are being educated with their nonhandicapped peers. Johnson, Smith, Bittle, and Nuckolls (1980) reported that information found by Congress resulted in amendments in 1978 of the Child Nutrition Act. The changes were based on research of children's knowledge of nutrition. They concluded that:

- Children's knowledge of nutrition was not up to par and that proper nutrition of children should be a high priority.
- Children who do not understand the relationship of proper nutrition and health are likely to eat less nutritious foods.
- Teachers and other school personnel are not trained to motivate students to learn about good nutrition.

Nutrition needs to be included within the school curriculum and should be covered in conjunction with the health and physical education instruction of both handicapped and nonhandicapped students. An in-depth, broad-based, correlated curriculum could be developed that includes nutrition, physical fitness, and weight management.

Weight Management

Obesity occurs when the desirable weight of the body is exceeded by 20 percent. This is the accepted standard for establishing the excess weight of someone considered to be obese. Underweight is said to exist when the body weight is under 20 percent below a person's desirable weight. As we have noted, these conditions exist among handicapped populations for several reasons. Many of them are similar to the causes for weight problems in the normal population.

Overweight may be a result of inactivity, overeating, or a combination of both. Fox, Rotatori, and Fox (1981) found from preliminary research that overweight and obesity is a prevalent problem in the mentally retarded population. These researchers report that major contributions to obesity among retarded populations are the same as in the nonretarded population. Their research suggested that only a small incidence of obesity is found among retarded populations based on their actual physical disorders. Retarded subjects with Prader Willi Syndrome often develop obesity by the second year of life. Children with this disorder were reported to show preferences for all foods and seemed to be unable to satisfy hunger (Fox, Switzky, Rotatori, & Vitkus, 1982).

Underweight, on the other hand, among the handicapped may result from poor feeding skills. Children with malocclusions or chewing and swallowing difficulties may be significantly underweight by having to eat restricted foods and reduce caloric intake. Some handicapped students may be underweight as a result of overactivity and preferences for nonfood items, commonly referred to as pica.

Malnutrition is often seen in underweight students. However, an individual may be overweight and malnourished also. Both conditions have undesirable and harmful effects on the body.

Briggs and Calloway (1979) report several increased risk factors that can accompany obesity. These range from heart disease, high blood pressure, diabetes, back strain, and other joint stress.

Handicapped persons may have a difficult time, as it is, with their disabilities. Allowing handicapped students to become obese will add to their disabilities. Obesity limits children socially and physically. The adapted physical educator is in a good position to aid students in developing good dietary habits and positive attitudes toward exercise that will eventually assist them in keeping their weight within desirable limits.

Individuals who are over- or underweight, lack physical fitness, and have poor nutrition are less likely to be good employees and good health risks. These same problems are also present among handicapped populations. Conditions such as these represent an additional burden or handicap to an individual with a disability.

The major purpose of this section is to provide the health and physical educator with knowledge regarding the importance of nutrition in weight management and fitness programs. Also, information will be provided about motivating and implementing weight management and good nutrition practices.

The Need for Good Nutrition

Proper nutrition is needed for all children. Martin (1973) reported that poor or improper nutrition is related to poor attention and inability to learn. Proper nutrition may also be effective as a preventive measure for some handicapping conditions (Wallace, 1971).

In a study by the Tennessee Department of Public Health (1977), developmentally disabled youngsters were reported to be significantly different from normative standards in weight, growth, and height. Inadequate diet and altered metabolism were reported to be major contributors to these conditions.

Stevens and Baxter (1981) have suggested that lowered nutritional status during pregnancy could result in lowered vitality, poor attention, decreased exploratory behavior, and reduced environmental contact in offspring. The impact of good nutrition on the prevention of mental retardation and other developmental delays cannot be overstated. Stevens and Baxter (1981) further reported that mothers who received nutritional supplements during pregnancy produced infants who showed significant differences in eye-hand coordination and gross motor skill development as compared with offspring of mothers who received no supplementation.

Stevens and Baxter's research also indicated that significant numbers of children had diets low in quality while consuming high quantities of foods. These children were classified as mildly undernourished. As a result, they were small for their ages and generally came from low-income families. The effects of these mild forms of malnourishment included reduced performance on developmental measures and intellectual tasks.

Poor Nutrition and Heavy Metal Absorption

Poor nutritional status is a significant factor in the absorption of toxic metals. Mahaffey (1977) reported that diets high in fat and low in proteins increased the absorption of heavy or toxic metals, particularly lead. Also, the presence of a subminimal level of certain essential trace minerals increases the absorption of toxic metals. Mahaffey (1977) further reported in her study that children with reduced calcium, iron, and zinc had higher incidences of toxic metal absorption than children with adequate levels of these minerals. Toxic metals should be considered as part of the nutritional evaluation of handicapped students.

Research on toxic metals has primarily centered around the heavy metal lead. Studies of the intelligence and performance of children exposed to lead have indicated that psychological, neurological, and other functional impairments can occur in young children with evidence of undue lead absorption who are otherwise asymptomatic of levels seen in clinical lead poisoning (Lin-Fu, 1975). As early as 1943, Byers and Lord conducted a study of the subclinical effect of lead in children. They concluded that children with lead poisoning, who presented no evidence of central nervous system involvement, often later showed visual and motor impairment in dealing with shape, directionality, and spatial orientation. Behavioral disorders associated with minimal brain dysfunction were also observed within this group of children (Byers & Lord, 1943).

Other studies have found similar results. Perino and Claire (1974) reported that as lead levels increased in black preschool children, general cognitive, verbal, and perceptual motor abilities decreased.

Another study comparing children exposed to lead and a control group reported that the exposed group had a higher incidence of gross and fine motor dysfunction, irritability, and impaired cognition at the age of 4 years. After retesting the groups at age 7 and 8 years, it was found that the impairment found in the exposed group had not improved.

Needleman, Gunnoe, Leviton, Reed, Peresie, Maher, and Barnett (1979) conducted a study of children from the suburbs of New England in which dentine lead was analyzed for body lead levels. They found that children with high dentine lead performed significantly less well on IQ tests than their counterparts with low lead content. There were differences in performance on measures of auditory processing, attention, and adaptive behavior in classroom settings.

Undue Lead Absorption and Mental Retardation

The findings of some recent studies suggest that handicapped and impaired children have functional and behavioral problems as a result of undue lead absorption. While it is impossible to conclude from studies of handicapped and impaired children that lead exposure and these conditions have a direct connection, the findings are highly suggestive that lead exposure may frequently be the causal factor (Graham & Graham, 1974).

Routh, Mushak, and Boone (1979) conducted lead level determinations on 100 children seen at an outpatient clinic for developmental and learning disabilities located in rural South Carolina. Most of the children had intellectual deficits of varying degrees. A statistically significant number of the 100 children had microcephally. The researchers suggested that the higher lead levels in children caused the microcephally and may have been related to prenatal exposure to lead. Folio and Marlowe (1980) reported that 60 percent of 47 handicapped children receiving special education services in Middle Tennessee screened for lead through trace mineral analysis of scalp hair had elevated lead levels, whereas only 9 percent of a nonhandicapped control group showed elevated lead levels.

In a similar study, Pihl and Parkes (1977) found significantly higher lead and cadmium levels in hair samples taken from learning-disabled children than those taken from a control group. Some studies have suggested that there is an association between hyperactivity and antisocial behavior and elevated lead levels (David, Clark, & Voeller, 1972).

Other Toxic Metals

Frequently, elevated lead levels are found in combination with elevations of other toxic metals such as cadmium, arsenic, and mercury (Lin-Fu, 1975). Pihl and Parkes (1977) found cadmium in combination with lead in a study of hair samples taken from 31 learning-disabled and 22 normal children. The highest levels of lead and cadmium were found in the learning-disabled group.

It has been found that even though two toxic metals may be present in the body below the tolerable limits, when combined they may produce an additive effect that causes adverse health reactions. This combined effect can be as detrimental as having only one toxic metal elevated (Doctor's Data, Inc., 1979).

Folio, Hennigan, and Errera (1982) reported the results of combined toxic metals found in a comparison of urban and rural special education children in Middle Tennessee. Their findings indicated that urban subjects had frequently and statistically higher levels of lead and cadmium than rural children. Children in rural areas had more frequent combinations of lead and arsenic.

Effects of Toxic Metals

Any toxic metal will affect various body parts and interfere with bodily functions when present in elevated amounts. Toxicity symptoms vary for each metal and depend on factors such as age and an individual's health and nutritional status. Rimland and Larson (1983), in their review of the nutritional status reports of studies conducted with specific handicapped populations, concluded that nutritional deficiencies and toxic metals appear to be highly correlated with specific handicapping conditions. They concluded that:

- High levels of lead and cadmium and, to a lesser extent, aluminum and mercury, tend to be correlated with several types of behavior pathology.
- Minerals such as copper, chromium, potassium, and sodium appear to be more associated with behavior disorders than other minerals.
- Learning disabilities are characterized by high cadmium, lead, copper, and manganese levels.
- Students with delinquent behavior have high cadmium, calcium, magnesium, and aluminum levels.
- Behavior-disordered students tend to have high lead, chromium, and molybdenum levels.

The studies thus far are not generalizable or conclusive. However, they do present sufficient evidence to warrant further investigation and consideration of toxic metals and nutritional deficiencies as contributors to learning and behavioral problems.

Other studies have found some emerging trends with respect to other specific populations. Folio and Brown (1982) reported the results of trace mineral and metal analysis of hair samples taken from emotionally disturbed adolescents. The samples taken from the disturbed population were compared with normal lab standards derived from healthy subjects screened by physicians. The results indicated that the disturbed adolescents were low in lithium, chromium, cobalt, phosphorus, and silicon and high in calcium, magnesium, potassium, copper, and selenium. The toxic metal found commonly to be elevated was cadmium.

Folio and Garrett (1982) reported the results of trace mineral and metal analysis of Down's Syndrome subjects compared with normal standards. Significant differences were found between the Down's population and normal lab standards. One important finding was that none of the Down's children had elevated levels of any metal or mineral. However, deficiencies of two standard deviations below the normative mean were found for several important minerals. These included:

- copper
- calcium
- zinc
- magnesium
- potassium
- sodium
- phosphorus
- lithium
- selenium

Sources of Toxic Metals

Knowing the sources of various toxic metals can assist in the reduced absorption of the metals by simply eliminating them from the child's environment or limiting exposure to them. Table 6–3 lists toxic metals and their sources.

The sources of toxic metals are numerous in the environment. Children are at a higher risk than adults because toxic metals tend to settle in the air in higher concentrations at the height at which young children breathe. This also is true for individuals in wheelchairs. Young children also are more susceptible to damage from absorption of toxic metals. Lead, for example, is stored more in the soft tissues of young children, such as the heart, kidneys, brain, etc., whereas in adults, lead seems to be stored more in hard tissue such as bone. The following are some additional effects of toxic metals listed by metal type.

Lead

Lead can interfere with many bodily functions. Anemia can result since lead interferes with the biosynthesis of heme (Chisolm, 1971). One of the most significant effects of undue lead absorption is the damage to the central nervous system. After a single large dose absorption of lead can cause acute encephalopathy resulting in severe mental retardation. Minimal damage can result in lead absorption at levels before clinical symptoms appear. Researchers are not sure at what levels in the body lead appears to cause changes in bodily functions and behavior. Marlowe, Folio, and Hall (1982) report that levels of lead that were once thought safe are now being investigated as causes of behavioral and intellectual impairments.

Mercury

Symptoms of elevated mercury levels include reduced memory capacity, fatigue, depression, and eventually antisocial behavior. Clinical symptoms can result in hearing loss, lack of coordination, and speech disorders (Lesser, 1980). In conducting research to determine the extent of toxic metals among specific handicapping conditions, an interesting, although unfortunate, discovery was made. A boy of 9 years old, who will be called Allen, was screened for

Table 6–3 Toxic Metals and Sources of Exposure

Metal	Sources
Lead	• lead-based paint in old housing, antiques, farm fences • imported toys with lead-based paint • imported pottery with lead paint • leaded gasoline • lead smelters • some clays • lead in plants from pesticides, herbicides, defoliants • illicit whiskey • industrial pollution • lead sinkers • newsprint and giftwrap • house dust in homes bordering high traffic patterns
Cadmium	• cigarette smoke • oxide dusts • contaminated drinking water • galvanized pipes • welding • pigments and paints • contaminated shellfish
Aluminum	• aluminum cooking ware, utensils • antacids • baking powders • foils • processed foods
Arsenic	• coal burning • pesticides, insecticides, herbicides • manufacture of glass
Mercury	• manufacture and delivery of petroleum products • fluorescent lamps • hair dyes • amalgams in dentistry • contaminated saltwater fish

minerals and metals by using scalp hair as a tissue. Very high levels of mercury were reported in the analysis of the hair sample. The lab rechecked the analysis to be sure of the results. It was confirmed that high mercury did exist. Allen, until age 6, was a normal healthy boy. Reports from his teacher indicated that he began to lose weight and appetite. Speech began to deteriorate and he had difficulty with memory tasks. Eventually, Allen lost his hearing and his behavior became rather aggressive. Evidence for sources of mercury were investigated. However, no conclusion could be reached. There were no diseases reported that would cause this type of damage in the boy. It is quite possible in Allen's case that high mercury absorption resulted in the disorders he now has.

Aluminum

Aluminum is often reported to be at elevated levels in students with delinquent behavior and memory loss (Lesser, 1980). Elevated aluminum primarily affects the stomach, bones, and brain. Gastrointestinal irritations can result. Also, aluminum absorption beyond levels the body will tolerate can result in memory loss, fatigue, and irritability. Lesser further reports that patients with Alzheimer's Disease have higher than normal levels of aluminum in the brain tissue and cerebrospinal fluids.

Cadmium

Cadmium at elevated levels in the body can affect the kidneys, heart, blood vessels, brain, appetite, and smell centers. Cadmium is becoming more evident as a causal factor in high blood pressure and heart disease (Lesser, 1980).

Arsenic

Arsenic interferes with cellular metabolism. As a metabolic inhibitor, it reduces energy production efficiency. Symptoms may include fatigue, low vitality, listlessness, dark spots on the skin, and gastrointestinal difficulties. At higher levels of absorption, hair loss can result.

A Word To The Wise

In many cases when students who are low in vitality, overly fatigued, listless, and doing poorly in school, the notion of toxic metal absorption as a contributing factor is rarely considered. In the course of screening and identification of handicapped students, a screening for toxic metals should definitely also be conducted. There are many possible interventions for students who are behavior disordered, learning disabled, mentally retarded, and low in vitality. The majority of approaches to intervention consist of psychodynamic and behavior models. Intervention should be aimed at the total student.

While the reduction and prevention of toxic metal absorption should be one intervention strategy, it should not be considered a panacea to any problem. This point can be illustrated by comparing the student's body to an automobile engine. There are many adjustments and changes that can be made to help an engine run smoothly; the carburetor can be adjusted, sparkplugs changed, timing can be reset, etc. Lowering the body's toxic metal levels can be thought of as filtering out particles that interfere with engine performance. Maintaining a good level of nutritional status can be compared to using high-octane fuel. Thus, it may take many adjustments to the car's engine to get it at peak performance. The same is true with handicapped students. Many adjustments and modifications may need to be made to help the handicapped student. Behavior problems have been associated with the following types of foods:

- reduced fiber content
- refined carbohydrates
- refined sugars
- overcooked and overprocessed foods
- high content of food dyes and artificial color

Dietary Changes to Aid Learning Problems

Cott (1977) explains that deficiencies in certain trace minerals can be detrimental to students with learning disabilities. Learning-disabled students have been found to be deficient in copper, calcium, magnesium, manganese, and zinc.

Mindell (1981) recommends that supplements be given to students with particular types of learning problems. (See Table 6–4.)

Essential Trace Minerals

There are basically two types of trace minerals. Macro minerals are present in relatively high amounts in body tissues. Trace minerals are present in the body and are essential to proper bodily functioning. Micro minerals are present in minute quantities. The majority of minerals are found in unrefined foods. Refined foods such as fats, oils, and sugars contain almost no minerals. The mineral content of food is found by burning the organic part of a known amount of food and weighing the resulting ash (Nutrition Search, 1979). Fortunately, persons who are deficient in certain trace minerals can be treated through mineral supplements and/or a diet that includes food rich in the particular minerals that are needed.

Table 6–4 Dietary Supplement for Learning Problems

Learning Problem	Increase Intake
Low Achiever	• eggs, poultry, fish, meats • citrus fruits • green and yellow vegetables (raw or barely cooked) • whole grain foods
Uncoordinated Student	• dark green vegetables • yellow vegetables • B complex vitamins • general vitamin and mineral supplement
Overanxious Student	• calcium and magnesium • vitamin B_6, pantothenic acid • vitamin C • multivitamin and mineral supplement
Student with Poor Memory	• vitamin B complex • Brewer's yeast • whole grains • vegetables
Hyperactive Student	• B complex vitamins • calcium and vitamin D • zinc

More in-depth studies are needed to determine the effect of mineral supplements on learning, behavior, and psychological changes in handicapped students. Folio (1982) reported that handicapped students when compared with normal controls and laboratory standards tend to have a greater incidence of trace mineral deficiencies.

NUTRITIONAL FITNESS

Nutritional fitness is as important to develop in handicapped students as physical fitness. When a child has a handicap imposed on the periods of growth and development, the physiological and psychological stresses can be detrimental to the child's overall health. The handicapping condition is a stress factor in itself. Smith (1979) reports that the need for additional nutritional supplements increases under times of stress in the normal child. This is even more true of children with handicapping conditions.

Of course, nutritional intervention is not a cure-all for handicapped students. As an adjunct to other forms of intervention, nutritional education and supplementation should be included in every handicapped student's IEP. It is quite predictable that, at some point in the near future, nutrition will become a larger component of the handicapped student's school curriculum.

A good analogy for understanding the concept of good nutrition and its benefits is physical fitness. Physical fitness can be viewed as having enough strength, energy, endurance, etc., to get through an everyday routine and still have enough

stamina to get through an emergency. Being nutritionally fit is very similar. Many students will get sick with colds and other ailments, usually right after some stressful event in their lives. This may be a result of using a large amount of their body's nutritional stores to meet stress and then not having enough to ward off illnesses.

There are many ways of testing for vitamins, minerals, and other nutritional stores in the body. One way is to take a survey of what foods the students consume. If diets consist of foods mostly composed of sugar, fats, carbohydrates, and little protein or whole grains, obviously, the students will not be nutritionally sound.

Mentally retarded students may be shown pictures of foods and asked to indicate the ones most often consumed. Parents can also be interviewed at the IEP meeting. The same procedure may be used with young handicapped students.

Blood Analysis

If nutritional problems are suspected, the student should be referred to a physician for further testing. The physician should be carefully selected since many receive little training in nutrition education in medical school. This trend is beginning to change, however.

Vitamins can be analyzed through blood analysis. Blood generally tells what is circulating in the body. Toxic metals and minerals may also be determined through blood analysis. However, blood does not provide an accurate picture of what is stored in the body at the cellular level. It tells what is currently available, but not what is in reserve. Urinalysis may be more accurate in revealing what the body is eliminating.

Trace Mineral Analysis Using Scalp Hair

Scalp hair is becoming recognized as an invaluable tissue for monitoring human environmental exposure to toxic metals and determining levels of nutrient minerals at the cellular level. Trace mineral and metal analysis of hair seems to be a better indicator of past exposure than blood serum or urine (Maugh, 1978). Blood concentrations may not reliably reflect the total body burden or give an indication of past absorption in relation to toxic metals. This is related to the fact that after exposure a toxic metal, such as lead, may leave the bloodstream fairly rapidly after absorption and become stored in soft or hard tissues or both. Conversely, scalp hair provides a continuous record of nutritional status and exposure to heavy metal pollutants (Chattopadhyay & Jervis, 1974). Research by Maugh (1978) indicates that there is a strong correlation between concentrations of metals and minerals in the hair and those in internal organs. The technology of trace mineral and metal analysis of hair has improved greatly within the last five years and is becoming an increasingly accurate diagnostic tool (Rimland & Larson, 1983).

A state-of-the-art laboratory for trace mineral and metal analysis is Bio-Medical Data, Inc., located at 130 W. 101 Roosevelt Rd., West Chicago, Illinois, 60185. Three primary instruments used to analyze the mineral and metal content of scalp hair are the atomic absorption spectrophotometer, the graphite furnace, and the induction-coupled plasma torch. This procedure is also being recognized by the Environmental Protection Agency as a valuable and reliable screening tool. When trace mineral analysis is performed under strict and controlled laboratory standards, it can be a highly reliable and accurate screening tool for determining the nutritional status of an individual. The average cost of a trace mineral analysis, which must be requested through physicians and public health officials, is about $25.00.

ALLERGIC REACTIONS TO FOODS

Hyperactive, irritable, and fatigued children may be showing signs of intolerance for certain kinds of foods. According to Crook (1980), hidden food allergy is caused by foods to which some people are hypersensitive, or have adverse reactions. The food then becomes an allergen. Histamines are released when allergens and antibodies come together. Symptoms from allergic reactions include:

- rashes
- swelling
- sneezing
- wheezing
- cramps

Some reactions may be hidden or delayed in onset. Hidden food allergies may produce symptoms, according to Crook (1980), that include:

- dark circles under the eyes
- sniffing and pushing up the nose with the hand
- nervousness
- overactivity
- fatigue

Mindell (1981) also describes symptoms of hidden food allergy to include:

- hyperactivity
- nosebleeds
- higher susceptibility to colds and respiratory infections
- ear infections

- poor school achievement
- muscle aches
- short attention span
- digestive difficulties

Crook (1980) suggests that by eliminating from the diet certain foods to which the person is allergic the symptoms should improve. The recommended diet developed by Crook includes the elimination of the following foods:

- wheat
- chocolate
- coffee and tea
- sugar
- foods with artificial color and additives
- corn
- eggs
- citrus
- dairy products

The foods may then be introduced one by one to see when the symptoms appear.

If providing camping experiences, outings, or picnics, those responsible for food preparation should be made aware of a child's food allergies and be understanding and cooperative with parents in keeping the child on a proper diet. Parents should also help by supplying some of the appropriate foods if they are not readily available.

Before using food as a behavioral reinforcer, teachers need to check to make sure the handicapped child is not allergic to it. Sugary foods and chocolate are used frequently as reinforcers.

NUTRITIONAL EDUCATION APPROACHES

Handicapped as well as nonhandicapped students need to be educated regarding proper nutrition. Techniques that appear to have motivated students to eat more nutritious foods have included fun-through-learning approaches.

1. One of the most effective methods is having students participate directly in preparing nutritional foods (Sloan, 1977).

2. Students enjoy taste parties where they can sample a variety of nutritional foods.

3. Involving students in games for learning about good nutrition is also motivating.

4. Other activities can be centered around art projects in which students can color, draw, and make objects to learn about good nutritional concepts.

5. Nonhandicapped students may be allowed to teach handicapped students and serve as models for good nutritional patterns (Johnson, Smith, Bittle, & Nuckolls, 1980).

Good weight management programs teach sensible eating habits and include various levels of physical activity. Fox, Switzky, Rotatori, and Vitkus (1982) reported that a behavioral approach to weight management has been very successful in reducing and maintaining desirable weight levels among obese populations. This approach includes the use of several techniques.

1. Self-monitoring techniques have been successful when the individual is allowed to record what he or she has eaten daily. Ultimately, this procedure allows the person to become aware of eating habits.

2. Association includes the teaching of events in the person's daily living that cause overeating, such as emotional difficulties, happiness, fear, and anger.

3. Stimuli often produce or lead to eating. Another technique is to reduce stimuli that are likely to cause individuals to eat. Individuals are asked to stop and substitute a fun activity other than eating when the stimulus appears. Stimuli can be observation of others eating, pictures or advertisements of food, smell or visual stimulation, or prompts from others.

4. Another effective technique is that of reinforcement for weight loss. The rewards are given by the individuals themselves or those teaching the techniques. This allows the person to be more in control of eating patterns and habits.

Rotatori (1978) developed a weight loss program for mentally retarded individuals. The program consisted of 14 weeks of intervention that included several major components.

- Students were involved by observing and recording their weight and food consumption on a daily schedule.
- Monitoring and controlling emotional responses that lead to overeating were emphasized.
- Instruction was provided on how to eat. This included having only one helping of food and reducing the rate at which food was eaten.
- Students were instructed to be aware of cues for eating and the techniques on how to eliminate them.
- Exercise was taught so that physical activity could be induced and maintained to burn calories.
- Education was also provided on how to eat healthy low-calorie snacks and eliminate eating between-meal snacks if possible.

Fox et al. (1982) reported a research review of weight loss programs for mentally retarded persons. Such programs primarily were successful through using instructional techniques on how to choose proper foods and applying reinforcement for losing from ½ to 1½ pounds per week.

Reinforcers ranged from special recognition, special activities, and peer reinforcement. Also, the involvement of school staff and parents seemed to be the most effective means of motivating weight loss among the mentally retarded persons.

The Adapted Physical Educator's Role in Weight Management

The adapted physical educator could serve as a coordinator for a school-based weight loss program. The program could be based on Rotatori's (1978) concepts since they appear to be successful and widely applicable. Other resources should be used in the program.

1. The school nurse should be involved to monitor students' progress.

2. The school dietitian or one from the public health department might provide some information or volunteer time in instruction about selecting proper foods.

3. The students' teachers need to be involved, to be aware of the program and provide support.

4. The parents or primary caregiver should be involved so that the diet or change in eating habits can be carried out in the home and school.

5. A volunteer physician would also be helpful to monitor students in terms of a physical exam at the beginning, during, and end of the program.

The adapted physical educator would have the following roles and responsibilities within the weight management program.

1. Select a parent, teacher, home economist, guidance counselor, or some other individual to assist with the program.

2. Inform parents and other significant persons about the program.

3. Set up a program coordinating instruction with the identified personnel.

4. Conduct the physical activity class at least two days a week.

5. Conduct sessions with parents, since they will be involved in menu planning and food purchasing.

In many cases, the mothers are the targets when trying to provide information on good nutritional habits. A study by Burt and Hertzler (1978) reported the effects of parental influence on their children's food preferences. The results indicated that the father's food preferences dominated the meal plans in the home. This study suggested that both the father and the mother should be included in any nutrition information programs.

Ways for Parents to Help in Weight Management

Parents need to provide ways to help their children control and manage their weight. Parents can assist by following these simple procedures.

1. A meal plan should be made each day and adhered to to the maximum extent possible.

2. Food should never be used as a reinforcer or offered as a form of soothing emotions.

3. Parents should provide snacks that are high in fiber and low in calories. Some examples include:

- sliced apples with a small dab of peanut butter
- carrot sticks, celery sticks
- small wedges of cheese on toothpicks
- banana slices
- pineapple chunks
- skim milk

To be avoided:

- cookies
- chocolate milk
- candy
- rich desserts

4. Children should be encouraged to drink plenty of liquids, especially water and unsweetened juices.

5. Foods should not be fried, fatty meats should be avoided, and sugar cut to a minimum.

6. Parents should try to have children avoid eating snacks before going to bed.

NUTRITION AND PHYSICAL PERFORMANCE

The amount of work that an individual can produce depends, to a great extent, on the energy available to the musculature. Carbohydrates seem to produce more energy output than fats or proteins. Briggs and Calloway (1979) recommend that carbohydrates should be consumed in larger amounts in addition to proteins a few days before athletic competition. This would apply to students participating in the Special Olympics. While most participants do not exert themselves as in a competitive track meet, still parents and teachers should try to see that children eat well before they go out all day and compete.

A meal before the day's events should include a carbohydrate breakfast and whole grains. Sugar should be avoided as much as possible. Protein-rich foods should include milk, eggs, and poultry. A good multiple vitamin and mineral supplement for children should also be given. Eating should occur about three to four hours before competition. A light carbohydrate snack might be given during the day.

POINTS TO REMEMBER

1. Physical, motor, and postural fitness are important components of a program designed for disabled students, both from preventive and corrective standpoints.

2. Students with disabilities have lower levels of physical and health-related fitness compared with their nondisabled peers.

3. Students whose fitness levels are extremely low or who have orthopedic problems should have their programs approved by a medical professional.

4. Exercise programs should be highly individualized.

5. Exercises should be modified where necessary to ensure that students are starting at a level that best fits their abilities.

6. Handicapped students should be screened for postural deviations and those with severe problems should be referred for further diagnosis and treatment.

7. Handicapped students may be found to have nutritional deficits and poor eating habits. Nutrition education must be included as part of a total health approach and should always accompany weight management and intervention.

8. An overweight status can adversely affect a disability by making movement difficult or by aggravating conditions such as diabetes and arthritis.

9. Weight management programs have been successful with disabled persons, particularly the mentally retarded.

REFERENCES

Briggs, G.M., & Calloway, D.H. (1979). *Nutrition and physical fitness* (10th ed.). Philadelphia: W.B. Saunders.

Burt, J.V., & Hertzler, A.A. (1978). Parental influence on the child's food preference. *Journal of Nutrition Education, 10,* 127–128.

Byers, R.K., & Lord, E.E. (1943). Late effects of lead poisoning on mental development. *American Journal of Diseases of Children, 66,* 471–494.

Chattopadhyay, A., & Jervis, R.E. (1974). Hair as an indicator of multi element exposure of population groups. *Proceedings of the University of Missouri's 8th Annual Conference on Trace Substances in Environmental Health, 8,* 31–37.

Chisolm, J. (1971). Lead poisoning. *Scientific American, 224,* 15–23.

Cott, A. (1977). *The orthomolecular approach to learning disabilities.* San Rafael, CA: Academic Therapy Publications.

Cratty, B.J. (1980). *Adapted physical education for handicapped children and youth.* Denver: Love.

Crook, W.P. (1980). *Tracking down hidden food allergy.* Jackson, TN: Professional Books.

Crowe, W.C., Auxter, D., & Pyfer, J. (1981). *Principles and methods of adapted physical education and recreation* (4th ed.). St. Louis: C.V. Mosby.

Dauer, V.P., & Pangrazzi, R.P. (1979). *Dynamic physical education for elementary school children* (6th ed.). Minneapolis: Burgess.

David, O.J., Clark, J., & Voeller, K. (1972). Lead and hyperactivity. *Lancet, 2,* 900–903.

Doctor's Data, Inc. (1979). Nutrient mineral level and toxic metal level laboratory chart. West Chicago, IL: Author.

Fait, F. (1978). *Special physical education*. Philadelphia: W.B. Saunders.

Fait, H.F., & Dunn, J.M. (1984). *Special physical education* (5th ed.). Philadelphia: Saunders College Publishing.

Falls, H., Bayler, A., & Dishman, R. (1980). *Essentials of fitness*. Philadelphia: W.B. Saunders.

Folio, M.R. (1982). Trace mineral comparisons of gifted students compared to normal laboratory standards. Final Report, Faculty Research Grant, Tennessee Technological University, Cookeville, TN.

Folio, M.R., & Brown, T. (1982). Trace mineral and toxic metal levels of emotionally disturbed adolescents compared to normal laboratory standards. Final Report, Faculty Research Grant, Tennessee Technological University, Cookeville, TN.

Folio, M.R., & Marlowe, M. (1980). Trace minerals and toxic metal status of mentally retarded children. Faculty Research Grant Final Report, Tennessee Technological University, Cookeville, Tennessee.

Folio, M.R., & Garrett, C. (1982). Trace mineral levels of Down's Syndrome children compared to normal peers. Final Report, Faculty Research Grant, Tennessee Technological University, Cookeville, TN.

Folio, M.R., Hennigan, C., & Errera, J. (1982). A comparison of five toxic metals among urban and rural children. *Environmental Pollution, 29*, 261–269.

Fox, R., Rotatori, A.F., & Fox, T. (1981). *The prevalence of obesity in the mentally retarded: A Pilot Study*. Paper presented at the annual meeting of the American Association on Mental Deficiency, Detroit, MI.

Fox, R., Switzky, H., Rotatori, A.F., & Vitkus, P. (1982). Successful weight loss techniques with mentally retarded children and youth. *Exceptional Children, 49*, 238–244.

Graham, A., & Graham, F. (1974). Lead poisoning and the suburban child. *Today's Health, 52*, 38–41.

Johnson, V.S., Smith, M.H., Bittle, J.B., & Nuckolls, M.A. (1980). *Nutrition education for retarded children: A program for teachers*. Memphis, TN: Child Development Center Department of Nutrition.

Kalakian, L.H., & Eichstaedt, C.B. (1982). *Developmental/adapted physical education: Making ability count*. Minneapolis: Burgess.

Lesser, M. (1980). *Nutrition and vitamin therapy*. New York: Grove Press.

Lin-Fu, J.S. (1975). Lead exposure among children: A reassessment. *The New England Journal of Medicine, 300*, 731–732.

Mahaffey, K.R. (1977). Quantities of lead producing health effects in humans: Sources and bioavailability. *Environmental Health Perspectives, 19*, 285–295.

Marlowe, M., Folio, M.R., & Hall, D. (1982). Increased lead burden and trace mineral status in mentally retarded children. *Journal of Special Education, 16*, 87–99.

Martin, H. (1973). Nutrition: Its relationship of children's physical, mental and emotional development. *American Journal of Clinical Nutrition, 26*, 772–774.

Maugh, T.H. (1978). Hair: A diagnostic tool to complement blood serum and urine. *Science, 202*, 1271–1273.

Mindell, E. (1981). *Vitamin bible for your kids*. New York: Rawson, Wade.

Needleman, H.L., Gunnoe, C., Leviton, A., Reed, R., Peresie, H., Maher, C., & Barnett, P. (1979). Deficits in psychologic and classroom performance of children with elevated dentene lead levels. *The New England Journal of Medicine, 300*, 689–695.

Nutrition Search, Inc. (1979). *Nutrition almanac*. New York: McGraw-Hill.

Perino, J., & Claire, B.E. (1974). The relationship of subclinical lead level to cognitive and sensorimotor impairment in black preschoolers. *Journal of Learning Disabilities, 7*, 26–30.

Pihl, R.O., & Parkes, M. (1977). Hair element content in learning disabled children. *Science, 198*, 204–206.

Rarick, G.L., Dobbins, D.A., & Broadhead, G.D. (1976). *The motor domain and its correlates in educationally handicapped children*. Englewood Cliffs, NJ: Prentice-Hall.

Rimland, B., & Larson, G.E. (1983). Hair mineral analysis and behavior: An analysis of 51 studies. *Journal of Learning Disabilities, 16*, 279–285.

Rotatori, A.F. (1978). The effects of different reinforcement schedules in the maintenance of weight loss with retarded overweight adults. *Dissertation Abstracts International, 38*, 4738–N.

Routh, D., Mushak, P., & Boone, L. (1979). A new syndrome of elevated blood lead and microcephaly. *Journal of Pediatrics Psychology, 4*, 67–76.

Schurr, E.L. (1980). *Movement experiences for children: A humanistic approach to elementary school physical education* (3rd ed.). Englewood Cliffs, NJ: Prentice-Hall.

Sherrill, C. (1981). *Adapted physical education and recreation* (2nd ed.). Dubuque, IA: William C. Brown.

Sloan, S.A. (1977). *A guide for nutra lunches and natural foods*. Atlanta: SOS Printing.

Smith, L. (1979). *Feed your kids right*. New York: Dell.

Stevens, J.H., & Baxter, D.H. (1981). Malnutrition and children's development. *Young Children, 36*, 60–71.

Tennessee Department of Public Health. (1977). *Printout of annual summary of Tennessee in nutrition surveillance*. Atlanta: Center for Disease Control.

Wallace, H.M. (1971). Nutrition and handicapped children. *Journal of the American Dietetic Association, 61*, 127–133.

Winnick, J.P., & Short, F.X. (1982). The physical fitness of sensory and orthopedically impaired youth. Project UNIQUE. (ERIC Document No. ED 240–764).

Wiseman, D.C. (1982). A Practical Approach to Adapted Physical Education. Reading, Mass.: Addison-Wesley.

Part III

Program Development

Chapter 7

Assessing Psychomotor Performance of Handicapped Students

Focus

- Defines and discusses the need and purposes of assessment in general and applies them to physical education in particular.
- Discusses methods of evaluating tests to determine their appropriateness for assessing handicapped students.
- Discusses procedures for developing a sound testing environment for students with handicapping conditions.
- Provides a model for reporting test performance and relevant information to be included in the student's IEP.

Assessment is an important beginning for program planning with handicapped students. The purposes of assessment are varied but the main goal is to enable the instructor to determine the unique needs of each handicapped student being served in the physical education program.

The results of assessment can provide a clear picture of the students major strengths and weaknesses. The assessment process should not be taken lightly. Planning and coordination of all phases of assessment is of utmost importance. Careful planning of the process will usually yield accurate and reliable results.

The term *assessment* will be used in this chapter to include testing and evaluation that will be applied to students and programs. The intent of this chapter is to provide an overview of assessment purposes and techniques useful with handicapped students. The chapter does not include a review of specific instruments for assessment. Tests commonly used in physical education for handicapped students are reviewed in Appendix 7–A. They are included in this form so the reader can quickly find a testing tool, rather than searching throughout the text. Tests are organized by the types of skill areas they are designed to measure.

P.L. 94–142 AND ASSESSMENT

P.L. 94–142 provides guidelines for assessment related to placing pupils for educational services and individualized program planning. The law clearly provides for protection of students and parents in terms of procedural safeguards against discriminatory testing of handicapped students. This is important for physical education providers to comprehend.

Included in the law are the following guidelines for nondiscriminatory testing, as outlined in the August 23, 1977 *Federal Register*.

1. Tests or other evaluation procedures must be administered in the child's native language or best communication mode.
2. Tests must be valid for the purposes for which they are designed.
3. Tests must be administered according to recommended procedures and by persons knowledgeable of the tests' uses.
4. A variety of tests must be used to determine levels of skills and abilities.
5. No individualized education program shall be based on a single test or evaluation criteria.
6. Students must be evaluated in all areas where there is a suspected disability.
7. If parents are not satisfied that the test has been fair, they are entitled to an independent evaluation at no cost to them.

8. Parents must be notified in writing in their native language about any testing of their children for placement or change in the educational program.

PURPOSES OF ASSESSMENT

Other than classification of students for services and determining their eligibility, assessment has several major purposes. These include:

- screening
- classification
- individual program development (IEPs)
- motivation
- reporting of achievement and progress
- program evaluation

Screening

Screening is usually completed for the purposes of determing if problems exist and more in-depth testing is needed. Several general skill areas are usually involved in the screening procedure. In some situations, screening may focus on one or two specific areas, such as vision, hearing, or posture. After screening, assessment of weaknesses may be followed by more in-depth testing and evaluation.

Screening devices are usually short and require less amount of time to administer than a full-scale test. Many tests have screening devices included with them. Screening is geared toward testing and evaluating groups, rather than individuals.

Classification

Assessment instruments used to classify students are more lengthy than screening tests and provide more in-depth information about the students' performance. Classification of students is based on standardized tests. Examples of standardized tests in physical education include the *AAHPERD Youth Fitness Tests, Peabody Developmental Motor Scales, Bruinicks Oseretsky Test of Motor Proficiency*, and the *AAHPERD Youth Fitness Test for Mentally Retarded*. These and other standardized tests are used to compare the student being tested with the population on which the test was standardized. This provides a relative picture of where the student stands in terms of other students within the same age category. For instance, the *Peabody Developmental Motor Scales* (Folio & Fewell, 1983) cover an age range of birth through 84 months. If the physical education teacher wishes to determine how a Down's Syndrome boy compares with normal developmental motor standards of other children, the teacher could administer the *Peabody* to determine the developmental age of the student. Generally, Down's children are from two to four years behind their normal peers in motor development. So, if the student was eight years old, most likely motor skills would be between four and six years. After testing and scoring, the teacher may find that the student is developmentally at a four-year level. The *Peabody* yields several scores, however, including raw, normalized *t* and *z* scores, and percentile ranks. Thus, one would be able to see where, along a chronological sequence, the student's motor skills compare with normal motor development.

Individualized Programming

Tests used to determine individualized programs may vary widely. They are more detailed than screening instruments and usually measure a more in-depth sequence of skills. These tests usually form the basis for the development of objectives in a hierarchical sequence and the planning of other instructional needs of the student.

Two essentials for individualized programming are sufficient data and appropriate interpretations about the student's individual needs. Criterion-referenced tests can also be used to develop objectives for the student. A discussion of types of tests will follow in this chapter.

Motivation

Frequent testing provides feedback to students regarding their progress. Knowledge of results can be a good means for motivating students to increase their skill levels. Documentation of the progress in the form of individual charts and communication to parents can keep interest high and increase parent involvement. This may also lead to more motivation on the part of the student.

Reporting of Achievement and Progress

Although P.L. 94–142 requires only an annual review of the handicapped student's individualized program, it is wise for the instructor to evaluate student progress on an ongoing basis. This will ensure that the objectives established are appropriate and serve as a way of communicating to all concerned that the student is progressing. Baumgartner and Jackson (1975) consider the assessment of the achievement of instructional objectives as one of the most important purposes of measurement.

Program Evaluation

Seaman and DePauw (1982) suggest that program evaluation include an assessment of the learning changes and the environment. The program evaluation should be broader and focus on its effectiveness in terms of all students.

Facilities, both indoor and outdoor, should be evaluated in terms of space, lighting, and safety. Safety is particularly important, since handicapped students may have a difficult time functioning and performing in a cluttered space. This is true for students who are blind and for the orthopedically handicapped.

Equipment needs to be evaluated, particularly in terms of a sufficient number of pieces and their adaptability for individual students. Lighter-weight equipment may be necessary for students with weak skills. For example, a student who has poor catching skills may need to begin with a lightweight foam ball, especially if the student is also fearful of catching.

The right teacher-pupil ratio is important. The more severe the handicaps that the students have, the smaller the teacher-pupil ratio will have to be. Ysseldyke and Algozzine (1984) report that studies have shown that as class size decreases, achievement increases when handicapped students are involved. Also, the quality of time allotted to the student is important. Thus, the ratio of students and teachers needs to be evaluated in terms of the amount of teaching time being allotted to students and the opportunity for them to engage in on-task behavior.

Changes in student behavior are good indicators of how successful the program has been in terms of skill acquisition. Changes in behavior need to be within the three domains of learning. While the physical educator may focus on the psychomotor domain, the cognitive and affective domains must also be included. Every motor skill has a cognitive and affective aspect associated with it. For example, Bob is a 15-year-old with a learning disability. Suppose that Bob's IEP goals included several physical education components such as:

1. Bob will be able to develop the motor skills to participate in at least two leisure sports.
2. Bob will be able to understand the rules of at least two leisure sports to the degree that he can play a game successfully.
3. Bob will show an appreciation for at least two sports to the degree that he participates in them at least twice a week.

In goal 1, the evaluation should focus on the motor skills developed by Bob. The second goal centers on the cognitive aspects of leisure sports. Evaluation should center on knowledge about rules and strategies of the sports. Goal 3 emphasizes the affective aspects, or the degree to which Bob is interested and likes the chosen sports. Evaluation should concentrate on how well Bob enjoys participating in the selected sports.

THE ASSESSMENT PROCESS

Some preliminary procedures should be followed before actual testing of the student begins. The more the instructor knows about the handicapped student to be tested, the more effective the testing process will be. The kind of information gathered prior to testing depends on the nature of the student's handicapping condition. Several methods may be used to find information prior to testing. The instructor should try to complete the following:

- review any previous data available about the student's prior performance
- interview others who have worked with the student
- review referral forms
- interview the student before formal testing

School records should provide some information about the student that may be valuable to know before testing. Information such as special health problems or medications the student may be taking may be noted. The condition or medication could affect test performance. Unfortunately, the extent of coverage ranges widely from one school district to another. Other information, if included in the school record, which might be helpful will include:

- developmental history
- social factors
- intelligence and achievement scores
- behavior problems
- handicapping conditions
- medical records

After reviewing the student's records, the instructor should have a good idea about how to arrange for testing so that the best results can be obtained.

Assessment Techniques

Observation

Observation is a good strategy to use after the student record has been reviewed. Observation in the physical education setting may provide more in-depth information than the student's record. In many cases, physical education performance may not be well documented in the student's record.

Observation may be structured or unstructured. Both have their merits. The instructor must have some purpose in mind during observation; otherwise, important information may be missed. Skills are needed to be a good observer of student performance. The instructor should have at least the following knowledge.

1. Whatever skills are being observed should be well known by the evaluator. A continuum of skill development should be firmly in the instructor's mind while observing the student perform the skills. This will allow the evaluator to determine if the student is in the immature phases or mature phases of a particular motor skill.

2. While observing the student's performance, the evaluator should be able to analyze each skill in terms of form and the sequence followed.

3. The tester should be able not only to analyze the performance but also to record any deviations noted. For example, if the student does not cover the expected distance while doing the broad jump, the tester should be able to recognize why and record the observation accurately.

Observation may be conducted first in an unstructured setting. The evaluator may place the student in a general physical education setting and simply observe several behaviors, interactions, and skill levels. The student's attitude toward physical education activities can also be noted. Other aspects that might be observed are the student's familiarity with equipment, use of equipment, general body coordination, interactions with other students, and posture.

The physical education teacher may want to set up particular situations in which to observe specific kinds of skills and abilities. In this case, the instructor may want to provide more structure for observation. This type of observation lends itself to circumstances such as:

- observation of specific skills or levels of skills
- determination of specific teaching techniques that might be successful with a student
- determination of the ability to follow specific directions

Van Etten, Arkell, and Van Etten (1980) suggest that structured observation include a task-oriented session. Someone who is familiar with the student's skills may interact and allow the student to perform so that a demonstration of some of the motor skills acquired can be observed.

Identification of Skill Deficits

Recording accurate descriptions of observed behaviors is extremely important in interpreting the program needs of each student. Vague descriptions of performance are difficult to interpret. For example, saying that throwing skills are poor is too vague. Loovis and Ersing (1979) developed an interpret-referenced motor assessment instrument to qualitatively assess 11 fundamental motor skills. Each skill is assessed on four functional levels. This allows more accurate descriptions of the strengths and weaknesses and errors in performance. The Ohio State University Scale of Intra-Gross Motor Assessment (OSU SIGMA, Loovis & Ersing, 1979), also includes a progressive instructional curriculum to aid in program development.

Scales of this nature greatly aid in the skill analysis while the student is performing. Another example might include a description of the student's jumping skills such as "Arms were not used to initiate the jump." This is more precise than saying that jumping skills were not coordinated. Or it might be noted that the student used one side of the body more than the other. Exact statements related to the student's particular problems in performance will provide the instructor with information for further decisions, including areas in need of more testing, or any adaptations needed for testing equipment.

After observations and initial data are obtained, more in-depth assessment can begin. At this point, the teacher needs to decide on the selection of tests that will be administered.

CHOOSING ASSESSMENT INSTRUMENTS

Careful thought must be given as to the types of assessment instruments that will be used. Several criteria should be considered.

- areas needing testing
- validity
- reliability
- utility of the test
- administration qualities
- appropriateness of the test
- cost

Areas Needing Testing

If the instructor knows the student to some degree, then the areas that will need to be tested will be known. For example, tests might include physical fitness measures, perceptual motor tests, sports skills tests, and posture screening.

Validity

Test Validity

Test validity refers to how well a test measures what it is supposed to measure. Validity is a very important criterion to consider when selecting a test. If the evaluator wishes to measure physical fitness the test should not be measuring something else.

Validity is usually determined by logical analysis of the test content. The types of validity to be discussed include content, construct, and concurrent validity.

Content Validity

Content validity, according to Baumgartner and Jackson (1975), is established by logical examination of the capacities to be measured. For instance, the 50-yard dash is considered as a valid measure of running speed since it can be

viewed as a measuring tool for the speed at which someone is able to run.

Construct Validity

Baumgartner and Jackson (1975) explain *construct validity* of a test as it relates to measuring the skills or traits that compose an attribute. For instance, soccer-playing ability may be made up of the constructs of dribbling, passing, trapping, and so forth. If a test battery includes these skills, it is most likely to measure soccer ability.

Another example might include a motor development test. Children who are older would be expected to have a higher level of motor skills than younger children or those with disabilities. Since, in theory, this is true, a test that would yield higher motor scores for older children could be measuring the theoretical construct of motor development. Likewise, handicapped students would also score lower on motor development. The test would then be a valid measure of motor development. Thus, a test of motor development should discriminate performance between a six-year-old nonhandicapped child and a four-year-old.

Concurrent validity involves the degree to which a test agrees with performance or scores on other similar tests. A method used to check concurrent validity is the degree to which a test agrees with a clinical judgment or some established criteria. A correlation coefficient is used to determine the extent to which two tests or a clinical judgment and the test agree. The closer the correlation coefficient is to "1" the closer the relationship is between the two tests.

Reliability

Reliability is another feature of assessment instruments that must be considered. Tests that are reliable will provide a stable and accurate measure of the student's performance level. Two important types of reliability are test-retest and rater reliability.

Test Retest Reliability

Test-retest reliability is established by repeating the test to the same group in a different testing period, usually with a one-week interval. If the test has test-retest reliability, scores should be relatively similar from one testing occasion to another if the retesting period is relatively short. This is particularly true of tests for younger children, where maturation can effect performance on a test. If the time lapse between the first and second administration of the test is too long, factors such as learning and maturation may affect scores.

Rater Reliability

Rater reliability is generally established by having two examiners independently rate a student's performance and then comparing the scores. The degree to which these scores correlate or agree will determine how reliable the test is in yielding similar measures when two different examiners test the same student. Correlation coefficients are used to determine the rater reliability of a test. The closer the correlation coefficients are to "1," the greater is the rater reliability.

It is very important that physical educators carefully evaluate the validity and reliability of all tests used to plan individualized physical education programs for handicapped students. Most tests have examiner manuals that include reliability and validity data.

Utility of the Test

When selecting or evaluating a test, the examiner needs to consider how useful the test is, particularly related to the information generated by the test. For example, if the objective of testing is to obtain information about the motor development of a mentally retarded five-year-old so that objectives and instructional strategies can be developed, a comprehensive motor development test should be administered. Consequently, the content and depth of the test would be important in this instance. If the child is five years old and moderately retarded, motor skills may be two to four years below the child's chronological age. A motor test would be needed with sufficient items plus a broad range of skills in order to be useful for program development.

Another factor to consider is whether or not the test can be individually or group administered. If several students need to be tested, group testing may be more economical.

Administration Qualities

The factors related to administration of a test need to be considered before purchasing it. The amount of equipment required should be evaluated. If the test items require much costly equipment, it may not be feasible to purchase it. Some tests provide all or most of the equipment while some provide none. If the equipment is too unusual, the test may not be useful.

Time is a factor to consider. A test that is too lengthy and time consuming may not be useful to a classroom physical educator, though it might be appropriate for a clinician. This is an important consideration when students need to be tested who tire easily or become distractable. Another factor is the preparation time for testing. A test may not be useful for the physical education classroom if elaborate and time-consuming preparation is required for administering many of the items.

Appropriateness of the Test

Age is one of the most important factors in viewing the appropriateness of a test. If students are more concentrated at

the adolescent age, then higher-level tests need to be considered, or tests that are standardized on the relative age group. On the other hand, if older students are severely retarded, a test used for young children may not be appropriate. A test must focus on skills that are age appropriate and yet be able to be used by the testing group. Adolescents who are severely retarded tend to be difficult to test since tests for this group sometimes have items that really do not fit with the physical and chronological age of the group. The test should also be easily understood by the students. One should avoid tests that result in poor performance motorically because students were not able to understand the items presented.

Cost

Tests will vary in their prices. Cost is an important factor to consider. A test that has a high cost may not provide much useful data for program development. On the other hand, if a test yields scores and other information that can be used in a broad sense for program development, the cost may not be a significant factor if considerable information can be generated. For example, the *Peabody Developmental Motor Scales*, published by DLM-Teaching Resources, costs, at present, $150.00. The test covers a broad age range, is both norm and criterion referenced, and has instructional objectives and teaching strategies included for motor programming. For the cost, a good deal of information can be generated.

Organizational Procedures for Testing

Being prepared for any testing session is of primary importance for the testing to proceed smoothly. The instructor needs to consider the following prior to testing:

- becoming familiar with the test/s
- having materials and equipment ready for administering the test
- arranging the testing environment
- establishing rapport

The instructor needs to be thoroughly familiar with the test in terms of procedures, materials, and method of recording performance. This will help the testing session to proceed smoothly. Furthermore, the tester will be able to pay attention to the student's performance rather than being concerned about the next item to be administered.

All materials and equipment necessary for administering the test should be collected well in advance of the testing period. While the materials need to be readily available, only those needed for the current test item being administered should be presented to the student.

Optimum performance may be affected by the testing location. This is extremely important to consider when testing handicapped students. The environment should be comfortable and free from distractions. Lighting needs to be adequate and seating comfortable. Proper safety precautions should be taken. For example, a mat should be used when students perform on a balance beam. Extremes in temperature should also be avoided.

Better test results occur when the instructor has the confidence of the student. First, the student's physical needs should be met. If the student is hungry or thirsty, performance can be significantly hampered. Students should be allowed to go to the restroom and to the water fountain before testing begins.

The instructor needs to alleviate any fears the student might have about being tested. A few minutes taken before testing to develop rapport with the student could make a significant difference in how the student performs.

Testing should begin with skills the student already knows. By starting at a successful level, the tester can instill confidence in the student.

TESTING SPECIFIC HANDICAPPED POPULATIONS

While there are general procedures to follow before testing and during testing, some specific considerations must be taken into account when testing students with particular handicapping conditions. The following section will provide some general considerations for testing specific handicapped groups.

Mentally Retarded Students

When testing mentally retarded students, the instructor should consider some of the characteristics of mentally retarded students. While each student is different, the following will serve as general guidelines for testing.

The mental age of the student is important to consider when giving directions, particularly if a standardized test is being used. Standardized tests require precise forms of administering items. The standard format for presenting items may have to be changed to the level of language that the student has achieved. Jansma and French (1982) report that mentally retarded students may not perform a motor task well if the directions are too complex for the students' cognitive and language skill levels.

Some mentally retarded students may have particular health problems. If the student tires easily, frequent rest periods should be offered and the testing time carried over to several testing periods. Brief rest periods may also be necessary if attention span is short. More motivation may be necessary. Encouragement and praise should be offered for attempts to complete test items.

Learning-Disabled Students

The particular suspected or confirmed learning disability should be known before testing the student. Nonverbal learning disabilities and behavioral characteristics may play more of a role in motor performance than verbal types of learning disabilities. The effects of the student's specific disability on communication and interpretation of requests during testing should be carefully noted by the tester. Particular behavioral difficulties must be considered while testing the student. The instructor should be aware of ways to handle problems during the testing period. The following suggestions are offered to provide a smooth testing period for both the evaluator and student.

Behavior	*Implications for Testing*
Hyperactivity	Provide a relaxation period when the student becomes fidgety.
Distractability	Minimize the amount of objects and distractions during the testing period.
Perseveration	Change test items slowly and remind the student when to stop.

Emotionally Disturbed Students

Before testing emotionally disturbed students, it is extremely important to establish rapport. The instructor must also exercise extreme patience. While testing the student signs of frustration should be noted and a rest period should be offered. The student should be encouraged to try hard and do a good job. The following summary will highlight testing procedures to use with emotionally disturbed students.

- Start on a positive note by giving the student items that can be completed easily to build self-confidence.
- Test in a more secluded environment.
- Be patient and wait for the student's responses.
- Offer encouragement such as "You can do it," "Good job," "You're really trying hard."
- Do not threaten the student's ego through repeated failures. If a student is really having difficulty, go on to another item.

Visually Impaired Students

The amount of difficulty in testing a visually impaired student will depend on the amount of residual vision that remains. Several strategies can be developed that will aid the evaluator in determining the skill levels of visually impaired students. The following suggestions should prove beneficial in testing psychomotor skills of visually impaired youngsters.

1. Lighting should be at the optimum level so the student can make use of any residual vision.

2. Remove any unnecessary clutter or unwanted objects within the testing area.

3. Orient the student to the testing area before the testing session begins.

4. Explain what the student is to do and be sure that the instructions are understood.

5. Use equipment that is brightly colored. Yellow or white is the most preferred color.

6. Sometimes kinesthetic input may be necessary when explaining a test item.

Hearing-Impaired Students

The severity of hearing loss will determine the methods of presenting test information. However, if the hearing impairment is not very severe, several procedures should be followed when testing. The following suggestions should be kept in mind while testing a hearing-impaired student.

1. Always make sure the student is able to see the tester clearly.

2. Do not have the student face a bright light while trying to see the tester's face.

3. Maintain eye contact while giving instructions.

4. If the test items permit, demonstrate what the student is to do.

5. Be sure the student understands the test item and what is to be done.

Orthopedically Handicapped Students

Test items may have to be presented and deviations in performance accepted according to the capabilities of the student with orthopedic disorders. For example, running speed may have to be accepted as speed in maneuvering a wheelchair. The teacher needs to be extremely flexible when testing the student who has orthopedic problems. Several points should be considered prior to testing:

- The teacher should note any medical conditions and medications that the student may be taking.

- Timed items may need to be modified or eliminated.

- Mats should be provided where appropriate for students who fall frequently.

Projects such as Project UNIQUE, directed by Joseph Winnick, provide modifications for physical fitness testing of orthopedically handicapped students. Information on Project UNIQUE can be obtained from Joseph Winnick, State University of New York, Brockport, New York.

WRITING TEST REPORTS

Reporting test results is a very important skill for the instructor to develop. Reports are used to communicate how the student performed and what needs to be done in terms of providing an individualized program. The accuracy and completeness with which the report is made will lead to sound recommendations.

It takes practice and skill in writing reports that will convey an accurate description and interpretation of what the student's strengths and weaknesses are. Several points should be noted when summarizing an evaluation and reporting results. Although many different formats may be used to present test results, the content is the most important and critical issue.

The following guidelines are offered for reporting evaluation results in physical education to be included as part of the student's individualized education program.

General Information

Statements about the tests used and the date/s on which the tests and other evaluations were made should be included. Pertinent information should be provided about the testing environment and the status of the student during testing occasion/s. For example, if the student did not feel well, some of the test scores may not be the best that the student could have achieved.

Test Results

The instructor may want to report scores in general. However, specific and accurate descriptions of the student's performance will be more practical. If the evaluator noted specific clusters of motor problems, it would be important to indicate this to the student's educational planning team. For example, a student may have difficulty with balance and locomotor skills and not do well at throwing and catching. Any other factors measured should also be reported, such as how cooperative the student may or may not have been.

Projections and Recommendations

Once the report of actual evaluation of performance has been made, the instructor needs to make some projections and recommendations. The instructor may project how well the student is able to learn motor skills and the rate of progress based on the data gathered at this point. General recommendations should also be made regarding how the physical education program might be best implemented. Actual placements may be discussed. The evaluation data may suggest that the student would be best served in a self-contained physical education classroom, or through mainstreaming, or combinations of both approaches. Recommendations will also depend on the services available within the school district

Goal Priorities and IEP Development

Once the general recommendations have been made, specific long-term goals and short-term objectives can be developed. When appropriate, the student should take part in the program development. Also, teaching strategies and equipment modifications can be included at this point, if necessary. Perhaps the student may require a strong behavior management program. The strategies for implementing the management program should be developed. Another example of a teaching strategy is that the student might need a peer teacher and more visual demonstration of specific skills. This type of approach will enable a well-developed physical education program to unfold and be implemented.

Other Considerations

Projected dates for beginning and reaching objectives need to be stated. An evaluation plan must also be provided. Though P.L. 94–142 requires only an annual review of the IEP, ongoing assessment of the student's progress is much more effective than an annual evaluation.

Periodic assessment or charting of progress serves to keep the student motivated. Frequent notes can be sent to parents to let them know how the student is achieving. This process also lets the instructor know if the stated goals and objectives are indeed appropriate for the student. Goals and objectives need to be changed if they appear not to be appropriate. IEPs are not written in granite. They may be changed whenever it appears that the goals and objectives are either at a level that is too high or too low for the student to achieve.

A MOTOR ASSESSMENT REPORT MODEL

Exhibit 7–1 is an example of how the evaluator may write a report of an evaluation of a referred student. If this model report is followed, the service providers should have a fairly good picture of the student's strengths and weaknesses in terms of gross motor functioning and perceptual motor skills.

The written report of a motor assessment can be used to develop an IEP for the child tested. The general recommendations can be translated into long-term goals and objectives. These can be included along with teaching strategies and adapted materials. The assessment data will indicate strengths and weaknesses in the child's motor performance and aid in deciding on the most appropriate placement for the child. In the example of Willy, an appropriate placement would include his regular physical education activities. However, three hours a week should be spent in a resource physical education setting to work on weaknesses defined. Placement decisions would not be made until all test data were provided and the IEP team conferred.

POINTS TO REMEMBER

1. Assessment is an ongoing process and serves a variety of purposes.

2. The purposes of assessment include measurement of a student's strengths and weaknesses, information for placement decisions, development of individualized education programs, documentation of student progress, and determination of program effectiveness.

3. P.L. 94–142 offers specific procedural safeguards for testing to avoid unfair tests and discrimination.

4. Careful consideration should be given in choosing assessment instruments, including several criteria such as test design, structure, cost, and feasibility of administration of the items.

5. It is important to establish rapport with each student being tested.

6. Test reports should be carefully compiled, with both strengths and weaknesses addressed. Examples of student's performance should be included.

Exhibit 7–1 Report Model

MOTOR ASSESSMENT REPORT

Child's Name: Willy L. School: J. Wilson
Date of Birth: 9/9/79 Grade: Kindergarten
Evaluation Instruments: Teacher: Mrs. Smith
    Cratty's *Body Image Test for Blind Children*
    Peabody Developmental Motor Scales

Examiner: Mr. Tim H.

Overview

Willy's motor skills and body image were tested over three 30-minute testing periods in one week. Willy was referred for testing because he had difficulty in playing with other children on the playground. He had difficulty catching and throwing a ball and when trying to engage in balance activities, seemed unsure and unsteady. He often avoided these tasks. He appeared to his classroom teacher to be behind other children in these areas. Willy was about average size, although a little underweight for children his age. Height was average.

The *Peabody Developmental Motor Scales* and the *Cratty Body Image Test for Blind Children* were administered in a resource room and gymnasium at J. Wilson Elementary School. Both testing sites were well lighted and excellent environments for testing. There was nothing at either site that distracted Willy from responding to the test items as accurately as possible.

The Body Image for Blind Children had to be administered twice because of the child's refusal to follow commands on the test. Body image and knowledge of body concepts were at the expected level for a child of Willy's age. Some inaccuracies were noted when identifying left and right and certain body parts.

Only the gross motor portion of the *Peabody Developmental Motor Scales* was administered. It yielded a percentile rank of 7, a *t*-score of 35, and a developmental motor quotient of 78. Percentile ranks for skill components were: balance, PR of 2; nonlocomotor, PR of 9; locomotor, PR of 8; receipt and propulsion, PR of 2. While Willy's chronological age was 69 months at the time of testing, his gross motor skills were clustered around the four-year level.

Body Awareness Evaluation

Identification of Body Planes

Willy displayed a good understanding of the three body planes on the administration of the *Body Image Test for Blind Children*. Body planes identified included the top of the head and back and the front of the body.

Body Part Identification

No difficulty was observed in identifying simple body parts such as the arm, hands, etc. When asked to "touch your feet," the leg was touched.

Objects in Relation to Body Planes

Objects were identified placed in front and back and Willy appeared to have the concepts of front and back learned. The side could not be identified when objects were placed either to the right or left.

Body Planes in Relation to Objects

Willy was able to place front and back sides next to objects. However, difficulty was noticed when asked to place his side next to an object.

Movements of the Body

Trunk Movement While Fixed

Movements requested were to bend forward, to the side, and backwards. Willy bent his knees, rather than bending at the waist. While bending occurred in the general directions of forward and backward, the movements were not accurate.

Gross Movements in Relation to Body Planes

Movements were jumping up, forward, and backward. No difficulty was encountered with movements in these planes. Willy was confused when asked to move sideways.

Limb Movements

No mistakes were made when asked to straighten the arms, bend the arms, lift arms at shoulders, rotate arms at the shoulders, straighten the legs, bend the leg at the knee, and lift the leg at the hip.

Laterality of the Body

Willy was able to touch and identify his right arm but not his right leg. There is some confusion about left and right. Balance on one foot was for three seconds.

Laterality in Relation to Objects

Placing the left or right sides next to an object was missed. The left and right sides were confusing for Willy to identify.

Other Portions of the Test

The rest of the levels on the body image test were missed. These are higher-level items and require the student to identify left and right sides of the body while moving in relation to an object, the left and right sides of objects, directionality of other people, relationship of objects to the laterality of others, moving objects in relation to other's laterality, and laterality of other's movements. Willy mostly guessed at these items and was not able to correctly identify laterality and directionality consistently. These items are above the level of six-year-olds.

Peabody Developmental Motor Scales

A developmental motor quotient (DMQ) of 78 was obtained on the PDMS gross motor section. A percentile rank of 7 was determined from the raw score and a *t* score of 35. Nonlocomotor and locomotor skill areas were the strengths, while balance and receipt and propulsion were the weakest areas, both with a percentile rank of 2. Most of the gross motor skills were clustered around the four-year level.

Table 7–1 is a summary of the strengths and weaknesses displayed by Willy on the administration of the PDMS.

Exhibit 7–1 continued

Table 7–1 PDMS Summary

Area	Strengths	Weaknesses
Balance	Standing on tip toes	Walking balance beam Walking on tip toes Standing on one foot
Nonlocomotor	Standing up Jumping up	Turning while jumping Jumping sideways Push-ups Sit-ups Standing agility
Locomotor	Jumping hurdles Galloping Rolling forward Running speed	Skipping Hopping speed Jumping forward
Receipt and Propulsion	Throwing ball Catching ball	Kicking ball Catching ball off wall

Balance

Walking on Balance Beam

Walking forward on a four-inch-wide beam was completed successfully. When asked to walk backwards, Willy fell off the beam after the second step. Most of the time Willy led with the right foot.

Standing on Tip Toes

The criteria of standing for eight seconds was met on this task. A distance of 15 feet was covered while walking on tip toes. However, one foot was kept flat during half of the steps.

Standing on One Foot

The criterion for ten seconds was met while standing on one foot with the free leg bent backward at the knee. Balance was maintained for only three seconds while standing on the left foot.

Nonlocomotor Skills

Jumping

Jumping up was accomplished with only a two-inch jump beyond the normal reach, as in the vertical jump. Jump turns were completed with no difficulty, with the body maintained upright and landing smooth. Jumping sideways occurred by jumping back and forth across a one-inch taped line. Difficulty was encountered with this task. Problems noted were not keeping the feet together, loss of rhythm during three jumping cycles, and loss of balance one of three times while landing.

Push-Ups, Sit-Ups, and Standing Agility

Only two push-ups were completed correctly, using a modified form with a chair. Only one sit-up in 30 seconds was accomplished.

Standing agility was measured by having the student lie on his back, stand up, lie back down, then stand back up for four cycles within 20 seconds. Only three cycles were completed.

Locomotor Skills

Jumping Hurdles

The right foot led in attempts to jump over a rope ten inches from the floor. A two-foot takeoff and landing was not observed within three attempts at jumping.

Galloping

No difficulty was observed during galloping. The same foot led and movements were smooth and well coordinated.

Rolling Forward

Somersaults were completed with fairly good form. The chin was well tucked in and the body balanced. Two consecutive rolls were completed instead of three.

Running Speed

Running speed was slightly below the criterion for Willy's age. A shuttle run between two taped lines was to be completed within 12 seconds. However, Willy completed the task in 14 seconds. The arms were coordinated while running, but the feet were kept somewhat flat, rather than the subject running on the balls of the feet.

Skipping

Skipping was difficult since the lead foot was not alternated. Skipping attempts were more like a gallop. Even after several demonstrations, Willy was still unable to alternate the lead foot.

Hopping Speed

Willy was unable to hop four consecutive steps before losing balance. A distance of six feet was covered in ten seconds.

Jumping Forward

A standing broad jump was completed for a distance of 18 inches. A two-foot takeoff and landing was not smooth. The left leg was used last in the takeoff portion of the jump.

Receipt and Propulsion

Throwing

A target on a wall 12 feet away was hit on only one of three trials. Throwing overhand was not well developed. Some shoulder rotation was observed, but no followthrough. A step forward on the opposite foot of the throwing hand was not taken.

Catching

A tennis ball was caught by using a corralling motion. When required to bounce a tennis ball on the floor and catch it, Willy made two out of three catches using both hands.

When asked to throw a ball against a wall and catch it after the first bounce, Willy missed on all trials. Difficulty was observed in plac-

Exhibit 7–1 continued

ing the body in position to catch. The proper throwing force was not used. The ball landed either too far from Willy or too short.

Kicking

While stationary, Willy was unable to kick a ball rolled slowly toward him. Timing appeared to be a major factor in missing the ball. While moving toward the ball and trying to kick it, Willy stumbled into the ball rather than making a smooth kick.

Conclusion

It appears that Willy is following a normal pattern of development regarding knowledge of body parts, planes, and movements. Laterality is weak, however, not greatly deficient considering the child's chronological age.

Gross motor development is following a normal progression. However, it is about a year behind overall. Weaknesses exist in locomotor and receipt and propulsion skills. Strengths are related to nonlocomotor skills and balance, even though all areas are delayed. Skills requiring timing and coordination present this child with the greatest amount of difficulty.

Recommendations

1. Activities should be included in Willy's daily motor program that utilize the integration of both sides of the body, such as jumping, hopping, climbing, running, etc.

2. Both static and dynamic balance should be increased using a variety of equipment beyond a balance beam.

3. Locomotor skills need to be improved in terms of timing and rhythm.

4. A mature pattern in throwing, catching, and kicking skills needs to be developed.

REFERENCES

Baumgartner, T.A., & Jackson, A.S. (1975). *Measurement for evaluation in physical education*. Boston: Houghton Mifflin.

Folio, M.R., & Fewell, R.F. (1983). *Peabody developmental motor scales and acitivity cards*. Allen, TX: DLM-Teaching Resources Corporation.

Jansma, P., & French, R. (1982). *Special physical education*. Columbus, OH: Charles E. Merrill.

Loovis, E.M., & Ersing, W.F. (1979). *Assessing and programming gross motor development for children*. Cleveland Heights, OH: Ohio Motor Assessment Associates.

Seaman, J.A., & DePauw, K.P. (1982). *The new adapted physical education: A developmental approach*. Palo Alto, CA: Mayfield.

Van Etten, G., Arkell, C., & Van Etten, C. (1980). *The severely and profoundly handicapped: Programs, methods and materials*. St. Louis: C.V. Mosby.

Ysseldyke, J.E., & Algozzine, B. (1984). *Introduction to special education*. Boston, MA: Houghton Mifflin.

Appendix 7–A

Recommended Assessment Instruments

The following descriptions include both standardized and criterion-referenced assessment instruments. These are widely used and will yield information for formulating goals and objectives for the student. The test or curriculum name is followed by information on the uses of the instrument, validity and reliability data if standardized, and the skills measured. The publisher is also provided. The information will allow the reader to determine if the instrument is appropriate for a particular student.

MOTOR DEVELOPMENT AND MOTOR ABILITY TESTS

Basic Motor Ability Tests

Purpose

This test is designed primarily as a screening test for motor ability. It measures:

- large muscle control
- static and dynamic balance
- eye-hand coordination
- flexibility

Format   4-12 yr.

The test is for ages ranging from four to twelve years. Children can be tested individually or in groups of five. The time required to administer the test is about 30 minutes.

Data

The test was normed on 1,563 children for the age range of the test. Percentiles are included in the norm tables. No validity data are reported; however, a .93 test-retest reliability has been established.

Evaluation

The administration of the items does not require unusual materials. Items can be arranged in a circuit format.

Source

Arnheim, D.D., & Sinclair, W.A. (1979). *The clumsy child: A program of motor therapy* (2nd ed.). St. Louis: C.V. Mosby.

Bayley Scales of Infant Development

Purpose   birth → 2½ yr.

The *Bayley Scales of Infant Development* (BSID) is a three-part evaluation of an infant's developmental status from birth to 2½ years. The three measures include a

- mental scale
- motor scale
- social orientation scale

Format

The BSID is individually administered. Materials for the test are included in the test kit. About 45 minutes are required to administer the test. Score sheets are included in the manual. Scores are expressed in mental and psychomotor indexes. A pass/fail scoring system is used with other responses including "refuse" and "parent report."

Data

Validity reports are addressed in terms of increases in scores with increases in age. The scores on the mental scale correlate from .47 to .57 with the *Stanford Binet* IQ scores. Reliability is reported in terms of split half coefficients ranging from .88 to .92. The BSID was standardized on 1,262 children representing varied ethnic, racial, and socioeconomic groups.

Evaluation

The *Bayley Scales* are used primarily by psychologists and other clinicians. Special physical educators should be familiar with this test, particularly the motor scale. The scale for motor development does not contain a large number of items.

Source

Bayley, N. *Bayley Scales of Infant Development* (1969). New York: The Psychological Corporation.

Brigance Inventory of Early Development

Purpose   under 7yr.

The *Brigance* is an inventory of basic skills designed for children under seven years of age. The areas included are:

- motor development
- speech
- language
- general knowledge

Format

The *Brigance* can be administered to individuals or groups of three or four. The physical educator may be the person to administer the gross motor portion of the inventory. Specific criteria are provided for items. The point along the inventory where the child misses two consecutive items is determined as the child's present level of performance. Directions for assessing the child are included, as are goals and objectives.

Data

No statistical validity data are available. Face validity is based on skills already established by previous scales and instruments. No reliability data are available.

Evaluation

No specialized training is required to use the *Brigance*. It is used widely by special educators and some adapted physical education programs. The *Brigance* provides good information for developing IEPs and a means for documenting classroom achievement. A computerized program is now available, which teachers find quick and effective for generating information on children. The *Brigance* is not standardized and does not serve as a test for placement.

Source

Brigance diagnostic inventory of early development (1978). Woburn, MA.: Curriculum Associates.

Bruninks-Oseretsky Test of Motor Proficiency

Purpose

The *Bruninks* is a standardized test designed to measure the components of

- running speed
- agility

- balance
- bilateral coordination
- strength
- upper limb coordination
- response speed
- visual motor coordination
- upper limb speed
- dexterity

Format   4.5 → 14.5yr

The test is appropriate for ages 4.5 to 14.5 years. The *Bruninks* is an individually administered test that requires about 45 minutes to an hour. A short form is available that requires only 20 minutes to administer. The short form is good for screening.

Data

The test was normed on 800 normal subjects from 4.5 to 14.5 years. Validity and reliability data are included in the test manual. Test-retest reliability is .86. Norms are available in tables with z-scores, percentiles, and stanines.

Evaluation

This test is excellent for testing motor proficiency. The test kit contains all materials needed to give the test. The *Bruninks* is well organized, with good scoring procedures and profile sheets for each student being tested. It is used frequently by school psychologists and less frequently in the classroom.

Source

American Guidance Services, Circle Pines, MN.

Denver Developmental Screening Test

Purpose   0 - 6

The *Denver Developmental Screening Test* (DDST) is a screening tool designed to measure developmental delays in children from birth to six years. Four areas are measured:

- personal social skills
- fine motor adaptive skills
- language skills
- gross motor skills

Format

The DDST is administered individually. The time required to test a child on all four components should generally not take over an hour. Some items may be reported by parents. The score sheet includes each item on the test and what percentage of children in the norming sample passed it at a particular age. A pass/fail scoring system is used to rate each item. Other ratings include "refusal to perform" and "no opportunity to observe the skill."

Data

The DDST was normed on over 1,000 Denver children from birth to age six years. A .97 validity coefficient is reported with the *Yale Developmental Scales*. Also, validity is reported in terms of the skills cited in the literature on growth and development. Test-retest reliability data range from coefficients of .66 to .93.

Evaluation

The DDST is a widely used screening instrument but normative data are restricted. No specialized materials are needed to administer any part of the test. The motor section taps only a limited number of skills at each age level.

Source

University of Colorado Medical Center, Denver, Colorado 80220.

Frostig Movement Skills Test Battery

Purpose

This test is a norm-referenced tool designed to measure sensory motor development in the following areas:

- bilateral eye-hand coordination and dexterity
- motor sequencing
- eye-hand fine motor coordination
- midline crossing skills
- aiming and throwing accuracy
- flexibility
- leg, abdominal, and arm strength
- agility
- static and dynamic balance

Format *6-12yr.*

The test is designed for children ages 6 to 12 years. The time required for administration is 25 minutes for an individual and 45-50 minutes for small groups of four or five persons. Some standardized equipment is required and none is included in the kit. The fine motor items, in particular, call for specified items of specified dimensions, such as beads, etc. Specifications for equipment are described in the test manual.

Data

The test was standardized on 744 white children in Southern California. Test-retest reliability coefficients range from .44 to .88. Validity was established using a factor analysis of intercorrelations of each age group. Means, standard deviations, and scaled equivalents are provided for raw scores for both males and females.

Evaluation

The norming sample is quite restricted in location and race. Test administration does not require any specialized training. The test covers a broad range of components and children seem to enjoy taking it.

Source

Orpet, R.E. (1972). *Frostig movement skills test battery.* Los Angeles: Frostig Center of Educational Therapy.

Geddes Psychomotor Inventory (GPI)

Purpose

The GPI measures a number of skill areas including:

- balance
- visual skills
- eye-hand coordination
- eye-foot coordination
- physical fitness
- throwing
- striking
- kicking
- apparatus skills
- fine motor skills

Format *all ages*

Age range standards are provided from neonatal to adult. Criteria are specified for items at each age level. Both short and long forms are provided. The GPI may be used with normal and handicapped individuals. The time required is about 30 minutes to evaluate a student. No reliability or validity data are provided.

Evaluation

The GPI is relatively easy to administer and can be used with a broad age range. The GPI provides a broad sampling of skills. The long and short forms also make it convenient to use.

Source

Geddes, D. (1981). *Psychomotor individualized educational program for intellectual, learning and behavioral disabilities*. Rockleigh, NJ: Allyn & Bacon.

Koontz Child Development Program

Purpose   0-4 yr.

The *Koontz* is designed to measure the following areas in children from 0 to 48 months:

- gross and fine motor skills
- language
- social behavior

Format

The manual is in notebook form with pages designed as flip cards for each category measured in the particular age level. The rating system is pass/fail. Children may be evaluated using observation and parent inquiry. The time needed to evaluate all four areas is about an hour. A score card is provided.

Data

Validity is based on developmental motor, language, and social skills included in other validated instruments. Reliability of raters is .82 on independent ratings of the same child.

Evaluation

The *Koontz* can be easily administered and does not require unusual equipment. Common motor equipment is used such as a pull toy, ball, tricycle, etc. It is best utilized as a developmental checklist and guide for parent training. The sampling of motor behaviors is somewhat limited.

Source

Western Psychological Services, 13081 Wilshire Blvd., Los Angeles, CA 90025.

Lincoln-Oseretsky Motor Development Scale

Purpose

The *Lincoln-Oseretsky Motor Development Scale* was developed from the original *Oseretsky Scale*. This version is shorter than the original test. Components measured include:

- finger dexterity
- eye-hand coordination

- gross motor ability using the arms, hands, trunk, and legs

Format   6-14 yr.

The test is designed for children ages 6 to 14. A kit and manual are provided for testing. Most items needed to administer the test are included in the test kit. Specifications are provided for items not included in the kit, such as a target. Specific directions are given for each item. Norms are reported in tables included in the manual. Some items are timed.

Data

The test was standardized on 380 males and 369 females ages 6 to 14. A split half reliability is reported to be .72 to .94 for boys and .82 to .93 for girls. Scores increase fairly consistently with age except at the 13- and 14-year levels. Validity coefficients are .32 with the *Brace Motor Ability Test* and .37 with the *Cowan-Pratt Test*. Norms are expressed in percentiles by age and sex.

Evaluation

The test is designed to be individually administered. The time required is from 45 minutes to an hour. It covers a fairly broad age range.

Source

American Guidance Service, Circle Pines, MN 55014.

Ohio State University Scale of Intra Gross Motor Assessment (O.S.U. Sigma)

Purpose

The *O.S.U. SIGMA* is designed to measure 11 fundamental motor skills:

- walking
- stair climbing
- running
- throwing
- catching
- jumping
- hopping
- skipping
- striking
- ladder climbing
- kicking

Format

Subjects are rated on skill performance in terms of the degree to which each criterion is approximated. The test may be used in formal or informal sessions. Testing time may vary in each setting. A *Performance Based Curriculum* is provided which includes activities for remediation of problems indicated by the test.

Data

At present no validity or reliability coefficients are reported. Face validity is reported in terms of the literature on motor development.

Evaluation

Children can be tested in informal settings. The test does not require much unusual equipment. The fact that is has an accompanying curriculum is good for program planning. It should be usable in a broad range of programs.

Source

Mohican Textbook Publishing Company, Loundonville, Ohio 44842.

Peabody Developmental Motor Scale and Activity Cards

Purpose $0 \rightarrow 7$ yr.

The purpose of the PDMS is to assess the gross and fine motor skills of children from birth to 84 months of age.

Format

The PDMS is divided into two scales. The gross motor scale has 170 items divided into 17 age levels, including 10 items at each age level. The fine motor scale has 112 items divided into 16 age levels including 6 or 8 items at each age level. The test is standardized and criterion referenced, with specific instructions to the examiner for administering each item. Each scale requires about 20 to 25 minutes to administer. A child can be tested with both scales within 45 minutes to an hour. The test kit contains the materials needed for the fine motor scale except for one or two items at the lower levels of the scale. A rattle and a pull toy are required for those items. No materials are supplied in the kit for the gross motor items. However, the items needed are commonly found, such as a ball, steps, etc.

A 0,1,2 rating is provided for each item to the degree that the child meets the specified criterion. A "0" score means that the child will not attempt the item or the attempt does not indicate that the skill is emerging. A "1" rating on an item means that the child's performance shows a clear resemblance to the item criterion but does not fully meet the criterion. A "2" rating means that the child performs according to the specified criterion.

Raw scores can be converted to scaled scores using the norm tables provided. Scores can be converted to z scores, t scores, and percentile ranks. The score sheet provides a good summary of performance, including the child's raw score, percentile, t and z scores, and a developmental motor quotient (DMQ). These scores can be total scores or scores for gross motor or fine motor skills. Skill scores can also be calculated for each of the skill categories in the gross and in the fine motor sections. A mean motor age can also be calculated by finding the average of the child's gross motor and fine motor age equivalents.

Special instructions are included for administering the PDMS to handicapped children. Examples from case studies are provided. Another feature of the test manual is the inclusion of teaching strategies for motor training with specific types of handicapped students.

A set of activity cards is included in the kit and contains instructional strategies for specific objectives related to each item on the PDMS. The cards can be easily arranged in the same developmental levels included on the PDMS and by item numbers. These activity cards provide instructional objectives that can be included in the IEP. The teaching strategies provide the teacher with a quick, easy reference for instructional programming. The activities can also be used in the home and implemented by parents or older siblings of the handicapped child.

Data

The PDMS was normed on a total of 617 subjects within the age range covered by the PDMS. Geographical region, sex, race, and SES were factors on which the sample was stratified. The four major U.S. Census Bureau Regions were represented by 20 states.

Validity data include content, construct, criterion-related and ethic and sex validity. Content validity is based on the logical sequence of motor development depicted by the literature. Construct validity is reported in terms of the theoretical development of motor skills that should improve with age. The PDMS shows significant improvement on the test with age. Regression analyses age-score correlations also demonstrate statistically significant improvement with age. Another source of evidence for construct validity is the comparison of the performance of children identified as having motor development problems with the performance of the norming sample. Concurrent validity may also be established in this way. When total scores on the test were compared using a t-test, significant differences occurred between the two samples at each developmental level in the test. The clinical group scored significantly lower than the norming sample.

The PDMS correlates well with the *Bayley Scales of Infant Development* and the *West Haverstraw Motor Development*

Test. The PDMS also produces valid scores for both males and females. No statistical differences in total scores were found for males and females, nor for blacks and Hispanics.

Reliability of the PDMS is reported in terms of test-retest and interrater reliability. Test-retest reliability coefficients were high. A .99 coefficient was determined when groups were tested one week apart. Two raters were able to achieve similar scores on groups, with a .99 coefficient established comparing total scores and a .96 coefficient on particular items.

Norm tables are provided in the manual for converting raw scores to standard scores. The tables can be used to compare scores in terms of z scores, t scores, percentiles, and developmental motor quotients.

Evaluation

The PDMS is a very useful tool that can be utilized to determine the placement of a handicapped child for motor programming or for a developmental criterion-related test and curriculum. The uses are varied, including a preschool motor curriculum for normal children, a diagnostic/prescriptive program for various types of handicapped children, and an adjunct to reflex testing by physical therapists.

Source

Folio, M.R., & Fewell, R.F. (1983). *Peabody developmental motor scales and activity cards*. Allen, TX: DLM-Teaching Resources Corporation.

Six Category Gross-Motor Test

Purpose

This norm-referenced test is designed to discriminate performance between normal and mentally retarded children. Areas measured are:

- body perception
- gross agility
- balance
- locomotor agility
- throwing
- tracking

Format

Individually administered, the test requires about 30 minutes. It is designed for normal children ages 4 to 11; mildly handicapped, 5 to 20; moderately retarded, 5 to 24; and trainable mentally retarded, 6 to 20 years. The test has a five-point rating scale with criteria provided.

Data

Test-retest reliability on 83 subjects is reported to be .91. No validity data are reported. Norming was on 200 children ranging in ages from 4 to 11 years.

Evaluation

The test is easy to administer and does not require an unusual amount of equipment.

Source

Cratty, B.J. (1969). *Perceptual motor behavior and educational processes*. Springfield, IL: Charles C Thomas.

PERCEPTUAL MOTOR TESTS

Body Image Screening Test for Blind Children

Purpose

This test was designed to measure body awareness of blind children. Other populations may also be screened with this instrument, including mentally retarded, sighted, and deaf children.

Format

The test is sequentially arranged beginning with body planes, parts, movements, laterality, and directionality. The test is generally individually given, but small groups can be tested. The time will vary, depending on the age and developmental level of the child. The test includes screening of one's own movements and the movements of others. Directionality and laterality relate to the concept applied to oneself, objects, and others.

Data

Items were chosen from current literature to ensure their validity. Test-retest reliability was established on 18 blind children with a coefficient of .81 reported.

Evaluation

This screening test can be easily administered with common items found in a classroom. It is quite detailed, containing 52 items arranged from the least to the most difficult.

Source

Cratty, B.J., & Sams, T.A. (1968). *The body image of blind children*. New York: The American Foundation for the Blind.

Developmental Test of Visual Motor Integration (VMI)

Purpose

The VMI was developed to measure the process of visual motor integration on a developmental continuum.

Format

Designs are provided that were established as appropriate for young children. The test requires that children being tested copy the geometric figures, such as a square or triangle on a score sheet provided. There are 24 figures included in the test in order of increasing difficulty. When the child misses satisfactorily reproducing three figures in a row, testing is stopped. Age-equivalent scores are provided for ages 2 years to 15 years and 11 months.

Data

The test is well standardized with a good cross section of rural, urban, and suburban areas; 1,039 subjects were used in the norming sample.

Reliability for one tester is .96 and .95 for two testers. Test-retest reliability ranges from .80 to .90, depending on the sex of the subject being tested.

Validity is highly correlated with the chronological age of the subject. Correlations of .53 to .79 were achieved comparing the VMI with subtests on the *Illinois Test of Psycholinguistic Abilities*.

Evaluation

The VMI can be easily administered in groups or with individuals. It is a good screening test for the perceptual integration of visual motor skills on a fine motor level. No data appear to be available related to visual motor integration on this test and gross motor skills requiring visual motor integration. The physical educator may use this test as a possible indication that a student may have problems with gross motor skills requiring spatial relationships and motor coordination.

Source

Beery, K.E., & Buktenica, N. (1967). *Developmental test of visual motor integration*. Chicago: Follett.

Frostig Developmental Test of Visual Perception (DTVP)

Purpose

The DTVP is designed to measure five aspects of visual perception:

- eye-motor coordination
- figure-ground perception
- shape recognition
- position of space
- spatial relations

Format

The DTVP may be administered individually in about 40 minutes. Small group testing is also possible. Group administration requires about an hour. Scores are reported as perceptual age scores.

Data

Normative data are provided on children ranging in age from four to eight years. Only California children were used in the norming procedures. Ethnic groups are not represented.

Reliability data include coefficients ranging from .80 to .98 for total test performance. Reliability of subtests is slightly lower than for the total test.

Validity data include construct and predictive validity. Content validity has not been sufficiently determined.

Evaluation

The DTVP is easily administered. The standardization is weak, however. Caution should be used in making generalizations and conclusions from the test. The test does not require many materials but a test booklet is needed for each child.

Source

Frostig, M., Lefever, W., & Whittlesay, J.R. (1966). *Administration and scoring manual for the Marianne Frostig Developmental test of visual perception*. Palo Alto, CA: Consulting Psychologists Press.

Milani-Comparetti Test of Reflex Development

Purpose

This test is designed to measure several types of reflexes, including:

- primitive reflexes
- righting reactions
- protective reactions
- postural control
- active movement

Format

The test is individually administered to infants 0-24 months, others functioning at that level, or anyone thought to have remaining immature reflexes. A checkoff system for scoring in months is provided.

Data

Normative data include the months that the reflexes are normally present. No validity or reliability data are reported.

Evaluation

This test is widely used by physical therapists. The adapted physical educator may use this as a screening device to refer students suspected of having primitive or poorly developed reflexes. Even though the test is not well defined in terms of reliability and validity, it is still widely used.

Source

Milani-Comparetti, A., & Gidoni, E.A. (1967). *Developmental Medicine and Child Neurology, 9*, 5.

Purdue Perceptual Motor Survey

Purpose

The *Purdue* was designed to measure several perceptual motor aspects, including:

- balance and posture
- body image and differentiation
- perceptual motor match
- ocular control
- form perception

Format

This survey provides a four-point rating scale with criteria related to problems in performance. The survey is administered individually in about 45 minutes to an hour. Age ranges are from 6 to 10 years for normal children. A manual is provided and some of the materials are included within the manual. A chalkboard, penlight, and yardstick are also needed to administer the test.

Data

Test-retest reliability coefficients are high, with .95 for testing children one week apart. Validity is described in terms of test scores and teacher ratings. A .65 coefficient is provided related to these two parameters. Norms are provided for grades 1-4 in terms of means and standard deviations.

Evaluation

The *Purdue Perceptual Motor Survey* provides a good screening overall for perceptual motor integration, particularly the visual achievement forms and imitation of body movements and positions. The item called "Angels in the Snow" helps the physical educator to determine if the student can control body movements of the limbs in particular. A few items are devoted to physical fitness. However, they are so few that they are really not worthwhile. A physical fitness screening test would be more useful, especially with students who are learning disabled or mildly and moderately retarded. It may not be very useful with students who have severe motor problems or who are visually handicapped.

Source

Roach, E., & Kephart, N. (1966). *Purdue perceptual motor survey*. Columbus, OH: Charles E. Merrill.

Southern California Sensory Integration Tests

Purpose

Measures include:

- position in space
- figure-ground perception
- form copying
- manual form perception
- kinesthesia
- tactile discrimination
- midline crossing
- right-left discrimination
- bilateral motor control
- stationary balance

Format

The test is individually administered to ages ranging from four through eight years. About 60 to 90 minutes are required to give the test battery. Scores are obtained from objective criteria. Raw scores can be converted to z-scores using a norm table. A scoring booklet is available and little equipment is required to administer the test.

Data

The test was standardized on children from four to eight years of age. The norming sample was 1,004. Test-retest reliability varies from .78 to .92. Reliability is higher among younger groups. Validity is reported in terms of a coefficient of .50 with the *Bender Gestalt* test.

Evaluation

This test is a good evaluation tool for sensory motor integration. It is a good adjunct to a complete battery of testing for overall motor integration when combined with motor skill achievement, physical, and motor fitness.

Source

Ayres, J.A. (1969). *Southern California sensory integration tests*. Los Angeles: Western Psychological Services.

PHYSICAL FITNESS AND POSTURE

AAHPERD Special Fitness Test for Mildly Mentally Retarded Persons

Purpose

This fitness test is designed to measure the following components of physical fitness for mentally retarded persons ranging in age from 8 to 18 years:

- arm and shoulder girdle strength
- strength of abdominal and hip flexor muscles
- speed and agility
- muscular power
- speed in running
- skill and coordination
- cardiovascular efficiency

Format

Items on the test are similar to the original *AAHPER Youth Fitness Test*. Some are modified and include the flexed arm hang, sit-ups, shuttle run, standing broad jump, 50-yard dash, softball throw for distance, and the 300-yard walk-run. The time required is about an hour if the teacher is prepared and students are cooperative. Objective scoring is used for time, number of repetitions, and distance for certain items.

Data

No validity or reliability data are available. The test has been normed on 4,200 mildly retarded persons throughout the United States. Norms are reported in percentiles for males and females ages 8 to 18 years.

Evaluation

The test is relatively easy to administer and does not require an unusual amount or type of equipment. Incentive awards may be given for achievement of specific percentiles. This test would be useful if a school district had several mildly mentally retarded youngsters.

Source

American Alliance for Health, Physical Education, Recreation and Dance. Reston, VA, 1976.

Motor Fitness Test for the Moderately Mentally Retarded

Purpose

The purpose of this test is to measure the following components of physical fitness among moderately mentally retarded persons:

- arm and shoulder strength
- abdominal strength and endurance
- muscular power (legs)
- speed and coordination
- flexibility
- height and weight
- skill accuracy

Format

The test takes at least one hour to administer, if not more, depending on the student's cooperation. No specialized equipment is necessary. Objective scoring relates to time, the number of repetitions, and distance for various items.

Data

Test-retest reliability coefficients range from .60 to .90 on the test items. Generally, reliability is .80 on the majority of items. No validity data are provided. The test was normed on 1,097 mentally retarded persons ages 6 to 20. The population was in an institutional setting. Percentiles are provided for each age level.

Evaluation

Since subjects in the normative study were in institutional settings generalizations cannot be made beyond these populations. The test does require time to administer, although parts can be used, rather than the entire test.

Publisher

American Alliance for Health, Physical Education, Recreation and Dance. Reston, VA, 1976.

BUELL Adaptation of the AAHPERD Youth Fitness Test for the Blind

Purpose

This test measures several aspects of fitness and is a modification of the *AAHPERD Youth Fitness Test* and measures blind students ages 10 to 17 years. Components include

- running speed
- arm and shoulder strength
- strength of abdominal musculature
- muscular power
- cardiovascular endurance
- body agility
- strength and power of the upper extremity

Format

Normed on blind children, the test includes items requiring running, such as the 50-yard dash, the 600-yard walk-run, and the shuttle run. Except for these items, the test is administered much like the regular *AAHPERD Youth Fitness Test*. Scoring is based on objective data such as times, distance, or number of repetitions completed by the student for a particular item.

Data

Normative data may be used for regular students on items that do not require running. No reliability or validity data are provided on the items normed for blind students.

Evaluation

No unusual equipment is required to give the test. Generally, not all items should be given in one day. Two or more classes should be used to give the test. Awards are available for various percentiles.

Source

Buell, C. (1974). *Physical education and recreation for visually handicapped.* Reston, VA: AAHPERD Publications.

Fait Physical Fitness Battery for Mentally Retarded Children

Purpose

This test is designed to measure the following physical fitness components of mildly and moderately mentally retarded boys and girls ages 9 to 20 years:

- running speed
- static muscular endurance of the arms and shoulder girdle
- dynamic muscular endurance of the legs and abdominal muscles
- static balance
- agility
- cardiorespiratory endurance

Format

The test can be given during one testing period. The running events may be separated and given on different days from the rest of the items. A large number of students may be administered the long-distance run at one time. Score cards are provided to record each student's times, repetitions, or distances.

Data

Norms are available for age groups of 9-12, 13-16, and 17-20. Validity is based on the selection of items based on other validated physical fitness measures.

Evaluation

The modified items on this test are reliable with retarded populations. The fact that the items can be easily and simply administered removes any performance difficulty because of intelligence.

Source

Fait, H.F., & Dunn, J.M. (1984). *Special physical education: Adapted, individualized and developmental.* Philadelphia: W.B. Saunders.

CURRICULUM

Behavioral Characteristics Progression

Purpose

The major purpose of the *Behavioral Characteristics Progression* is to identify skills and behaviors a child has or does not have. There are 59 behavioral strands that include various behaviors. Strands useful to the adapted physical educator include:

- health
- self-identification
- sensory perception
- auditory perception
- visual motor skills
- gross motor skills
- adaptive behaviors
- impulse control
- self-confidence
- outdoor skills
- posture
- ambulation
- swimming

Format

The BCP can be used as an assessment tool to determine skills in a large area. The assessment is not a standardized assessment, however. Objectives for developing the nonexisting skills are included in the BCP. No specific criteria are provided to determine when a skill has been learned.

Evaluation

The total administration of areas is time consuming. The BCP is a good classroom evaluation tool and covers a broad age range. Most curricula of this nature do not provide normative data or research as to effectiveness with intervention. Thus, the BCP must be used as a guide and not a diagnostic tool for placement.

Source

Behavioral Characteristics Progression (BCP). (1973). Palo Alto, CA: VORT Corporation.

Callier Azuza Scale

Purpose

The *Callier Azuza Scale* was designed to measure skills in five areas for deaf-blind children. However, the scale can be used with severely handicapped children as well. The five areas include:

- motor development
- perceptual skills
- daily living skills
- language
- socialization

Format

Items are arranged by developmentally sequenced behavior descriptions. The rater selects the developmental description that best fits the child's response. The scale is very good to use with low-functioning children and does not require an unusual amount of time to assess the child. The scale can also be used to monitor the child's progress after an instructional period. There are numerous motor items.

Evaluation

This scale is a good guide for use with multi-impaired children or young handicapped children. The fact that the measures are in terms of behavioral descriptions is useful in planning objectives for the child.

Curriculum and Monitoring System (CAMS)

Purpose

The CAMS is designed for monitoring and evaluating the progression of young handicapped children. A motor component is included with other areas such as self-help skills and social and emotional development. The CAMS may be used for programming in educational settings and in the home.

Format

The curriculum states particular skills to be learned in a developmental sequence. Then procedures are included for teaching the skills. Specific criteria indicate a mastery level for each skill. A training manual aids in teaching and positioning the child to achieve the desired outcomes. Summary sheets are provided to record pupil progress during the teaching sessions.

Evaluation

The CAMS provides a good method for identifying missing skills in a child's repertoire and a management system for teaching and recording progress. The fact that it is designed for use in classrooms and the home setting makes it a useful tool when parents are needed to aid in the instruction of the child.

Source

Jones, J., Hoagland, V., Peterson, A., Sedjo, K., Casto, H., Baer, R., & Douglas, V. (1977). *Curriculum and monitoring system.* New York: Walker Educational Book Corporation.

Developmental Profile

Purpose

The *Developmental Profile* is a scale designed to measure the child's progress from birth to preadolescence in five areas:

- physical development
- self-help skills
- social adjustment
- communication
- academics

Format

The scale has 217 items included within the five areas. Each is arranged at six-month intervals with three items included at each interval. An age-equivalent score can be obtained after administering each area.

Evaluation

This is a good screening tool for the classroom but should be used in conjunction with other curricula and tests.

Source

Aplern, G.D., & Boll, T.J. (1972). *Developmental profile*. Aspen, CO: Psychological Development Publications.

I CAN Series

Purpose

I CAN is an individualized physical education program that includes an instructional management system for children whose developmental growth and motor skills are generally below average or who have specific learning disabilities. The *I CAN* system has instructional packages for the following areas:

- fundamental skills
- body management
- health and fitness
- aquatics
- team sports
- dance and individual sports
- backyard and neighborhood activities
- outdoor units

Format

The *I CAN* series was established around a sequential set of behavioral objectives. Each performance objective contains a developmental sequence of skill levels. The materials include an age span from elementary through adolescents and adults. Within each module are curriculum guides, assessment records, game books, and an implementation guide. The curriculum guides contain the performance objectives, assessing activities, and instructional activities. Assessment records are for recording and monitoring student performance. The game book contains games and activities to reinforce the social components of each skill. The implementation guide shows school personnel how to develop daily, monthly, and yearly program plans.

Data

The materials have been field tested with educable, trainable, and severely mentally retarded student populations. Significant changes were demonstrated in student performance during teaching sessions over a period of time. The program is valid for improving the skills it is designed to teach in handicapped populations.

Evaluation

The *I CAN* series is an excellent resource for a physical education program for handicapped students. It is particularly useful for developing motor objectives for IEPs and monitoring student progress. The programs can be used in a variety of settings that provide services to handicapped individuals. The broad age range covered makes it particularly useful.

Source

Wessel, J.A. (1976). *I CAN adaptive physical education program*. Northbrook, IL: Hubbard Publishing Company.

Chapter 8

Developing Individualized Educational Programs

Focus

- Defines purpose of the Individualized Education Program.
- Describes the IEP process and content.
- Delineates physical educator's role as an IEP committee member.
- Discusses developing goals and objectives for handicapped students.
- Explains IEP documentation and review.

Individualized educational programs (IEPs) are mandated by P.L. 94–142 and serve as an agreement between the local education agency, the handicapped student, and parents that an appropriate education is being provided. Often the IEP is developed so that local school districts can demonstrate their compliance with P.L. 94–142. This should be the last reason for developing an IEP.

Almost every handicapped student can achieve skills and success when appropriate skills are taught within the framework of the learning styles of handicapped students. When IEPs are developed with the intent of actually providing appropriate educational experiences for handicapped students, they become a means to accountability. Actual documentation of teaching effectiveness can be accomplished through IEP development and implementation.

Some teachers say that they develop goals in their heads, such as "Students will increase in fitness, or students will learn three team sports." These are excellent goals. However, they do not focus on specific individuals. The needs of handicapped students are actually brought into focus through a coordinated effort among professionals, parents, and handicapped students themselves, when appropriate. As a result, everyone benefits.

In the past, educators merely fitted students into the existing curriculum. The IEP changes the focus to students so that they will have a curriculum and teaching emphasis designed to meet their unique needs. Those responsible for physical education must gear their thinking toward designing the curriculum for handicapped students, rather than trying to fit the students into the curriculum. Many failures on the part of handicapped students are a result of not having appropriate educational experiences provided for them. The IEP should be viewed as a road map for achieving educational outcomes. Educational experiences can result in achievement if the teacher and students know where the destinations are and how to get there.

The January 19, 1981 *Federal Register* provides an interpretation of the IEP as a monitoring device to be used by state and local school districts to see if students are receiving an appropriate educational program. If the IEP committee has functioned well, most school districts have no difficulty with monitoring.

If teachers accept the idea that the IEP provides a structure and clearly designed steps for instruction, they will find it a very useful tool. Some find the IEP an unpleasant chore. However, as practice in developing IEPs accumulates, they become increasingly less difficult. Computers are aiding in the development of IEPs through software that can quickly generate goals and objectives from information supplied. Still, a good deal of team input is required. Many school districts have not been able to purchase and utilize extensive computer assistance. This section will discuss the IEP process with only brief mention of computer-assisted IEP development.

Most school districts have procedures for completing the IEP. Although these procedures may vary slightly from one district to another, they all must comply with guidelines specified in P.L. 94–142. Turnbull, Strickland, and Brantly (1978) provide an extensive amount of information on the IEP process. The steps they recommend include the following, after formal assessment of the student's abilities has occurred.

- IEP development
- IEP implementation
- IEP monitoring
- IEP review

IEP DEVELOPMENT

Development of the IEP is an extension of the assessment process, findings, and results. Data gathered during assessment can then be used to develop an educational program individually tailored to the needs of each handicapped student who will be receiving special education services.

P.L. 94–142 specifies the content of the IEP. It must include at least the following information:

- present levels of the handicapped student's functioning
- annual long-term goals
- short-term objectives for achieving goals
- special education services to be provided
- related services that are needed and will be provided
- extent to which the regular student will participate in the regular classroom
- dates when services will begin and their duration
- procedures for evaluating the goals and objectives, at least on an annual basis

Other relevant information may be included in the IEP such as:

- actual test information
- special health problems
- list of the IEP committee members
- a checklist of procedures followed
- special materials such as modified equipment for physical education (Turnbull et al., 1978)

The IEP Committee

The IEP committee is responsible for developing the IEP. Physical educators should serve on the committee to assist in developing the handicapped student's physical education portion of the IEP. If physical educators will have the responsibility for teaching handicapped students, whether in regular or modified classes, they should have the opportunity to develop and tailor programs to meet the student's needs.

After assessment has been completed and data summarized, goals and objectives can be developed and discussed at the IEP committee meeting. During this information sharing and planning meeting, the physical educator's role would be to give a summary of the student's psychomotor assessment results. The oral summary should include at least the following information:

- names and types of tests used
- other assessment techniques utilized, i.e., observation
- present levels of student performance including strengths and weaknesses
- other information the physical education teacher wishes to share, such as the student's motivation, behavior, rate of learning physical skills
- statements concerning goals and objectives based on the assessment results

This information can be combined with other assessment information. The committee can then prioritize goals and objectives and make recommendations for placement and the amount of time to be spent in regular classes. If a student is to spend all or a portion of time in the regular physical education class, the physical education teacher should assist in making the decision. Once the IEP is agreed to by the parents, responsibilities can be assigned and preparation for implementation initiated. The physical educator should be responsible for implementing the physical education portion of the IEP and documenting student progress.

IEP Implementation

The implementation of the IEP strives to aid the student in achieving the annual goals and short-term objectives agreed upon by the IEP committee. The goals and objectives that are developed for each handicapped student should specify the instructional program and how it will be delivered.

GOALS

Goals involve long-range outcomes for the student and usually pertain to a one-year period in the IEP. Goals are based on the student's present level of functioning and skills that can be expected to be achieved. Many goals can be envisioned for students. However, only the most important and relevant goals must be developed. Physical education goals for the student, while long term, should be developed in terms of their attainment within a school year.

All goals do not have to be achieved in one year, and most likely some will not. Even after assessing a student, teachers

Table 8–1 Goal Statements

General Goal	More Precise Goals
Improve fitness	Increase shoulder girdle strength
Appreciate fitness	Express a desire to participate in fitness activities
Learn about team sports	State the rules of two team sports

and other professionals are still providing only best professional estimates of what is reasonable for students to try to achieve within a one-year period. P.L. 94–142 does not specifically hold teachers accountable when students do not achieve goals. Generally, if the goals are reasonable and appropriate, some progress toward their attainment can be observed and documented. Turnbull et al. (1978) recommends that three or four annual goals be included for each curriculum area. This allows for priorities to be established.

Goal statements need to be broad but at the same time specific. The following are examples of goal statements that may be part of a student's educational program.

- Increase cardiovascular fitness levels.
- Develop coordination in throwing skills.
- Express a desire to participate in fitness training.

Sometimes goals can be too broadly stated. Compare the goals in Table 8–1. The goals on the left would be considered too general. The goals on the right present a more precise statement. Stating goals to be achieved as precisely as possible leaves little room for misinterpretation.

SHORT-TERM OBJECTIVES

While goals can be specific, they are too general to be measured directly. Objectives provide the means for measuring if goals have been achieved. Objectives also provide a mode of communication between parents, educators, and the handicapped students themselves. Ryan, Johnson, and Lynch (1977) indicate that objectives may also provide a guide to sequencing instruction and curricula. When objectives are clearly sequenced, documentation and evaluation of instruction may be systematically managed.

Writing Short-Term Objectives

Mager (1962) emphasizes that behavioral objectives must have three important components before they can be considered measurable. Ryan et al. (1977) suggest that behavioral objectives contain the components mentioned by Mager as well as an indication of who the objective is for. Combining what Mager and Ryan have to suggest for behavior objective components, a measurable objective should contain:

- for whom the objective is written
- what will be displayed by the learner
- conditions under which the behavior will occur
- specific criteria indicative of successful performance levels

Observable Behavior

The behavior must be specific and observable, not only to one person but to others as well. Objectives are sometimes written with nonspecific behavior and become ambiguous. An example of an ambiguous objective is "John will learn to jump." The behavior is jumping, but still nonspecific as to the type or distance involved. No two people could clearly measure whether John has learned to jump. Davis (1973) explains that objectives in the psychomotor domain should be relatively easy to write since motor skills, by their very nature, include observable behavior. Action words usually denote observable behavior, such as *run, jump, walk, defines*, etc.

While the physical educator is primarily concerned with the psychomotor domain, the affective and cognitive domains should also be considered. Dauer and Pangrazzi (1979) recommend the development of objectives in the cognitive, affective, and psychomotor domains for each physical education behavior. The following example illustrates objectives in the three domains for jogging.

Psychomotor: John will be able to jog at least 200 yards without stopping to rest.

Cognitive: John will be able to state at least two good effects of jogging.

Affective: John will demonstrate his appreciation for jogging by recording how many times he jogs in his leisure hours.

Criteria for Acceptable Performance

Even though observable behavior may be specifically stated, the objective is still not measurable unless the criteria for acceptable performance is established. Davis (1973) notes that criteria for acceptable performance may be stated several ways, depending on the skill to be developed. Van Etten, Arkell, and Van Etten (1980) recommend that criteria must be realistic and based on the handicapped student's ability to achieve the skill level. Two handicapped students may be working on the same objective but each may require different criteria. For example, two students may be trying to develop overhand throwing skills. However, the physical education teacher may reduce the throwing distance for the

handicapped student who has lesser arm strength than the other. If throwing accuracy is the goal, the number of times a target is hit may differ from one handicapped student to another. The accuracy level may need to be less, for example, if a handicapped student is having eye-hand coordination problems.

Criteria can be expressed in different ways. Usually, criteria can include percentages, allotted time to complete a task, number of repetitions, and form. The following are examples of objectives including the criteria or degree of performance:

Percentage: John will score at least 70% on a knowledge test on the rules of basketball.

Allotted time: John will complete the 300-yard walk-run, with the aid of a peer within four minutes.

Number of times: John will be able to make at least three baskets unguarded during each practice session.

Number of repetitions: John will jump rope independently three consecutive jumps.

Form: John will be able to throw at least three softballs overhand using shoulder rotation and followthrough.

Conditions

The conditions under which the behavior will occur must also be specified. Van Etten et al. (1980) explain that the same objective might include different conditions for different students. For instance, two handicapped students may be trying to develop batting skills. The objective for both students may be to bat the ball at least three out of five times the distance to second base. The students may differ in physical and coordinated abilities. It is important that the conditions under which the batting will occur be geared to each student's ability. For example, John may bat the ball from a batting tee or cone stand. Jeff, on the other hand, may bat the ball as it is rolled by a pitcher because Jeff has more skill at this point than John. In this case, the objectives specify conditions that are geared to the skill level of each student so that each can experience success while at the same time improve batting skill. Here is how the objectives might be written for each student.

- John will be able to bat a six-inch playground ball from a batting tee so that it travels at least the distance to second base three out of five times.
- Jeff will be able to bat a six-inch playground ball rolled by the pitcher so that it travels at least the distance to second base three out of five times.

Examine the following examples of goals and objectives based on a sample skill deficit or weakness.

Benny
Benny is a 15-year-old high school student with cerebral palsy. Crutches are used to aid with walking. Arm movements are not well coordinated. Benny loves baseball and basketball. He needs a batting tee and lightweight bat to hit. A designated runner must also be used. Thus, he can participate to a limited extent in a game. Benny really wants to know the game and be a knowledgeable spectator. In addition, he wants to maintain flexibility in his musculature and maintain endurance. He really tries hard in physical education and enjoys the class. Goals for Benny might include the following examples followed by specific objectives.

Goal: By the end of the first term, Benny will be able to improve his knowledge of the game of baseball.

Objectives
1. Given a typewriter, Benny will be able to answer questions on baseball strategy and rules getting at least 21 out of 30 correct.
2. Benny will be able to define, with no errors, the following baseball terms found in the sports section of the newspaper: RBIs, batting average, runs, hits, errors, stolen bases.
3. Benny will complete a log of his favorite team's progress including at least five different types of information about the team.

Lucy
Lucy, an emotionally disturbed tenth grader, has difficulty following class routines in physical education after changing clothes. She tends to loiter, not complete the exercise course, and is late for roll call.

Goal: Lucy will be able to attempt each exercise station and be on time for roll call.

Objectives:
1. Lucy will be able to attempt three out of six of the exercise stations with the aid of the teacher.
2. Lucy will be on time for roll call at least two out of five days each week with the aid of her peer model.
3. Lucy will independently attempt three out of six exercise stations two out of five days each week.

Note that it is important to set objectives in the beginning that are achievable. It is not appropriate for Lucy to be able to complete the entire exercise circuit and be on time for roll call in the very beginning. Her behavior has to be achievable in small steps and objectives should be sequenced that way. In fact, it may take the entire year to achieve the goal of getting Lucy to complete the exercise circuit and be on time.

Jerilyn
Jerilyn is an eight-year-old elementary school student who is mildly retarded. She has basic skills developed to the point that she can participate in basic games and lead-ups to sports. Her concept of team interaction is poor and she does not relate well to other players. Specific problems include keeping the ball instead of passing it to other players in some lead-up games. Other examples include arguing and fighting when her team loses.

Goal: Jerilyn will be able to share the ball with her teammates in game situations.
Objective
1. Jerilyn will be able to complete an exercise drill and pass the ball to her teammates in three out of five trials.
2. Jerilyn will be able to pass the ball to a teammate during a lead-up game at least twice during the game without the aid of the teacher or peer.

Translating Student Data into Meaningful Goals and Objectives

Preceding this section information was provided on developing goals and objectives with specific exercises. In reality, teachers will be viewing assessment data and then developing goals and objectives for each handicapped student. This section provides actual data on students and demonstrates how the goals and objectives are prioritized and developed for students.

The following summary describes the strengths and weaknesses of a nine-year-old female with Down's Syndrome.

Suzie
Suzie is a nine-year-old moderately retarded child with Down's Syndrome. She transferred from another school district. Information concerning her physical and motor skills was sketchy. Suzie's previous school did not have a physical education program of any structure. An assessment was made by the physical education teacher in Suzie's new school, using the *Geddes Psychomotor Inventory, Primary Level* (Long Form), and the *Motor Fitness Test for the Moderately Mentally Retarded*. Results indicated that Suzie has some basic locomotor skills and beginning perceptual motor abilities. She understands basic body parts and planes and basic spatial relationships. Games skills are weak and need improving, particularly throwing, catching, and striking. Observa-

tions of Suzie during testing indicate that she enjoys motor activities, however, tends to have a short attention span. Suzie appears to respond best to visual rather than verbal cues.

Physical development is below average, particularly related to endurance and strength. Suzie's parents are concerned about keeping her weight appropriate and would like for her to receive regular exercise for weight control. Her parents would also like for her to learn to swim.

Based on information about Suzie, a program tailored to her needs should be developed. The following are sample goals and objectives that could be developed.

Goal: Accurately throw and catch a lightweight ball with another person.

Objectives
1. Using the throw of her choice, Suzie will pass a 16-inch playground ball to another person standing 8 feet away so the ball lands within arm's reach three out of five times.
2. Suzie will be able to pass a 16-inch playground ball to her teammates in simple relays involving passing a ball, so that it lands within arm's reach two out of four times.
3. Suzie will be able to catch a 16-inch playground ball passed by another student from a distance of 5 and 8 feet two out of five times.
4. Suzie will be able to catch a 16-inch playground ball passed by another student from no more than 8 feet three out of five times.

Goal: Strike different-sized balls with the aid of a batting tee in a lead-up game.

Objectives
1. Using a plastic bat, Suzie will be able to strike an 8-inch playground ball placed on a plastic cone, making contact three out of four times.
2. Using a plastic bat, Suzie will be able to strike an 8-inch playground ball placed on a batting tee three out of five times.
3. Using a plastic bat, Suzie will be able to strike an 8-inch playground ball placed on a batting tee so that it travels at least 10 feet in bounds three out of five times.

Goal: Increase attention span while performing motor tasks while in a group.

Objectives
1. Suzie will be able to complete five trials of a task with the aid of a peer tutor before changing or stopping the task.
2. Suzie will be able to complete at least five trials of a task with only three praises or urgings from the peer tutor before changing or stopping the task.

3. Suzie will be able to complete five trials of a task in a small group (three to five) with only verbal encouragement from a peer tutor.

Goal: Complete an endurance walk-run without showing signs of undue fatigue.

Objectives
1. With the aid of a peer model, Suzie will be able to walk 300 yards, stopping only once for rest.
2. Suzie will be able to walk with a group with no more than one rest time a distance of 300 yards.
3. Suzie will be able to walk and run at least 100 of 300 yards with one rest period of no more than 30 seconds.
4. Suzie will be able to walk and combine running a distance of 300 yards with no rest period.

Goal: Demonstrate basic fundamental swimming skills for drown proofing.

Objectives
1. After ten swimming lessons, Suzie will be able to combine breath control, floating, kicking, and arm movements to propel herself at least a distance of 5 yards in the pool.
2. Suzie will be able to jump into the pool feet first, return to the surface, and float for at least one minute.
3. Suzie will be able to jump into water at least 6 feet deep, and return to the pool edge unassisted.

Goal: Lose weight by exercising and eating proper food.

Objectives
1. Given an exercise routine to follow, Suzie will be able to complete the routine at home with her family at least three times per week.
2. Select a between-meal snack that is nutritious and reduced in calories at least three out of five times.
3. Lose at least 10 pounds by the end of the first semester by completing exercise routines at home and physical education activities at school.

THE IEP FORM

The IEP form in Exhibit 8–1 contains a sample of goals and objectives developed for Suzie based on the assessment results. Also included is other relevant information such as materials that might be used and instructional techniques. Again, it must be remembered that goals need to be prioritized. The IEP committee should decide which goals need the most attention and work on those first. Suzie's short attention span is an area of immediate concern. Physical fitness is another area that should also be a priority.

Exhibit 8–1 Sample IEP Form

Student's Name: Suzie Q.   Grade: Self Contained   Teacher: T. Smith

Program Entry Date: 9–10–81

Curriculum Area: Physical Education   Includes: Physical, gross motor and perceptual motor skills

Evaluation Instruments: Geddes Psychomotor Inventory—Primary level (long form); Motor Fitness Test for Moderately Mentally Retarded

Current level of educational functioning: (Include strengths and weaknesses)
  Suzie enjoys motor activity. Basic locomotor skills are developed. Needs work on throwing, catching, and striking. Has good body awareness and spatial relations. Needs to increase muscular strength and endurance. Has good flexibility. Parents would like to see weight control and swimming instruction.

Annual Goals	Short-Term Objectives	Teaching Strategies	Materials	Start	Finish
1. Improve physical fitness levels	1. Complete the 300-yard walk-run at the 50th percentile using the norms for mentally retarded	Vary activities for short attention span Keep directions short Use peer teachers to complete running-walk laps with Suzie Use much positive reinforcement	*Geddes Profile* *Motor Test for the Moderately Mentally Retarded*	9–20–81	2–30–8
	2. Maintain flexed arm hang for at least 3 seconds with chin above the bar			9–20–81	2–30–8
	3. Complete the vertical jump at least 3 inches			9–20–81	2–30–8
Least Restrictive Instructional Environment Special physical education class	Procedures for Evaluating Progress for Short-Term Objectives Keep weekly trials and scores on motivational chart and in Suzie's folder. Give post-test on pretest instruments.				

Source: From *Adaptive Physical Education: A Resource Guide for Teacher, Administrator, and Parents* (p. 28) by John M. Dunn, 1979, Mental Health Division, Salem, Oregon. Adapted by permission.

IEP RESPONSIBILITIES

The IEP committee will decide who is responsible for implementing the different portions. In Suzie's case, the parents have some responsibility for her physical fitness and nutritional goals. The physical education teacher will provide instruction related to the physical education portion.

The time spent in the regular classroom or the least restrictive environment must also be decided. In Suzie's case, the IEP committee has decided that her program should be delivered in a special physical education classroom. This is due to her short attention span at this point and her lack of skills to participate in a variety of activities.

DOCUMENTING PROGRESS

There are many ways of documenting the student's progress. Many of the commercial curricula, such as *I CAN*, provide forms for recording student progress. Teachers can also make their own forms. A folder should be kept on each student and progress noted each week or during a specified time period. Ongoing progress recording will aid the teacher in documenting whether or not the established goals and objectives are being met. This will allow the teacher to determine if the instructional procedures are effective. In some cases, the goals and objectives may be too high for the student. If documentation has occurred, they can be changed.

This procedure aids in keeping parents informed of their child's educational progress. It is much more effective and professional to say that "Suzie has completed the 300-yard walk run by herself" and "The home fitness activities are really helping." Parents really appreciate hearing specific information and enjoy knowing that they are providing assistance with their child.

Many forms of documenting student progress are possible. These can be as simple as a brief recording of observations, checklists, or noting the date an objective was reached on the IEP form itself.

Observational recording of student progress does not require much time. Suppose that Suzie has begun to rely less on a peer to help her through a task. The teacher might note this and record it in Suzie's folder. Observational recording can include specific data, such as the number of times Suzie, in this case, was able to complete a task without the aid of a peer. Or the teacher might make notes about the type of equipment that works best for Suzie. For example, she may attend to the skill longer if a brightly colored ball is used.

Checklists provide a quick method of recording progress and achievement. Numerous commercial curricula are available that have specific skills listed in a developmental sequence next to which the teacher can make quick checks as each skill is achieved. Some teachers prefer to make their own checklists or individual task cards that contain each objective and can be used to record progress and make notes about equipment or teaching methods that were effective in achieving the objective.

IEP REVIEW

As we have noted, while P.L. 94–142 requires only an annual review of the IEP, periodic documentation allows for ongoing review. It is not wise only to post evaluate a student at the end of a year since the objectives developed in the beginning may not have been appropriate. A periodic review with ongoing documentation assists in truly measuring the educational program's appropriateness.

IEPs should be monitored internally by the school staff. Teachers can pinpoint their strengths and weaknesses in terms of their ability to provide adapted physical education programs and to provide services within the least restrictive environment.

POINTS TO REMEMBER

1. The development of the IEP is a "team" approach and must follow guidelines specified by P.L. 94–142.

2. The IEP helps assure that handicapped students are being provided an appropriate educational program based on their particular strengths, weaknesses, and specific deficits.

3. IEPs aid in accountability and provide a means for monitoring the educational program of handicapped students.

4. Goals and objectives should be based on data gathered from assessment. This ultimately results in data-based documentation of student progress.

5. Objectives *must* be written so that they are measurable, including a specified behavior, conditions under which the behavior will occur, and the criteria or level of performance.

REFERENCES

Congress (96th). Final rules and regulations on P.L. 94–142. *Federal Register*, August 23, 1977.

Dauer, V.P., & Pangrazzi, R.P. (1979). *Dynamic physical education for elementary school children* (6th ed.). Minneapolis: Burgess.

Davis, R.G. (1973). *The effect of perceptually oriented physical education on perceptual motor ability and academic ability of kindergarten and first grade children*. Doctoral dissertation, University of Maryland.

Federal Register. (1981, January 19). Interpretation of the individualized education program (IEP).

Mager, R.F. (1962). *Preparing instructional objectives*. Belmont, CA: Fearon.

Ryan T., Johnson, J., & Lynch, V. (1977). So you want to write objectives. In N.G. Haring (Ed.). *The experimental education training program: An inservice program for personnel serving the severely handicapped*. Seattle: University of Washington.

Turnbull, A.P., Strickland, B.B., & Brantly, J.C. (1978). *Developing and implementing IEP's*. Columbus, OH: Charles E. Merrill.

Van Etten, G., Arkell, C., & Van Etten, C. (1980). *The severely and profoundly handicapped: Programs, methods, and materials*. St. Louis: C.V. Mosby.

Chapter 9

Goals, Program Support, and the Least Restrictive Environment

Focus

- Compares goals of physical education for handicapped and nonhandicapped students.
- Determines support methods for attaining the goals of physical education programs for handicapped students.
- Explores methods of developing program awareness and support.
- Explains how to achieve the least restrictive environment.
- Lists and discusses activities and teaching techniques that enhance learning in the least restrictive environment.

Goals provide direction to programs or other kinds of functions. Without goals ultimate outcomes of programs may be vague and left to chance. Also, by predetermining program goals, the outcomes can be measured.

Communicating the needs and directions of a program can be achieved by setting goals. This makes it easier for the physical educator to explain and demonstrate the purpose and direction of the program. Support may be less difficult to obtain if goals and priorities are known. This will lead to understanding from the support systems for the broad range of physical education services required by handicapped students.

PROGRAM GOALS

The goals of physical education for handicapped students are very similar to the goals of physical education in general. There are some differences, particularly when specific types of disabilities are involved.

Crowe, Auxter, and Pyfer (1981) include several aims of physical education for handicapped students. These authors contend that general goals of physical education should include:

- improvement of conditions that can be corrected
- protection, as much as possible, against further deterioration of disabilities
- development of skills that will enable handicapped students to participate in leisure-time activities
- assistance in helping students understand and accept their disabilities
- activities that will aid the student in achieving a sense of dignity and self-worth
- development of an appreciation for a variety of physical activities and one's maximum potential for participation

Additional goals should include the development of:

- cooperative attitudes among handicapped and non-handicapped students in physical activity programs
- appreciation for one's body in spite of a disability
- appreciation for health and exercise

FACTORS AFFECTING PROGRAM GOALS AND DEVELOPMENT

Even the most well-planned special physical education programs can be negatively affected by several factors. These may significantly influence the success of physical education programs for disabled students. They include, for the most part:

- administrative support for the program
- financial support
- qualifications of personnel
- facilities and equipment
- parent and community support

Administrative Support

One of the most important factors in the success of any special physical education program is the support of administrative personnel, including the principal, the supervisor, and members of the school board. Without administrative commitment, programs lose their impact and may be the first to be cut when financial levels are reduced. Administrators may fail to lend full support to special physical education programs for several reasons.

1. They do not fully understand laws and regulations mandating physical education and recreation for handicapped students.
2. Negative attitudes toward physical education and handicapped students may exist.
3. The goals and services special physical education can provide may be misunderstood.
4. Physical education may not be a priority, even if funds do exist.

Financial Support

Funding is often the deciding factor for maintaining or ending programs. However, in some instances, programs have been ruined even when money has been available as a result of misconceptions and negative attitudes on the part of those who control the financial purse strings. Financial support for programs does not necessarily have to reach huge dollar amounts. In some cases, financial support from local education agencies may require only the funding of a well-qualified teacher. Project PERMIT, a once federally funded program, demonstrated a model physical education program for handicapped students for the amount of the teacher's salary. Sometimes money is not an excuse for not having quality programs in special physical education.

Personnel Qualifications

Qualified personnel make successful programs, given financial support and administrative assistance. A well-trained and qualified teacher is a must for developing and conducting a special physical education program.

Personal Qualities

Personal qualities are important as the special physical educator will no doubt come into contact with a variety of personnel including those in the medical field, other teachers, counselors, administrators, and a variety of children with varying disabilities.

Children with disabilities require a teacher with excellent skills in relating to all types of children, including the mentally retarded, emotionally disturbed, and physically handicapped, to mention a few. In all cases, the physical educator must be able to genuinely care and show empathy and understanding.

Patience is a must when working with handicapped students since progress may be slow. Optimism is often necessary in terms of expecting positive results when working with handicapped students.

Creativity on the part of the physical educator will often be used in adapting teaching strategies and modifying equipment and materials for handicapped students. Creative means are also needed occasionally to motivate students.

Education

Educational training is important for developing physical education programs for handicapped students. All states do not provide or specify the competencies necessary for teaching special physical education. P.L. 94–142 also does not specify the qualifications of those persons who implement special physical education. This is left up to individual states. While most specialized training in adapted physical education or special physical education is conducted through advanced degree programs, there should be some emphasized preparation at the undergraduate level. Since more handicapped children are being mainstreamed, many physical educators are left unprepared to handle handicapped students in their regular classrooms.

A survey conducted by Durley (1981) showed that 92 percent of teachers responsible for providing physical education activities and programs for handicapped students were inadequately prepared to handle the situation. Professional preparation of undergraduate physical education personnel will need to change to produce teachers who can deal with handicapped students mainstreamed in the regular physical education classroom.

Professional preparation programs are beginning to provide preservice training in special physical education. Jansma and French (1982) reported that introductory courses in special physical education are being required by states for teacher certification. Several competencies have been addressed by Jansma and French (1982), which they believe other professionals such as elementary school teachers, special educators, and regular physical educators should have in order to provide at least adequate physical education for handicapped students. Their suggestions are related to those defined by the *Guidelines for Professional Preparation Programs for Personnel Involved in Physical Education and Recreation for the Handicapped* (1973). The competencies include:

- ability to assess motor and physical skills
- skill in developing programs and their implementation
- activity in interprofessional preparation

These competencies appear to be rather broad. The following specific competencies were developed for teachers participating in Project PERMIT inservice training for providing physical education for handicapped students:

- Relate to the notion of what it is like to be handicapped.
- Assess motor and physical abilities of handicapped students.
- Develop individualized physical education programs related to the handicapped student's physical education needs.
- Apply instructional strategies appropriate for the student's disability.
- Modify and adapt activities and equipment so that handicapped students may participate to the maximum extent possible.
- Determine mainstreaming strategies and implement a mainstreamed physical education program where possible.
- Affect positive attitude change toward handicapped students by their nonhandicapped peers.
- Develop a continuum of physical education services from the most restrictive to least restrictive environment (Folio, 1983)

Experience

Experience with a variety of disabled students will provide the physical educator with in-depth understanding of developmental delays, varied learning rates, individual learning styles, and interaction with handicapped students in realistic teaching situations. More training programs are providing early experiential skill training with handicapped youngsters via practical and direct field experiences. Model programs, such as Project PERMIT, have provided the opportunity to have preservice experiences with handicapped youngsters in a mainstreamed and self-contained physical education program.

Facilities and Equipment

Facilities may range from ideal to inadequate. Whatever the facility, programs may still exist that provide handicapped youngsters with well-developed physical education programs. Facilities may vary from one school to another.

Ideally, combined with good teaching, a physical education facility to meet the needs of handicapped students should include a gymnasium or other large, open space to allow for free movement of 25 to 30 children. Adequate storage space should be located adjacent to the open space so that equipment can be made available easily to students. Another room should be available for working with small groups of handicapped students. This might serve as a resource physical education room to assist students needing more individualized help with motor and physical development.

Access to a swimming pool is an added plus, since swimming is an excellent activity for many handicapped students. Many schools are fortunate enough to have a swimming pool or access to a community pool. Also, an open area outside is ideal for providing outdoor activities. This may include a court or grassy area.

An obstacle course designed for physical fitness, which is permanently set up, may be used and modified to develop physical conditioning. The court area can be arranged for a variety of activities from drills to specific sports and games. Figure 9–1 provides an illustration for arranging an outdoor area.

Before purchasing equipment for the physical education program, the teacher needs to be aware of the level of student and groupings. This will give the teacher some idea of what equipment can be teacher-made, purchased, or modified. For mildly handicapped youngsters, equipment may not need to vary a great deal from what would normally be used with nonhandicapped students.

Equipment can be categorized by the type of skill areas to be developed and the motoric levels of students. However, some equipment may be applicable to several levels of students. General equipment may include:

- mats for exercise, stunts, tumbling
- carpet squares
- ropes
- weights (dumbbells and ankle weights)

Figure 9–1 Outdoor Area

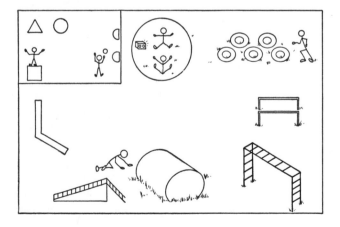

- parallel bars
- bicycle
- stationary bicycle or rack for converting a standard bicycle
- tricycle
- balls of various sizes (playground ball, wiffle balls, beach balls, medicine ball)
- balance beams of various widths
- incline boards
- triangular plastic flags for markers

Equipment can be further organized according to the motor and mental ages of the students thereby enabling it to be used with older students functioning on a lower level and regular students at the particular age level. Table 9–1 illustrates how equipment might be organized by levels.

Equipment for secondary-level students will basically consist of recreational and sports skill types of articles. If skills are at a lower level, the equipment may be modified or the upper elementary level may be used.

ORGANIZATION AND COORDINATION OF THE SPECIAL PHYSICAL EDUCATION PROGRAM

A well-defined program may take the coordination and cooperation of several individuals. As mentioned in Chapter 1, a continuum of services in special physical education should be offered along the same lines as special education service options. Organization needs to occur at each level of service delivery.

The special physical education teacher will have a major responsibility with teaching alone. There may be times when the physical educator will be asked to assist the special education teacher with implementation of motor activities with handicapped students in addition to teaching in the regular physical education program. Some students will require more motor activity programming than the physical educator can provide. The service options will depend on the number, variety, and severity of the disabilities of the students involved. Some of the options in service delivery that may be offered for physical education instruction for handicapped students are discussed in the following sections.

The Self-Contained Physical Education Classroom

The self-contained classroom in physical education is primarily for those students who are so severely handicapped that mainstreaming is an inappropriate placement. The self-contained class may be taught in the same location as a regular class, indoors, outside, or in another large, open

Table 9–1 Equipment for Special Physical Education

Preschool and Early Elementary Grades	
Throwing and Catching	yarn balls
	balloons
	bean bags
	boxes
	hoops
Balance	vestibular board
	balance board
	balance beam 4–6 inches in width
	portable stair set
	bamboo poles
	pull toys
	small trampoline
Rhythm and Movement Exploration	drum
	tape or record player
	lummi sticks
	laminated cardboard shapes, footprints, handprints
	tires
	hoops
	large boxes

Middle and Upper Elementary Level	
Throwing and Catching	suspended balls
	plastic scoops
	sock balls/frisbees
	NeRF® balls/tennis balls
	softballs
Striking and Kicking	large plastic bats
	batting tee
	paddles
Rhythm and Exploration	commercial records
	lummi sticks
	tambourines
	record or tape player
Miscellaneous	bicycle inner tubes
	targets made from 3-M tape
	weighted potato chip cans for markers or weights
	poster board
	cage ball
	wands with paper streamers

space. For some types of handicapped students, a large carpeted room would be more appropriate, particularly for students who might fall frequently. Not more than 8 to 10 students should be accommodated at one time. At that point an aide or two peer teachers would be necessary. In the self-contained classroom, students would need instruction in very basic kinds of motor patterns and skills. Equipment would be more for preschool and elementary level students. In some cases students may be taught in a very small group or individually.

The Physical Education Resource Room

The resource room for physical education is a new approach in providing services to handicapped students. It can be used as an academic resource room is used. The major purpose of the resource room for physical education is to provide extra help for students who may be having difficulty with a particular motor pattern or skill, such as balance, kicking, jumping, hopping, throwing, etc. In addition, difficulty in perceptual motor skills may be remediated or improved through utilization of a physical education resource room.

Another purpose of the resource room would be to provide a combination motor therapy program and mainstreaming. In addition, specialized motor assessment could be conducted within the resource room. The physical educator could provide prescriptive motor programs and a special education classroom aide may work with the student for short periods during the day within the resource room setting. Figure 9–2 illustrates how a resource room might be arranged.

The Mainstreamed Class

Unless a school has a variety of service options for physical education, mainstreaming is more difficult to achieve. Fewer students are mainstreamed successfully if the regular classroom is the only physical education placement. Mainstreaming should be viewed as a continuum. By having self-contained, resource, and regular class placement options, the least restrictive environment is more easily structured.

Mainstreaming does not necessarily have to occur on a full-time basis. Students may be mainstreamed for a particular activity or for some periods each week.

Figure 9–2 Physical Education Resource Room

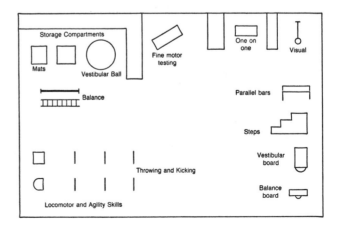

PARENT AND COMMUNITY SUPPORT

Under P.L. 94–142, parents have the right to fully participate in their handicapped child's educational program planning as a member of the multidisciplinary team. Working with parents and having them involved in the handicapped student's physical education program is an important plus. The physical educator will need to develop some skills for working with parents.

- The physical educator needs to be a good listener.
- Parents should be involved in the planning of their handicapped child's physical education program.
- Interpretation of the student's physical and motor development needs is necessary so that parents understand the purpose of physical education.
- Parents should be invited to see the student's participation in physical education.
- If parents wish to volunteer time in the physical education program, they should be encouraged to do so.

Parents can be powerful advocates for physical education if they truly see the benefits for their handicapped children. In addition, parents can be an excellent vehicle for developing community awareness for the physical education program.

Community awareness can result in many positive benefits for the special physical education program. Often, community groups will provide financial aid, volunteer assistance, sponsor special events, and donate equipment. Wiseman (1982) suggests that program awareness activities should be ongoing and well planned throughout the year. This approach will generally result in gaining long-term support and commitment from the community.

A quality program should be visible and well publicized. A variety of methods may be utilized to create community awareness and support.

Demonstration days can be used at special public events, such as half-time shows at athletic events, or at key locations such as shopping malls, spots on local television, and other special events. During these demonstrations, pamphlets or flyers can be distributed that provide further information about the physical education program.

News media announcements provide a means for publicizing special program events, the Special Olympics, and other program achievements. The physical education teacher should get administrative approval to write announcements or news releases and submit them to news media.

Newsletters to parents and other groups may also be used to tell about the program. Posters and pictures of students in action can also provide publicity. These serve as an open line of communication between the program and interested groups.

PTA night can be used to demonstrate several aspects of the special physical education program. Folio and Norman (1982) used this approach very successfully. Demonstrations of students mainstreamed and in self-contained groups were provided with students showing different activities. The resource room was open for demonstrations of how individual students were taught motor skills.

Also during PTA night, special awards may be given to students, such as the most-improved student, the good peer teacher award, and other special notes. Approval from the principal should be obtained before doing this activity.

Annual yearbooks or special reports are also effective for communicating the overall successes of the year. The publication does not have to be large or fancy. It may be shared with special interest groups who have helped and supported the program, parents, other teachers, and administrators.

Professional presentations at local, state, and national meetings allow for dissemination of program ideas. Articles are also another means for sharing ideas in special physical education that work. Part of professional presentations include workshops and special clinics. These may also be conducted at local and state meetings. Clinics should offer demonstrations and allow for interaction and dialogue. Often this approach is more effective than any other method of finding new skills and strategies for working with handicapped students in physical education settings.

Review teams are a method of selecting and advising the special physical educator on new ideas as well as evaluating the program. The review team is also another method of generating program support. Review team members should be carefully selected. A good review team should include the following members:

- school board member
- supervisor of physical education and special education
- regular physical educator
- community leader
- physician
- parent of a handicapped child.

Individuals who commit time to serve on review teams are willing to be of help. Their services should be highly utilized.

IMPLEMENTING THE LEAST RESTRICTIVE ENVIRONMENT

As we have noted, the least restrictive environment refers to the placement of handicapped students, to the maximum extent possible, so that they may be educated with their non-handicapped peers. Educators often refer to this notion as mainstreaming. P.L. 94–142, however, uses only the term "the least restrictive environment," and does not refer to mainstreaming. Many individuals and professionals use this term interchangeably.

In order to place students with disabilities in educational settings with nondisabled students, a system of services needs to be provided. These must range from alternatives from the most to least restrictive settings. Otherwise the least restrictive alternative cannot be fully implemented. This requires commitment to students with disabilities and the notion that education should focus on individual needs.

Because of familiarity with the term "mainstreaming" and the use of it in the literature, it will be used interchangeably with the "least restrictive alternative," or "environment."

The integration of handicapped students into settings with their nonhandicapped peers has met with both success and failure across many educational settings. Woodward (1981) cites some reasons why mainstreaming sometimes doesn't work. Three main factors can be noted:

- lack of parental involvement
- lack of adequately prepared teachers
- lack of administrative support

Where integration of the disabled has been successful several factors have prevailed, such as

- communication and cooperation among school personnel
- parental involvement
- accepting regular physical education teachers
- support for the program

A cooperative and working plan followed by all those involved can contribute to a successful mainstreaming program. The last step in mainstreaming should be when the handicapped student enters the regular or least restrictive setting. Unfortunately, in some cases, this is the first step. Several activities should preceed the day of the disabled student's arrival into the classroom with regular peers.

The physical educator should take time to prepare for students to be included in the class with peers and to be active participants. While some careful thought and preparation will be necessary in the beginning, the long-range outcomes will beneficial to all. The preparation time will aid the handicapped and nonhandicapped students in developing an understanding of each other and in successful social interaction. Handicapped students are often not accepted by their peers for reasons that include behavior differences, lack of knowledge about the handicapping condition, a general fear of those who have disabilities, and negative attitudes on the part of the regular teacher. The more familiar the regular teacher is with handicapped students and methods for teaching them, the more successful mainstreaming will be. The teacher can set the tone of acceptance or rejection within the regular physical education class.

ATTITUDES AND THE LEAST RESTRICTIVE ALTERNATIVE

Everyone has attitudes about handicapped persons. Values, experience, culture, and expectations are a few of the factors that affect those attitudes. Negative attitudes toward disabled persons have changed to the positive. As scientific knowledge about handicapping conditions has increased, more positive attitudes have been generated toward persons with disabilities. Glass, Christiansen, and Christiansen (1982) reported that the early work of Itard, demonstrating that even those who were thought to be severely retarded could be taught some skills, changed the notion that such persons were not teachable. The human rights movements also had a positive effect on attitudes toward the handicapped. In fact, P.L. 94–142 is often referred to as the civil rights movement for handicapped persons.

Teacher Attitudes

The teacher serves as a role model for students to follow. Students will behave in the same manner toward disabled peers as their teachers do. There is no doubt that negative attitudes toward those with disabilities do exist to some degree among regular educators (Johnson & Cartwright, 1979). A major reason for this is the fear of disruption of the regular classroom routine by having handicapped students present (Shotel, Iano, & McGettigan, 1972). Another major fear of teachers about mainstreaming has in the past been their lack of training concerning the instruction of handicapped students. Coupled with this fear, as reported by Thurman (1980), was the notion that all handicapped students would be mainstreamed. Obviously, this is not possible since P.L. 94–142 clearly states that only whenever and wherever appropriate handicapped students shall be educated along with their nonhandicapped peers. Placing a severely handicapped student full time in the regular classroom may not be appropriate.

Choosing the Right Classroom

If several regular physical education classrooms are available, some consideration should be given to the one that is most receptive to mainstreaming. Some of the features of a receptive classroom include:

- the class size
- the attitude and teaching skills of the regular physical education teacher
- the behavior and personalities of the students
- the number of handicapped students already mainstreamed within the class

Classes that have 35–40 students may not be ideal for mainstreaming. Classes of 25–30 students may be more suitable, although a great deal of research is not available related to the success of mainstreaming and class size. The average class size in Project PERMIT was 25 students.

Folio (1983) reported that five mild to moderately handicapped students was a sufficient number to mainstream in any class of 20–25 students. More than five mainstreamed at one time appeared to create management difficulties. In addition, if too many handicapped students are mainstreamed into one class, they tend to become isolated and form their own group. Such an arrangement actually creates more social isolation for handicapped students. This is probably more true of mentally retarded students and those with behavior disorders. Sometimes school districts make the mistake of sending an entire class of mildly retarded students to the same regular physical education classroom. Teachers participating in inservice training have reported little success in programming physical education activities with this type of arrangement.

While the attitude of the regular physical education teacher is an important factor to consider when choosing an appropriate class for mainstreaming, the class chosen for mainstreaming must also be one in which the handicapped student will feel accepted and allowed to try new skills in a nonthreatening atmosphere.

Changing Attitudes

Where negative attitudes exist, efforts to change them should be initiated. Numerous attempts at changing attitudes have been made within the last five years. These have been geared toward school personnel, nonhandicapped students, and other significant service providers for the handicapped student. As a result of these efforts, mainstreaming has become more easily accomplished within the public school setting. These efforts have also extended beyond the school building and out into the community, resulting in more normal living environments for disabled persons. The mainstreaming concept is also finding its way into recreational settings.

Johnson and Cartwright (1979) suggested that attitudes toward disabled persons are best modified through direct positive experiences with disabled persons. A second and effective method for changing attitudes toward disabled persons is through the provision of information about specific disabilities (Krech, Crutchfield, & Bellachey, 1962). Also, as teachers gain knowledge about methods for teaching handicapped students, they become more self-confident and increase their acceptance and expectations for handicapped students (Stephens & Brown, 1980).

Children's attitudes toward disabled peers may be improved by openly answering their questions about disabilities. Also, the more the teacher treats students as individuals, the more tolerant they become toward those who are different. In fact, differences tend not to be so extremely viewed (Barnes, Berrigan, & Biklen, 1977). Programs that are able to successfully demonstrate mainstreaming were reported by Folio and Norman (1981) to be effective in creating positive attitudes toward disabled persons by students, parents, teachers, and administrators. In Project PERMIT, a model program for mainstreaming in physical education, parents of both handicapped and nonhandicapped children were the strongest supporters of the program.

Once the classroom has been chosen for mainstreaming, the nonhandicapped students need to be prepared. Students, just like teachers, have fears about persons with handicapping conditions, as a result of little or no experience and knowledge about various disabilities. Information provided to students about different disabilities will help alleviate fears, stereotypes, and bring about understanding of handicapping conditions. Physical education is an important area of development for all students. In addition, the physical education curriculum and setting provide an atmosphere for social enhancement through sports, games, dance, and other activities. The teacher should try to achieve specific goals toward acceptance. These might include the following examples.

- Disabled persons are more like their nondisabled peers than different.
- All students are different and have some limitations.
- People with disabilities are people first.
- Disabled persons can achieve.
- Different handicapping conditions require specialized instructional techniques and adaptations of materials.

The following activities may prove helpful in fostering more positive regard for handicapped students.

- *"Just Like Me"*

This activity is designed to acquaint nonhandicapped students with their feelings and the fact that handicapped students experience the same feelings as they do. The teacher should try to focus on different feelings. Students can be asked to talk about how they felt their first day of school, or the first time they tried something new, when they moved to another town, or went to the dentist for the first time. These feelings of fear or uncertainty should then be related to the handicapped student coming to the mainstreamed class for the first time.

Students can also be asked how they would feel if they thought they did not have any friends. The discussion can focus on loneliness. The next topic should be concerned with how to make others feel welcome and not be afraid. Students can usually come up with good ideas.

- *"Limitations"*

The concept that everyone has limitations is the purpose of this activity. The teacher should ask the physical education class to name a sports activity that they have difficulty doing. Ask those who cannot do a cartwheel to raise their hands, or play golf, run fast, jump a specific height, and so forth. Eventually, everyone will have raised their hands as the tasks mentioned become increasingly difficult. The major point is that all have some limitations and that in spite of limitations all have something to contribute.

- *"Handicapped Persons Can Achieve"*

Persons with disabilities have achieved and can participate in many activities. The teacher may want to find and provide literature to students about people with disabilities and what they are able to do. There are some well-known persons with achievements to their credit in spite of their disabilities. The teacher can then ask a person with a disability to come to the classroom and talk about his or her particular condition. The person should then participate in a physical activity with the students to demonstrate that a disabled person can participate, though in a different way. For example, the person who is in a wheelchair might participate in a free throw contest or another activity.

- *"Simulations" or "What's It Like"*

When nonhandicapped students experience the simulation of being disabled, they tend to be more sensitive and understanding of handicapped persons. It is similar to the notion of walking in someone else's shoes. Bookbinder (1977) suggested several simulations that will aid in understanding different types of handicapping conditions.

1. As an assignment, ask the students to watch a sports program on television with the sound turned all the way down. This experience can then be discussed in class.

2. Ask students to wear mittens and manipulate small objects to simulate tactile deficits.

3. Let students try out different equipment used by handicapped persons to aid with their disability. Students can try to do a physical education activity in a wheelchair or using crutches.

4. Ask students to play a short game but use only gestures to communicate with one another.

5. Have someone knowledgeable about sign language come to the class and show the students the different signs for terms used frequently in physical education.

6. Blindfold every other student and let a sighted partner lead a blindfolded student around the gym. Ask students to try to identify equipment with their blindfolds on or to try to shoot a basket. Be sure to stress safety.

7. Have students hold one hand behind their back and play catch using only one arm.

- *"Kids on the Block"*

One of the newest and most exciting methods of presenting information about disabilities to people, particularly children, is through the medium of puppetry. This is the purpose of a group of puppets called Kids on the Block, Inc. This concept of puppets telling about disabilities was created by Barbara Aiello (Kids on the Block, 1983). One of the main purposes of the group was to aid in the mainstreaming process. Nonhandicapped students generally did not understand the disabilities of some students who were in their classes. Because they are puppets, Kids on the Block can relate to children and adults in a nonthreatening way. As a result, they are able to make difficult subjects easier to deal with for children. Kids on the Block dress and act just like real children through the trained puppeteers. The puppets are nearly life size. Each puppet speaks candidly about his or her fears, hopes, disability, family, and interests. Some of the puppets are nondisabled and participate as friends of the disabled puppets. There are several puppets with specific disabilities such as cerebral palsy, spina bifida, emotional disturbance, diabetes, impaired hearing, and blindness. The puppeteers need special training to use and purchase the puppets. Almost every state has puppeteers with a set of puppets. They are also in some foreign countries. More information may be obtained from Kids on the Block, Inc., 822 North Fairfax Street, Alexandria, VA 22314.

Teacher Behavior

There are many ways in which teacher behavior can positively affect mainstreaming. Lilly (1975) suggests some behaviors that might prove beneficial to handicapped students in the mainstream:

1. Specify exactly what the students are to do.

2. Apply sound and consistent behavior management principles.

3. Avoid assumptions that students are being defiant when they do not respond to instructions.

Experience with Project PERMIT indicated several other teacher behaviors:

1. Model the behavior toward handicapped students that is expected from nonhandicapped students.

2. Be relaxed around handicapped students and treat them as any other student.

3. Do not be overly helpful when a student is trying a new skill. Allow time for practice.

4. Try not to focus on disabled students all the time.

5. Emphasize individualization within the class.

Communicating with Parents

Parents may have fears of their child being injured in physical education, or of being teased. An open line of communication can help to alleviate some of the fears parents may have regarding mainstreaming. Hardman, Egan, and Landau (1981) suggest that the following guidelines be used when meeting or communicating with parents. The physical educator needs to:

- Be a good listener, actually listening to what parents are trying to say.
- Speak in language that the parents can understand and feel at ease with.
- Emphasize that the parents are a part of the team and that their input is valued.
- Key discussions as much to the positive as possible.
- Compliment parents for taking an interest in their child's physical education program.
- Be specific about how the parents can be of assistance with the child's physical education program.

Bennett and Henson (1977) further suggest methods of preparing for a parent meeting. Their suggestions can be applied to adapted and regular physical education teachers. They recommend the following procedures:

- Decide on the purpose of the meeting and clearly state it to the parents.
- Review the physical education progress and status of the handicapped student.
- Be prepared to present information about the student's performance.
- Specify precisely how parents can aid in the implementation of their child's program.

These points are illustrated in the following example:

Shelly

Mr. and Mrs. Corey and the multidisciplinary team decide that their daughter, Shelly, a 12-year-old Down's Syndrome girl, could be mainstreamed for conditioning activities, dance, rhythmics, and the special exercise program for overweight students to meet her physical education goals and objectives. The rest of the physical education program would be within a self-contained physical education class conducted by the adapted physical education teacher. Shelly is a very pleasant and cooperative girl and most students enjoy having her in class. The priority goals for physical education in Shelly's IEP are to increase physical fitness levels and reduce her weight by 15 pounds, as advised by the family doctor.

Both the regular and adapted physical education teachers realized that unless Shelly's parents helped with the program at home, it would be difficult for them to meet the priority goals. The physical education teachers decided to have a parent conference with Shelly's parents. Shelly had participated in her M-Team meeting and did not like the idea of having to lose weight since she enjoyed eating snacks. All knew this would not be an easy goal to attain.

The objectives of the meeting were decided by the physical education teachers. They concluded that the main objective was to provide Shelly's parents with ideas for implementing the program at home. The parents needed some guidelines in helping with the conditioning and weight management program.

The teachers prepared a report of Shelly's current status in physical education which included her physical fitness progress, weight, and her performance thus far in the mainstreamed class.

The adapted physical education teacher arranged an after-school conference with Mr. and Mrs. Corey. The meeting was held in the teacher's office. Chairs were arranged in a semicircle so that participants could openly communicate with one another. The physical education teachers and Shelly's parents felt that if the conditioning and weight reduction program were to be successful, the parents would have to implement some activities at home and provide low calorie snacks for Shelly. Also, a system of rewards would be developed to motivate Shelly to eat low calorie snacks and to do some exercises at home. The parents agreed that this should be done and requested some ideas from the teachers. They decided that a contract system would be the best motivating approach. The contract would be helpful in specifying exactly what the parents would need to do and what the teachers would do. The contract was discussed and agreed upon by both the parents and the teachers.

Exhibit 9–1 Sample Parent Contract

PARENT CONTRACT

Teacher: I, Mr. Martin, will continue with conditioning exercises and provide an award chart for completing the exercises.

Parents: We, Mr. and Mrs. Corey, will take at least four afternoon walks of one half mile each with Shelly, and provide low calorie snacks after school.

Teacher Signature ⎯⎯⎯⎯⎯⎯⎯⎯⎯

Parents Signature ⎯⎯⎯⎯⎯⎯⎯⎯

Date ⎯⎯⎯⎯⎯⎯⎯

Exhibit 9–1 shows the contract developed between the teachers and Shelly's parents.

The contracting system can provide an open road to communication since the contract can be discussed and revised if both parties agree. This also helps the parents feel more of a part of the educational team. Such an approach is much more effective than telling parents what to do and not giving them any part in the decision making about their child's program.

Parents can also be involved in developing materials and activities for simulations. This is a chance for parents to have an active role in preparing the regular physical education class before the handicapped student is actually mainstreamed.

Once handicapped students have been mainstreamed, an end-of-the-year demonstration can be given to show what the classes have accomplished.

Teaching Strategies

Good attitudes and good intentions are not enough. They need to be put into practice. Grosse (1978) recommends several strategies for working with handicapped students in the mainstreamed classroom.

1. Make handicapped students aware of safety procedures.

2. Keep expectations high regarding the achievement of handicapped students.

3. Be sure that handicapped students have even amounts of drill, practice, and play activities.

4. Note everyone's contribution to an activity.

5. Practice positive behavior management strategies.

6. Have a variety of equipment available to meet individual needs.

7. Stress the importance of participation rather than winning.

8. Be ready to change a teaching method when one is not working.

9. Modify rules in games where appropriate.

10. Increase the number of players in an activity.

11. Decrease the playing areas.

12. Emphasize games that allow successful noncompetitive experiences.

POINTS TO REMEMBER

1. The goals of special physical education are similar to the goals of regular physical education.

2. The attainment of program goals may be affected by several variables, including administrative support and qualifications of the special physical education service provider.

3. Facilities and equipment are important but good programs can exist and be developed with minimal facilities and with teacher-made equipment. Support for the program can be expanded with public relations.

4. Continued communication and information about the special physical education program lead to public support.

5. Participation in the least restrictive environment can be a very successful experience if preplanning and communication among professionals and parents occur.

6. Teachers should take the initiative and responsibility for developing a receptive environment for disabled students.

7. Providing students with knowledge and straightforward answers to questions will have a positive effect on attitudes toward disabled students.

8. Each school should have a plan for implementing the least restrictive environment once the amount of time to be spent in the regular classroom has been determined.

9. Parents are more likely to get involved in the implementation portion of their handicapped child's physical education program if an open line of communication exists between the parents and the school.

10. Once the disabled student has been placed in the least restrictive setting with regular peers, strategies that focus on individual achievement versus group comparisons should be implemented.

REFERENCES

Barnes, E., Berrigan, C., & Biklen, D. (1977). *What's the difference? Teaching positive attitudes toward people with disabilities.* Syracuse, NY: Human Policy Press.

Bennett, L.M., & Henson, F.O. (1977). *Keeping in touch with parents: The teacher's best friend.* Austin, TX: Learning Concepts.

Bookbinder, S. (1977). What every child needs to know. *The Exceptional Parent, 7,* 31–35.

Crowe, W.C., Auxter, D., & Pyfer, J. (1981). *Principles and methods of adapted physical education and recreation* (4th ed.). St. Louis: C.V. Mosby.

Durley, M.W. (1981). *A resource guide outline for mainstreaming in physical education.* Unpublished Master's thesis, Tennessee Technological University, Cookeville, TN.

Folio, M.R. (1983). Project PERMIT annual report. Tennessee Technological University, Cookeville, TN.

Folio, M.R., & Norman, A. (1981). Toward more success in mainstreaming: A peer teacher approach to physical education. *Teaching Exceptional Children, 13*, 110–114.

Folio, M.R., & Norman, A. (1982). Strategies for obtaining physical education program support. Unpublished manuscript. Tennessee Technological University, Cookeville, TN.

Glass, R.M., Christiansen, J., & Christiansen, J.L. (1982). *Teaching exceptional students in the regular classroom.* Boston: Little, Brown.

Grosse, S.J. Mainstreaming the physically handicapped student for team sports. *Practical Pointers* No. 8. Reston, VA: American Alliance for Health, Physical Education, Recreation and Dance.

Guidelines for professional preparation programs for personnel involved in physical education and recreation for the handicapped. (1973). Washington, DC: American Alliance for Health, Physical Education, Recreation and Dance.

Hardman, M.L., Egan, M.W., & Landau, E.D. (1981). *What will we do in the morning? The exceptional student in the regular classroom.* (2nd ed.). Dubuque, IA: William C. Brown.

Jansma, P., & French, R. (1982). *Special physical education.* Columbus, OH: Charles E. Merrill.

Johnson, M.J., & Cartwright, C.A. (1979). The roles of information and experience: Improving teachers' knowledge and attitudes about mainstreaming. *Journal of Special Education, 4*, 453–462.

Kids on the Block. (1983). Washington, DC: Kids on the Block, Inc.

Krech, D., Crutchfield, R.S., & Bellachey, E. (1962). *Individual and society: A textbook of social psychology.* New York: McGraw-Hill.

Lilly, S.M. (1975). Special education—A cooperative effort. *The Education Digest, 3*, 11–15.

Shotel, J.R., Iano, R., & McGettigan, J. (1972). Teacher attitudes associated with the integration of handicapped children. *Exceptional Children, 38*, 637–683.

Stephens, T.M., & Braun, B.L. (1980). Measures of regular classroom teachers' attitudes toward handicapped children. *Exceptional Children, 46*, 292–294.

Thurman, R.L. (1980). Mainstreaming: A concept general educators should embrace: *The Education Forum*, 285–288.

Wiseman, D.D. (1982). *A practical approach to adapted physical education.* Reading, MA: Addison-Wesley.

Woodward, D.M. (1981). Mainstreaming the learning disabled adolescent. Rockville, MD: Aspen Systems Corporation.

Part IV

Methods and Strategies of Good Teaching

Chapter 10

Noncategorized Teaching Methods

Focus

- Provides methods of teaching that may be applied across categories of handicapped students.
- Discusses organizing and structuring the physical education classroom to allow for maximum participation.
- Explains the use of task analysis for teaching disabled students.
- Discusses behavior management strategies.

Some characteristics overlap among handicapped students, although the causes of disability may be different. This is particularly true among mild to moderately handicapped students. Since similar behaviors and characteristics may be present in several students at the same time, there are general teaching methods and strategies that can be used across categories of handicapping conditions.

Strategies that can be used with a number of different handicapped students include the use of behavior management, task analysis, peer tutors, and relaxation approaches. This chapter is designed to provide the reader with the techniques of these strategies and their application across handicapping conditions.

Teaching strategies are those methods, adaptations, and modifications that teachers may employ to assist handicapped students in learning a motor or physical skill. Strategies can be applied in general. However, some are best suited to a particular type of disabled student. Thus, there are two major approaches to be used. A noncategorized approach deals more with behaviors. In this instance teaching can be applied in a more generalized approach. On the other hand, children with severe disabilities or a disability, such as blindness, that is more unique, will require a specific strategy, such as large print when visual aids are used. This approach to teaching is more categorized in nature, where strategies are selected and implemented based on the unique characteristics of a particular handicapping condition. Ideally, an approach using both is most effective. For instance, a visually impaired student may need a sighted guide while running (a strategy unique to the disability) but also several behavior managment strategies (a strategy unique to his or her behavior).

The teacher should take into account both approaches to teaching and employ the strategies that are best suited to the disabled student. This chapter concerns itself with the noncategorized approach, while Chapter 11 deals with categorized strategies of teaching.

ORGANIZING AND STRUCTURING THE PHYSICAL EDUCATION CLASSROOM

The structure and organization of the physical education classroom are keys to effective teaching and to beneficial participation by handicapped students. Sometimes standard methods of classroom organization may require modification to allow for individual differences in students.

Classroom Environment

Whether physical education is taught indoors, outdoors, or both, the environment should be attractive and as clutter free as possible. Playing areas should be clearly designated with ample room to accommodate the class size. All physical education facilities need to be accessible by students in wheelchairs. All students should be able to feel that the physical education class is an accepting and successful place to go. Lighting should be adequate and ventilation functioning properly.

Classroom Organization

A classroom that is well organized will allow the handicapped student to have successful experiences in physical education. Many ways of organizing the classroom are available. The key to success is flexibility. If the teacher sees that one form of organization is not working, other forms should be tried until the right combination of organization and procedures is discovered.

Personal Space

Personal space is a form of organization where students are free to move in their own personal areas, where they can sit, stand, lie down, or move without touching another student. This eliminates having to keep students in lines or other formations. When students learn the concept of personal space, formations such as lines and circles are less difficult to manage. There are several benefits of using the personal space concept:

- Students appear to feel less self-conscious when trying new skills.
- Students feel more secure when in their personal space than in lines or other formations.
- Students feel freer to explore movements and skills while in their personal space.
- The teacher can work with students individually with less observation from other students.
- Students can work more at their own pace, since they feel more confident.

Peer Teachers

Peer teachers provide an excellent way for modeling behavior and skills for handicapped students. They also offer a wide variety of resources for the physical education teacher.

The Peer Teacher as a Model

The importance of providing a model in the learning of motor skills cannot be overstated. Bandura (1969) has researched the effects of modeling on learning behaviors and skills. Findings support the notion that when modeling techniques are used correctly, they can enhance learning. Children are great imitators. Thus, using peers as models has significant implications.

To use modeling effectively, the "model" demonstrating the desired behavior or skill should be reinforced for his or her behavior. This is true particularly when the student who is to copy the behavior is watching. The following example illustrates this point.

Suppose the teacher wishes to reward practicing skill drills. First, students must be paired. A student who "goofs off" should be paired with a good peer model, one who listens and does the task. When the model student is working hard on the drill, a reward should be given, particularly when the other student is paying attention to the model. The reward should be something that is meaningful to the students who are watching. If other students begin to copy the model, they should be rewarded. This connects what is desired and its reinforcement. Students will soon get the idea that if they copy the model, they can be reinforced.

Bandura suggests several benefits for modeling and some guidelines for its use:

- Students can learn a behavior or skill that they do not have.
- The models, or peer teachers, should have appeal to the other students. Otherwise, they are unlikely to be imitated.
- Give the student praise or other reinforcement for modeling.
- Modeling is beneficial only if those who are to copy understand the concept of imitating.
- Students who are to imitate the peer need to feel comfortable with the model.

Once modeling has been established with students, peer teachers can be effectively utilized in the following ways:

- one-on-one instruction
- assistance with distributing equipment
- setting examples of acceptable behavior
- relating to students with severe emotional problems
- assistance with record keeping and recording information

Peer Teacher Selection

Selecting peer teachers should be planned and well organized. Not every student is capable of being a peer teacher. Folio and Norman (1981) provide the following guidelines for selecting peer teachers.

- Peer teachers should be able to accept all types of handicapped students.
- A genuine desire to be of assistance to other students and the teacher needs to be present.

- The peer tutor's academic grades should be at a level where short absences from the classroom routine can be allowed for about two 30-minute periods per week.
- The peer teacher should provide assistance to the handicapped student without being overly helpful.

Peer teachers need to be selected using a standard procedure. The physical educator can ask 4th-6th graders in the elementary school, or 11th-12th graders in high school to apply for peer teacher positions.

Students interested in becoming a peer teacher can be asked to write a one-page letter concerning why they want to be peer teachers. The letters should be reviewed and selections made based on the criteria mentioned above. Applicants should then be reviewed in terms of behavior, grades, and parental permission.

After those selected have been notified and permission has been obtained, a training session should be developed to orient the peer teachers.

The teacher should try to involve as many students as possible in the peer teacher program. No peer teacher should be scheduled for more than two 30-minute periods per week.

Peer Teacher Preparation

Peer teacher training sessions should be used to orient the student about several factors. These points should be covered:

- Types of handicapping conditions that will be encountered should be discussed.
- Experiences of teaching some of the activities the physical education teacher will be presenting should be provided.
- Basic teaching strategies should be reviewed and practiced.
- Behavior management techniques to be used should be reviewed.
- Safety procedures should be taught.

The teacher will find that eager peer teachers will not need intense instruction. They generally will follow the teacher's behavior and ask many questions. They also seem to have a natural feel for working with handicapped students.

Long, Irmer, Burkett, Glasenapp, and Odenkirk (1980) described a nationally recognized program to aid handicapped students in physical education known as Project PEOPEL (Physical Education Opportunity Program for Exceptional Learners). This program is designed to provide a successful physical education experience for exceptional learners. The major goal of Project PEOPEL is to provide exceptional learners with an equal opportunity for health, social, and recreational benefits of physical education through individualized instruction. This is made possible by using trained student assistants. The main features of Project PEOPEL include:

- trained student aides to assist handicapped students in physical education activities
- small class sizes
- regular physical education equipment and facilities, instead of adapted approaches
- individualized instruction
- progress at the student's own rate without segregation into self-contained classrooms

Volunteer Aides

Volunteer aides are not the same as peer teachers. These include adults who may or may not be involved in actual teaching. Aides may volunteer their time for one event or be ongoing for specified activities and times. Some of the activities in which aides may be involved include:

- assisting with bulletin boards and adapting equipment
- preparing materials
- making motivational charts and posters
- assisting with special events, i.e., Special Olympics, PTA shows, and field trips

Stations Teaching

Stations teaching is a modification or adaptation of circuit teaching, in which students move from station to station performing sets of specified skills or exercises. Stations teaching includes a broader range of activities than exercise alone.

Stations teaching has many benefits for the student and the teacher. Students can work at their own rate, peer teachers can monitor stations, and students may return to a particular station to master a task.

Some organization and time is involved in designing and planning stations but the benefits are well worth the effort. This approach may be used with almost any level of student. Older students will not require as much supervision at each station. Handicapped students may need only a peer teacher or a buddy assigned to aid at each station. Severely handicapped students can also be taught using this format. However, one-on-one teaching is necessary.

Several factors need to be considered before designing and developing stations. These include:

- adequate space to accommodate from six to eight stations for a class of 20 to 24 students
- adequate room for safety
- ample equipment for each station

- enough personnel or aides to manage students needing individual attention
- creativity in designing stations to motivate students
- instruction about what is to be done at each station before beginning

Winnick (1979) suggests that stations for young students have a theme such as a "trip to the woods." The same idea can be used with older mentally retarded students whose mental ages are at a preschool and first grade level.

Stations need to have a purpose, such as development of fundamental motor patterns, problem solving, practice in specific motor skills, physical fitness, or whatever the teacher deems appropriate. It is wise to sketch on paper what stations are needed and their arrangement. Each station should then be arranged at an appropriate location and be clearly marked. Markers can be of a variety of materials including numbers, letters, cones or cans filled with dirt or gravel, flags, colored cards. Brief instructions or illustrations of what is to be accomplished at each station can be included. Also, recordings of instructions can be provided. Taped music can be used if necessary. Pictures of students also are helpful, particularly for motivating students.

Tape and/or footprints on the floor should be used to indicate the direction in which the students should move to proceed to the next station (*Practical Pointers*, 1977). Activity checklists can be provided so that students can check off the activity completed.

Stations can be changed by adding a variety of activities at the same stations. To accommodate handicapped students, equipment of various forms that the handicapped student can use successfully should be included at each station. Simplified instructions should be posted and instructions for those with sensory losses should be available.

Stations can be used with aquatics instruction as well. The possibilities for their use are unlimited. Teachers should use their imagination and creativity to attract students to stations teaching.

TASK ANALYSIS

An excellent skill for successful teaching with handicapped students is task analysis. The physical educator needs to be able to task analyze motor skills into their components or small sequential steps in order to teach the skill to the handicapped student. Usually, the more severely handicapped the student, the more subtasks are necessary in teaching the skill. Task analysis also involves the establishment of prerequisite skills for a particular task. This enables the teacher to:

- determine entry levels for handicapped students, or where to begin teaching

Table 10–1 Task Analysis of Hopping

	Goal: Develop Skill at Hopping on One Foot	
Prerequisite Skills	*Body Position*	*Initiation of Movement*
• Vestibular functions intact • Balance (static/ dynamic) • Jumps on two feet • Leg strength	• Leg positions • Body alignment over base of support	• Arms used to begin movement with legs • Body elevation • Force absorbed on landing • Leg bent slightly to absorb force • Arms used for balance • Balance maintained

- develop a sequential skill progression
- establish and pinpoint behavioral objectives for mastering a goal
- measure and document progress in small gains
- observe and note where weakness in performance of a particular skill exists

Table 10–1 explains how a task analysis of a particular skill might be accomplished. Since the implementation of computers in schools, many forms of software are now becoming available with many kinds of skills already task analyzed. Special education teachers are beginning to be familiar with this new software. The physical education teacher will no doubt have available all types of task analysis of motor skills in software for computer use. Several curricula are available also that have been task analyzed. Dr. Janet Wessel has produced a series with the skills task analyzed. These are available from Hubbard Publishers, P.O. Box 104, Northbrook, IL. Included in the series are:

- *I CAN: Aquatics*
- *I CAN: Fundamental Skills*
- *I CAN: Health and Fitness*
- *I CAN: Sport, Leisure and Recreational Skills*

Another example of a curriculum where skills are task analyzed is the *Ohio State University Scale of Intra Gross Motor Assessment* developed by Loovis and Ersing (1979). Included is the *Performance Based Curriculum,* which has a series of progressive instructional activities related to 11 basic motor skills. This is available from Ohio Motor Assessment Associates, Cleveland Heights, OH.

An illustration might be helpful for understanding how task analysis is applied. After identifying entry levels, or what skills the student presently has, the teacher should delineate the terminal behavior or goal, then derive a sequence of the components of the skills.

Bob

Bob is a tenth grade student with mild learning problems and some coordination difficulty, particularly with complex movements and speed. He dearly loves basketball. After assessing basketball skills, the instructor finds that Bob can dribble while stationary, pass accurately within 10 feet of another player, and make about 50 percent of two-handed shots within 10 feet of the basket.

The instructor should identify some terminal goals. These might include:

- Makes a lay-up shot.
- Shoots foul shots.
- Dribbles while running.
- Rebounds.

After a goal has been identified, the sequence of components for this goal should be developed. The teacher should ask what steps are necessary to master this skill. The components for, say, making a lay-up shot may include:

- Grasps ball properly.
- Dribbles and bounces ball while stationary.
- Dribbles the ball while moving.
- Shoots ball one handed.
- Dribbles and shoots ball one handed.
- Releases ball with followthrough.

If the teacher will actually go through the task, an analysis of the skill can be made by carefully noting all the components.

Prerequisite skills should be established. These might include, in this case:

- Is familiar with a basketball.
- Is familiar with the game.
- Knows and recognizes a basketball.

Tasks can be broken into as many components as are necessary for the student to learn the task. In this case, the actual sequence for shooting can be included.

Once the prerequisite skills are considered and the sequence has been arranged, instruction can begin, precisely at the point at which the student has mastered each component. Using the task analysis approach, the teacher is able to pinpoint an exact starting and ending point for instruction. In the example provided, Bob already knows some components of the task. Shooting a lay-up in terms of the form for the lay-up are his weak points. Thus, the teacher might want to select the lay-up in a backward chaining approach. This means that the actual shot itself is the beginning point, with the instruction proceeding backward. The lay-up is done first, then two steps, then a dribble is added. The procedure is repeated until the student can complete a dribble and lay-up shot.

TEACHING SEQUENCE

The proper teaching sequence for motor skills involves planning, knowledge, and organization. First the teacher must be able to plan effectively.

Planning includes several steps:

- assessing needs
- establishing priorities related to needs
- designing activities
- developing a behavior management strategy

Knowledge that the physical educator has related to content and handicapping conditions aids in pulling together the plan developed. This broad general knowledge provides the basis for implementation of the plan.

Organization provides the basis for keeping the teaching sequence in order and running smoothly. A plan can appear to be well designed but if it is not organized, it will not run smoothly. Organization requires consideration of:

- class structure
- equipment
- regular and/or modified activities
- teaching strategies

BEHAVIOR MANAGEMENT STRATEGIES

Students can, at one point or another, cause disruptions in the classroom or become unmotivated to learn. Some types of handicapped students for one reason or another can have disturbing behavior problems. This is not to suggest, however, that all handicapped students are a problem to the physical education teacher. Consistent classroom management also provides structure, which some handicapped students need to be successful. A point to remember is that not all behavior problems or lack of motivation are the student's fault. In some instances of failure, behavior problems are initiated and sustained by the teacher.

Essentially, positive classroom management, if properly applied, will extinguish undesirable behavior and performance and increase desirable student behavior.

"What Goes Here"

Undesirable behavior may occur unintentionally by students because they do not understand what is expected by the teacher. Sometimes students become confused when they

have two or more teachers, particularly if expectations are different from teacher to teacher. Other factors that affect behavior and performance include:

- family-rearing practices
- cultural styles
- organic or medical conditions
- psychological disorders
- learning and reinforcement for inappropriate behaviors

Whatever the cause, there is little that the physical educator can do to change it in many cases. There are, on the other hand, many management strategies that may be used to elicit and maintain desirable behavior and motivation among handicapped students.

Once the physical educator understands and can consistently implement a classroom management program, more favorable conditions occur for learning in physical education. Some of the techniques of classroom behavior management involve principles of reinforcement, motivation, contingency management, and contracting.

Management Guidelines

Affleck, Lowenbraun, and Archer (1980) recommend procedures that will lead to students' understanding of expected behavior in the physical education setting. These principles have also been applied in a mainstreaming model physical education program by Folio and Norman (1981). Another method of classroom management, similar to that of Affleck et al. was developed by Madsen, Becker, and Thomas (1968). It is called the RAID model of behavior management. RAID stands for Rules, Approval, Ignoring, and Disapproval. From an examination of the RAID model its applications for behavior management in the physical education class can be understood.

Rules

Rules in the physical education classroom help students to learn what behavior and tasks the teacher expects. Madsen et al. (1968) suggest several principles that should be applied when making rules.

- Rules should be briefly stated and in positive form.
- Rules should be stated in language that is appropriate for the mental age of the student. Signs and symbols can be used if necessary along with each rule.
- The behavior or rule that is desired should be stated precisely. For example:
  Try to do each activity.
  Put equipment away after use.
  Complete all drills and activities.

Work with other students.
Listen when others have permission to talk.
Follow all safety rules.
Work in your personal space.

- Rules should not be too long, nor should there be too many.
- Rules should be posted where students can be reminded of them.
- The teacher should go over the rules.

Rules have to be reinforced by the teacher to motivate students to follow them. It is important not to state rules negatively since this form only tells the student what not to do. The student needs to know what exactly gets reinforcement.

Approval of Desired Behavior

Van Etten, Arkell, and Van Etten (1980) explain that an event which follows a behavior and increases its occurrence is known as positive reinforcement. Many forms of reinforcement are available, such as smiles, verbal praise, attention, food, etc. The physical educator should be aware that what is reinforcing to one student may not be reinforcing to another. Thus, it is very important to determine what reinforcers work with specific students.

Finding the Right Reward

The physical education teacher may need to do some detective work to establish what rewards are effective with different students. Several clues may be obtained by:

- observing the students and what they respond to that increases their behavior: smiles, hugs, attention, points, etc.
- asking the students what they like
- surveying the students by helping them complete a rewards checklist
- asking other personnel and parents what works with particular students

Reinforcers can be classified in several ways, depending on the level of the reward. Reinforcers typically fall into four categories: social, activity types, tangible, and edible. Combinations of reinforcers may need to be used with various levels of students. Social rewards should always be paired with other types of reinforcers. Table 10–2 lists types of reinforcers.

It is very important for the teacher to reward behavior frequently in the beginning and then less frequently once the behavior is learned. Essentially, with this method the purpose is to go from teacher-directed behavior to student self-

Table 10–2 Classifications of Reinforcers

	Social	Tangible	Activity	Food
Preschool or elementary level	Smile Hug/pat Tickle "Great!"	Paper Crayons Toys	Helper Choice of activity Leader Free time	Fruit Cereal Drink
Upper elementary or secondary level	"Thumbs up!" "Good job!" "Way to go!" "Terrific!" "You are super!"	Rental of equipment Sports Magazine Certificate Good note to home	Choice of activity Listening to a record Game tickets Peer teacher	Juice Milk Fruit Peanut butter Popcorn

directed behavior. It is best for the student to be internally motivated. Table 10–3 illustrates the teacher-directed to student-directed model.

Walker and Shea (1980) emphasize that a social reinforcer should always be paired with other types of reinforcers. Also, as the behavior is learned, reinforcement needs to be varied by giving it only after so many behaviors or responses or after variable intervals of time have passed.

Contracting

Another method of establishing desired responses from students is contracting. Written contracts are concrete and tend to motivate students somewhat better than verbal contracts (Walker & Shea, 1980). Contracts are particularly good for students who have difficulty with the expectations and rewards. Lewis and Doorlag (1983) define a contingency contract as a form of agreement, in writing, between the student and teacher that specifies exactly what the student is to do to receive a reward. Contracts must be carefully developed. Some steps for the teacher to follow include:

Table 10–3 Teacher-Directed to Student-Directed Behavior

Teacher-Directed Behavior	Student-Initiated Responses	Student-Directed Behavior
Desired behaviors are defined Reinforcement applied	Student initiates desired behavior Reinforcement continuous/ partial	Student does the behavior for self-satisfaction

Exhibit 10–1 Sample Contract

Date: _____

Contract for Gymnastics

___Student's Name___ agrees to complete a routine on the balance beam that includes at least five different skills.

_____   _____
Start Date   End Date

___Teacher's Name___ agrees to let Student's Name be a student helper for one week.

_____   _____
Teacher's Signature   Student's Signature

Exhibit 10–2 Sample Certificate

HAPPY GRAM

TO TOMMY SMITH   FROM (Teacher's name)

MRS. SMITH,
TOMMY REALLY TRIED HARD TODAY IN PHYSICAL EDUCATION CLASS AND I AM VERY PROUD OF HIM!

_____   _____
TEACHER'S NAME   DATE

- setting a time to discuss the contract
- explaining that the contract is to help the student be more successful
- negotiating and developing the agreement

The contract itself should have several characteristics:

- The contract should be simple and to the point.
- The reward in the contract should immediately follow the specific behavior or task in the contract.
- The contract should be fair and reasonable.
- A time period should be specified for completing the contract (Lewis & Doorlag, 1983).

Exhibit 10–1 illustrates a sample contract that might be developed in a physical education class. Remember that contracts can be developed to motivate a student, to obtain good behavior, to decrease behavior, or for completing a specified number of tasks. Contracts may also be developed between the teacher and the student's parents when necessary, as we noted in Chapter 9.

Certificates

Everyone enjoys being told they are doing a good job. However, messages given by the teacher are even better! These do not have to be elaborate and the teacher should have several on hand to distribute to the student or to the parents. Suppose that a student is having difficulty with a particular sport and does not wish to participate because of embarrassment. To motivate and reward the student for trying the teacher might give the student a certificate for trying, even if the student did not perform successfully. A certificate might look like the one in Exhibits 10–2 to 10–7.

Exhibit 10–3 Sample Award

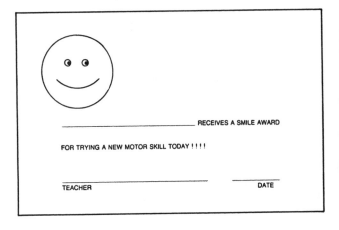

_____ RECEIVES A SMILE AWARD

FOR TRYING A NEW MOTOR SKILL TODAY ! ! ! !

_____   _____
TEACHER   DATE

Exhibit 10–4 Sample Reward

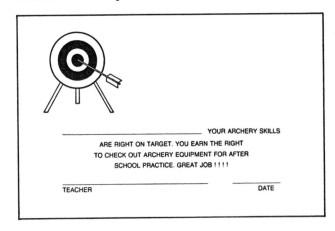

_____ YOUR ARCHERY SKILLS

ARE RIGHT ON TARGET. YOU EARN THE RIGHT
TO CHECK OUT ARCHERY EQUIPMENT FOR AFTER
SCHOOL PRACTICE. GREAT JOB ! ! ! !

_____   _____
TEACHER   DATE

Exhibit 10–5 Sample Helper Award

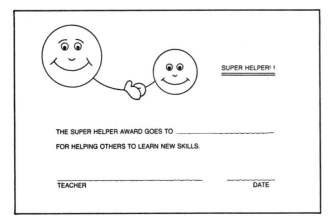

Exhibit 10–6 Sample Weight Management Award

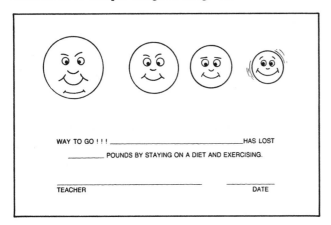

Exhibit 10–7 Sample Parent Notice

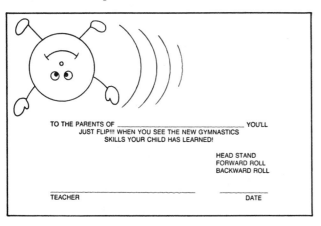

Tangible and Token Rewards

Tangible rewards are usually based on earning a token or specified number of tokens that later can be traded in for a tangible reward or activity. Tokens can take the form of check marks, stars, points, poker chips, marbles, or whatever is available. Points or check marks are easier to manage in a large physical education setting. These can be used with individual students or the entire class. Lewis and Doorlag (1983) recommend several pointers for using a token system.

- Students should know precisely what behaviors will earn them a token.
- Tokens should be used that are commensurate with the students' mental ages.
- A list should be developed of tangibles for which tokens can be cashed. Some activities on the menu should be worth more tokens than others and they should be arranged from the least cost in tokens to the highest.
- Students should be asked for suggestions regarding the tangibles to be included in the selection.
- Students should have frequent opportunities to trade in their tokens. Once or twice a week is best.
- The token needs to be given immediately following the desired student response.

This system can be used with both special needs and regular classroom students. It will take some time to develop, particularly if it was not begun at the beginning of the school year. The teacher will have to be patient and above all consistent. Otherwise, the system will not be effective. Table 10–4 provides an example of a token selection that is often referred to as a menu.

Table 10–4 Sample Token Menu

Reinforcement	Number of Checks or Points
10 minutes of free time	10 points
Leader of an activity	15 points
Leader for a week	25 points
Choice of an activity	35 points
Teacher's Helper	50 points
Check out piece of equipment	50 points
Tickets to a game	100 points
Play game with a friend	100 points
Listen to records	100 points
Physical Education Student of the Week	250 points

Exhibit 10–8 Rental Menu

RENTAL MENU

FRISBEE

BASKETBALL

FOOTBALL

ARCHERY EQUIPMENT

TETHER BALL

SOCCER BALL

HORSESHOES

SOFTBALL AND GLOVES

RECORD PLAYER AND RECORDS

SPORTS MAGAZINE

Ignoring Undesirable Behavior

Teachers are attuned to giving attention to undesirable behavior more than rewarding appropriate kinds of behavior. There are several problems with this approach. First, it establishes a negative environment. Second, the nagging of students who are behaving in an inappropriate way may actually be reinforced by the attention from the teacher and peers. The RAID model suggests that inappropriate behavior be ignored as much as possible. More important, teachers need to indicate exactly what behavior they wish to see decreased or stopped. Generally, behaviors that teachers view as needing to be decreased are:

- fighting, hitting, swearing
- talking out
- inattentiveness
- distractability, hyperactivity
- unsportsmanlike conduct
- abuse of equipment
- not practicing drills
- wearing improper clothing for physical education
- breaking other rules

A teacher might say, "I wish Sue would behave." "Behave" is vague and does not pinpoint what is to be decreased. Perhaps Sue argues constantly during a game. The teacher might define "behave" as decreasing arguing during game play. When the behavior is defined it is more easily changed.

Once the behavior is defined, the teacher can selectively ignore inappropriate responses. However, ignoring cannot occur by itself. While ignoring of inappropriate behaviors is occurring, approval of appropriate behavior must also take place. By approving of the appropriate behavior, the teacher is providing a model for getting rewards. Unfortunately, if the teacher has been nagging a student to "get busy" and then decides to ignore the student, the likelihood of the appropriate behavior occurring is minimal. Actually, the inappropriate behavior is likely to increase for awhile. The teacher will have to be patient at this point and continue to approve of on-task behavior. The following example will illustrate how this might be accomplished.

Teacher: Requests that students practice throwing and catching in small groups. Billy stands and does not participate.

Teacher: Responds by ignoring Billy and goes to Will who is practicing close to Billy. The teacher says, "Will, you are working hard and I like that!"

If this procedure is repeated often enough and in a consistent manner, Billy should eventually get the message that if he wants the teacher's attention, he will have to practice the drill.

Not all inappropriate behaviors can be ignored. Intervention needs to occur immediately when:

- students are endangering themselves
- equipment is being destroyed
- students are so disruptive that the instructional process is impeded
- safety rules are being ignored
- a student is endangering another student

Disapproving Strategies

Various options for showing disapproval of behaviors are available for teachers to use. When the teacher wishes to disapprove, several procedures may be followed that will cause the least amount of disruption.

1. Call the student to the side and tell him or her that you do not approve of the behavior. Specify the exact behavior.

2. Ask the student to tell you what the appropriate behavior should be.

3. Send the student back to the activity and look for positive behavior. As soon as it occurs, reinforce the student.

4. Let the student know that it is the behavior that you do not approve of and the student is O.K. Avoid statements like, "You are my worst-behaved student." "No one is going to like you because you......."

5. Avoid arguing with the student in front of the class.

Timeout is another method of disapproval. Walker and Shea (1980) explain timeout as a method of removal of students from a situation in which reinforcement was being received. Timeout needs to be carefully planned by the teacher and carefully used. When students cannot improve their behavior after other forms of disapproval have been tried, timeout may be necessary. This should be used only when appropriate and not simply to get rid of students for a period of time. To be effective, timeout should be developed with the following conditions in mind:

- The location should be secluded from the classroom but somewhere where the teacher can easily keep an eye on the student.
- There should be no objects or equipment that will keep the student entertained when in a timeout setting.
- Options for a timeout setting can be a corner of the gymnasium, a blocked off area of the court or other outside playing area, first or second row of the bleachers.
- Timeout should not occur for more than five minutes. If the student is in timeout too long, chances of earning positive reinforcers are decreased.
- The teacher needs to know the students before using timeout. Some students prefer to be alone and timeout will become reinforcing in itself. Timeout works well with students who like to participate in physical education activities.
- Above all, like other methods of managing behavior, timeout must be used consistently.
- When the teacher gives the student permission to return to the activity, reinforcement should be given when the student returns and behaves appropriately.

Other Methods of Management

The RAID model is effective when used as a general ongoing classroom procedure. However, if the teacher wishes to focus on individuals with more intense needs for behavioral change, other procedures should be followed. There are several principles of behavior change and steps that should be followed in order to modify a student's behavior. (See Table 10–5.) These are recommended when the teacher wishes to be more intense in changing behavior with one or two students.

The following example can be used to illustrate these steps.

Table 10–5 Modifying Student Behavior

Step	Analysis
Step 1	• Identify the behavior to be changed. • Be very specific. • The behavior should be in measurable terms.
Step 2	• Let the student try out the task or objective. • Note errors and successful portions of the task. • Determine, after observation, what the student's skill level is related to the task.
Step 3	• Determine the steps, in sequence, that the student could do in relation to the task.

Objective: The student will be able to kick a goal in soccer, including the elements of the task, five out of five times.

Step 1. The objective has been specifically stated.

Step 2. The student is asked to perform the skill of kicking the ball. The student can kick the ball, but not accurately, has difficulty controlling the ball, dribbles, but cannot put the movement sequence together.

Step 3. The teacher should develop the sequential steps to be learned to kick the goal. The student has some of the elements of the task but cannot put them together. The student needs to practice the following steps:

- Receive a pass and control the ball with the feet.
- Student already dribbles.
- Practice kicking goal.

The student can practice each sequence in the task that is unknown, then put the elements together to complete the task. These include:

- Moves toward goal.
- Receives pass.
- Controls ball.
- Dribbles toward goal.
- Aligns body and ball.
- Kicks goal.

Each of the elements can become subobjectives of the objective. This allows the teacher to measure the student's skill level in precise steps. This works well for any student, but where progress is slow, the subobjectives can be used to document progress toward achieving the target objective.

Linking Skill Components

As we have seen, chaining is a technique used to link together components of a task. This is used when students have some degree of skill related to some task components.

Chaining can occur from the beginning to the last step in the task, or from the last step to the first step. Both methods are effective. The FIRST to LAST step approach is used when the student has some of the elements, as in the example noted. The LAST to FIRST step approach can be used if the student can do the last step but few or none of the other elements of the task. This technique would apply if a student could stand at a basket and do the last part of the lay-up shot. The teacher could then work backward because the task has fairly discrete steps that can be taught, such as:

- Extends arms and shoots lay-up portion.
- Teach two steps, add shot.
- Teach dribble, add step, then shot.
- Dribbles, steps, then shoots.

Prompting

Rowbury, Baer, and Baer (1976) suggest several methods of using prompts to teach a skill. Prompting is a procedure that uses cues to bring about the desired behavior. The cues used in prompting can be strong or weak. Physical prompts are considered strong, where the teacher actually moves the body parts or physically guides the learner in the task. Verbal prompts or gestures are weaker than physical prompts. Prompts can be paired for students having difficulty learning a new task. A verbal prompt (telling the student), a visual prompt (demonstration), and a manual prompt (guiding the student's movement) can all be paired. Eventually, prompts should be faded or reduced. An example of fading is beginning with a manual prompt, then using only a verbal prompt.

This method of changing behavior and skills can be used with any student. The more severe the handicapping condition, however, the more structured fading and prompting have to be.

Shaping

Shaping is a systematic process of providing reinforcers for behavior or skill levels that come closer and closer to the end result or desired result. Shaping behavior is used more frequently with students who have more severe disabilities. This method works well when students do not pay attention to a stimulus, such as a ball or the teacher's voice or make eye contact.

For instance, the teacher may want a student to look at a ball in order to get ready to catch it. The student, however, prefers to attend to other objects, or not look at all. The teacher may call to the student, and if the student looks toward the teacher or the ball the student gets a reinforcer. Then, the student gets reinforced for looking more closely toward the ball, then for focusing on the ball, then for focusing for so many seconds. This way, each successive attempt to look at the ball is rewarded.

Shaping is a slow procedure and should be used carefully. The teacher should not expect fast results with this method of instruction. If another method of behavior management can be used more effectively, it should be employed. Sometimes shaping may not work because the teacher reinforces the wrong behavior or isn't distinct enough in applying it.

Punishment

Punishment may be effective in decreasing inappropriate behavior. However, it is often used ineffectively in physical education classrooms. Teachers may tend to punish on an inconsistent basis and confuse students. Walker and Shea (1980) define two forms of punishment that are commonly used. One is the addition of some adversive condition such as physical manipulation. Physical educators sometimes make students do a large number of exercises as a punishment. It seems very unwise to use in this way activities that you want students to appreciate.

The other form of punishment is removal of a desirable or pleasurable condition, event, or activity. The teacher may not allow the student to play a game or to participate in a special class activity. Points that have been earned may be taken away.

Often, punishment is too severe or not severe enough. Or the teacher may decide to punish one student and not another for the same behavior. In some instances, punishment may actually be reinforcing because attention in some form is better than no attention at all.

The physical educator needs to think carefully before administering punishment. Punishment is effective in decreasing undesirable behavior but only on a short-term basis in most cases. If punishment is decided upon as the means for dealing with inappropriate behavior, the physical educator should follow these guidelines.

- Punishment must immediately follow the behavior to be stopped or decreased.
- Students must know precisely what behavior is being punished.
- Punishment should not be administered when strong emotions by the teacher are active.
- The punishment should be readily available so that it can be administered quickly and easily.
- The person who gives the punishment should also be the one who provides positive reinforcement.

If punishment is used properly, and as a last resort for managing behavior, it will be effective. The teacher should keep in mind that punishment can produce undesirable side effects for several reasons.

- It may make the punished student behave toward others in a punishing way.

- Punishment that is too severe may cause anxiety and emotional fears, particularly among the primary- and elementary-level student.
- Punishment will stop inappropriate behavior but possibly also other behavior associated with it. For example, if a student is punished for not following directions for doing a headstand, the student may withdraw from other gymnastics activities.

RELAXATION ACTIVITIES

Arnheim and Sinclair (1979) explain that relaxed musculature is a prerequisite for executing coordinated movements. Stressing relaxation also can help the students to become more aware of tension and methods for reducing it. This ultimately enables the student to gain control and management of his or her body.

Many students who are emotionally disturbed, overly excitable, or neurologically impaired may have an abnormal amount of muscular tension that can interfere with coordinated movement. Eventually, these students need to learn internal control and management of tension. By providing the students with relaxation techniques, the physical educator will enable them to feel more in control of their own emotional reactions. In addition, a relaxation activity that follows a vigorous activity will aid the students in regaining control. If students who are prone to excitability can learn to recognize tension, they may be allowed to practice relaxation in a quiet corner and maintain their own control. This can eliminate many teacher-student conflicts.

When having students go through relaxation activities large amounts of equipment are not necessary. A carpeted space or mats need to be provided. A record or tape player is a plus, although not totally necessary. The location should be uncluttered and relatively free from noise.

Visualization

Using visualization of various scenes can provide a set mental attitude for the student to begin relaxation. The teacher will need to have the students try to imagine or pretend relaxing scenes that they can understand. The teacher can ask the students to visualize and imagine the following:

- rocking slowly in a swing
- rocking in a boat
- floating on a raft in a pool
- gliding like a bird
- swinging in a hammock
- riding on a cloud
- watching a candle flicker

Breathing Techniques

As students are visualizing relaxing scenes, they should be told to breathe deeply and slowly. Ten inhales and exhales is a good amount. Breathing will help students to focus on their own bodies. After the students have visualized for two to three minutes, the teacher can begin to focus on tensing and relaxing the entire body, then specific body segments, and eventually body parts.

It will be difficult to reach all levels of relaxation with every student. The important point is to teach students to control and manage themselves whenever possible. Some students will not be able to relax totally on their own after training due to the severity of the handicapping conditions. In these cases, the instructor will need to take a more active role.

Relaxing the Entire Body

The instructor will need to ask students to do the following activities. If verbal instruction is not sufficient, demonstration may be necessary. The teacher should try these activities:

1. Have students make their bodies stiff like a board and hold the posture for five to ten seconds, then repeating two or three more times.

2. As students learn tensing and releasing, let them practice individually until they can tense and relax the musculature smoothly.

3. Ask students to tense only the lower extremities, then repeat with only the upper extremities.

4. Have students focus on one body part, an arm or leg and so forth until all limbs and the head are tensed and released.

5. Have students think about how good it feels to be relaxed.

Other Activities

In addition to tensing and releasing, students may try other movements and activities that will aid in relaxation:

- swinging or swaying the upper trunk while standing or sitting
- rolling their heads from side to side
- listening quietly to soft music
- rotating ankles and wiggling toes
- rocking (severely handicapped students) on a rocker board, suspended hammock, or swing
- remaining quiet while the limbs are being massaged (severely handicapped students)

POINTS TO REMEMBER

1. Behavior should be thought of in terms of wanting to see it increased or decreased.

2. Most behavior can be systematically changed by applying several types of behavior management techniques.

3. Organization of the classroom is a method of managing behavior by providing the appropriate structure and environment.

4. Peer teachers can be an effective means of modeling the appropriate behavior for students to imitate.

5. Models should be individuals that students will want to imitate.

6. Task analysis is an effective means for providing a measurable teaching sequence.

7. Positive classroom management planning and implementation will be effective in reducing unwanted behavior and increasing desired behavior or skill levels.

8. Relaxation training for anxious or overactive students helps them to manage their own tense feelings.

REFERENCES

Affleck, J.Q., Lowenbraun, S., Archer, A. (1980). Teaching the mildly handicapped in the regular classroom. Columbus, OH: Charles E. Merrill.

Arnheim, D.D., & Sinclair, W.A. (1979). *The clumsy child: A program of motor therapy* (2nd ed.). St. Louis: C.V. Mosby.

Bandura, A. (1969). *Principles of behavior modification.* New York: Holt, Rinehart & Winston.

Folio, M.R., & Norman, A. (1981). Toward more success in mainstreaming: A peer teacher approach to physical education. *Teaching Exceptional Children, 13,* 110–114.

Lewis, R.B., & Doorlag, D.H. (1983). Teaching special students in the mainstream. Columbus, OH: Charles E. Merrill.

Long, E., Irmer, L., Burkett, L.N., Glasenapp, G., & Odenkirk, B. (1980). PEOPEL: Trained student aids provide exceptional learners equal opportunities for successful physical education experiences. *Journal of Physical Education and Recreation, 51*(7), 28029.

Loovis, E.M., & Ersing, W.F. (1979). *Assessing and programming gross motor development for children.* Cleveland Heights, OH: Ohio Motor Assessment Associates.

Madsen, C.H., Becker, W.C., & Thomas, R.D. (1968). Rules, praise, and ignoring: Elements of elementary classroom control. *Journal of Applied Analysis, 1,* 139–150.

Practical Pointers. (1977). *Individualized education programs: Methods for individualizing physical education.* Washington, DC: AAHPER Publications.

Rowbury, T.G., Baer, A.M., & Baer, D.M. (1976). Interactions between teacher guidance and contingent access to play in developing preacademic skills of deviant preschool children,. *Journal of Applied Behavior Analysis, 9,* 85–104.

Walker, J.E., & Shea, T.M. (1980). *Behavior modification: A practical approach for educators.* St. Louis: C.V. Mosby.

Winnick, J.P. (1979). *Movement experiences and development: Habilitation and remediation.* Philadelphia: W.B. Saunders.

Van Etten, G., Arkell, C., & Van Etten, C. (1980). The severely and profoundly handicapped: Programs, methods, and materials. St. Louis: C.V. Mosby.

RECOMMENDED READING

Kerr, M.M., & Nelson, C.M. (1983). *Strategies for managing behavior problems in the classroom.* Columbus, OH: Charles E. Merrill.

Popovich, D. (1981). *Behavioral programming for severely and profoundly handicapped students: A manual for teachers and aides.* Baltimore, MD: Brookes.

Walker, J.E., & Shea, T.M. (1980). *Behavior modification: A practical approach for teachers.* St. Louis: C.V. Mosby.

Chapter 11

Methods and Strategies for Categorized Teaching

Focus

- Emphasizes teaching methods that are more specifically geared to the characteristics of specific disabilities.
- Provides explanations and/or examples of the suggested method.

As discussed in Chapter 10, teaching physical and motor skills to exceptional children needs to be approached from two perspectives. The noncategorized method is used when students have similar needs and mild disabilities. Noncategorized teaching cuts across all disabilities and uses approaches that can be applied to all types of exceptional students. These approaches include behavior management and classroom structuring, for example, and they involve techniques that can be used with any disabled student. How they are administered depends on the severity of the disability.

Categorized teaching as discussed in this chapter includes methods and techniques that are more suitable for a specific type of handicapped student, such as learning disabled, moderately retarded, visually impaired, etc. Both approaches can be combined. Behavior management, for example, can be combined with specific techniques more relevant for visually handicapped students. The point is that the teacher needs to have a number of general and specific teaching techniques ready to be implemented with disabled students.

MILDLY RETARDED STUDENTS

Mildly retarded students respond well to general approaches and those geared to their specific physical and mental abilities. While most mildly retarded students can be integrated into regular physical education settings, specific teaching techniques geared to their particular needs will be more effective in enabling them to achieve. The following techniques and methods should be used with mildly retarded youth:

1. Directions and social expectations should be geared to the student's mental age. Physically, the student may not differ significantly from peers, but mental age and social maturity may require that activities be presented in smaller sequences or that the student be placed in a smaller group.

2. Motor activities should be coordinated with academic concepts. For instance, if the classroom teacher is working on measurement with a ruler, yardstick, or tape, the student should be allowed to help measure jumps, throws for distance, etc., in the physical education class. If the academic teacher is working on addition, the student should be allowed to help add scores in a game, etc.

3. Cooperative play should be emphasized. Peer models should be used to provide examples of sharing equipment, practicing good sportsmanship, helping other students, or following instructions.

4. Students should be taught how to be on time and start and complete a task. Models can be used for this behavior.

5. Leisure-time activities should be taught to retarded students. They should be asked what they like to play in their leisure time and units of instruction should be based on their choices, such as horseshoes, table tennis, darts, etc.

MODERATELY RETARDED STUDENTS

Moderately retarded youngsters will need more instruction in basic fundamental motor patterns and skills. These students will most often receive instruction in self-contained and regular physical education programs. The following techniques and methods should be used with moderately retarded students.

1. The instructor should present a stronger cue when teaching skills, i.e., brighter colored equipment, lighter weight equipment. For example, a batting tee and lightweight bat may be needed to teach striking.

2. Instructions should be communicated in ways that the student can comprehend. The teacher should use short verbal cues, demonstrate the key elements of a task, and have the student repeat the sequence with assistance.

3. Gestures should be paired with short verbal instructions. If the teacher wants to emphasize hand position in catching a ball, a verbal hint should be paired with the hand position.

4. Task analysis needs to be applied more in depth than with mildly retarded students since the moderately retarded student will most likely be missing more elements of a fundamental task, such as jumping, hopping, etc.

5. Moderately retarded students will need more teaching of how to anticipate oncoming objects, such as in catching, where to place the body, getting ready to catch, etc. The process of deciding when to respond and how needs to be practiced in addition to the elements of the skill. The teacher can help by asking questions or giving cues like "Get ready," "Put your hands up," "Here comes the ball."

6. Behavior management reinforcers need to be more tangible than those applied with mildly retarded students. Touching or a pat on the back is more effective than verbal praise alone.

7. The social aspects of an activity also need to be practiced. For example, waiting one's turn may have to be taught, or sharing a piece of equipment.

8. Manual or kinesthetic teaching should be used to help the student feel the correct movement. Moderately retarded students can be given additional instructional cues using this technique. Verbal cues, such as "Hands ready," for example, should be used when manually guiding the student's hands in position to catch a ball.

9. The instructor should present one activity at a time to the student but have one or two more that are similar ready to teach. This helps maintain attention.

10. About ten minutes should be spent on an activity. Then it should be changed or varied. A rest period should be given by offering additional instruction or highlighting what was accomplished.

11. Equipment that the student can safely and successfully manage should be used. A NeRF® ball may be more appropriate in the initial stages of catching to prevent injury.

12. A definite and consistent set of class routines should be provided that includes a definite place to be during the beginning of class, personal space, a marker on the floor, etc. A warm up should be accompanied by a record or definite set of exercises.

13. The goal is transfer of skills from one situation to another. Students should practice in different parts of the gym or playing area, practice with different students, with a variety of equipment, such as different sized balls, and incorporate the skill in many different activities.

14. The student should be allowed to try the skill many different ways to foster adaptability. Dynamic balance, for instance, can be made adaptable by having the student try to walk on different width beams, up inclines, down inclines, and on different surfaces. This approach helps the student learn to adapt the skill.

15. Rewards should be very meaningful to the moderately retarded student, such as tokens or physical contact. Verbal praise used along with tangible rewards is more effective.

SEVERELY RETARDED STUDENTS

Severely mentally retarded students will be functioning at levels significantly below their chronological age. Many will need training in motor skills at the preambulatory level. The setting will need to be mostly self contained, with peer tutors brought to the self-contained classroom to assist with instruction. The following techniques and methods should be used with severely mentally retarded students:

1. The teacher must be aware of any physical limitations or activities that should be avoided, consulting with the special education teacher, physicians, parents, and physical therapists if necessary.

2. Sensory stimulation may be necessary before beginning activities. Sensory stimulation is used with severely handicapped students to train them to recognize different sensations and use them with motor skills. Senses of touch, vision, kinesthesis, and auditory awareness should be developed.

Tactile sensations may need to be stimulated to get the student to use touch, the needed skills to use the hands and move. Students may not like to be touched or to touch things. They should be allowed to explore on carpeted surfaces by rolling, creeping, or sliding to use their hands to explore furry stuffed animals, which can be incorporated into exercises. For example, the teacher can ask the students to lift the animal way up high. Thus, stretching can be incorporated into a tactile activity.

Visual stimulation is needed in order to find cues in the environment. Pinlight tracking or other visual stimuli can be used to attract the student's visual attention.

3. *Kinesthetic sensory development* is useful in assisting students with body positioning. Trampolines, inner tubes, and vestibular swings are helpful in arousing the kinesthetic senses. A hammock has also proved to be adequate in training vestibular sensations.

4. *Auditory stimulation* includes sounds made by instruments and the teacher's voice. Implements such as drums, cymbals, toys that make noise, bells, and animal sounds are helpful to respond to in training auditory stimulation.

5. Equipment may have to be specifically designed to meet the motor needs of severely handicapped students.

6. Skills should be broken down into small sequential steps and taught accordingly. Each step should be reinforced. The teacher should choose tests that are designed at a level low enough for low-functioning students and that have accompanying curricula to sequence instructional skills. The *Peabody Developmental Motor Scales* are designed in this manner. Curriculum and criterion-referenced tests of motor development are useful with severely handicapped students. Tests such as the *Peabody Developmental Motor Scales and Activity Cards* provide the standardized as well as criterion-referenced measure needed to develop the type of motor program severely handicapped students require.

7. Table 11–1 is a section of test items on the gross motor section of the *Peabody Developmental Motor Scales* at the six-month level. This measure works well with low-functioning students.

8. The activity cards included can provide the sequential programming needed by this population.

9. The teaching environment should not be overstimulating, especially if the teacher is trying to develop a particular sensory modality.

10. Students in the severely handicapped category will often need physical therapy. Most likely, a therapist will complete an initial assessment and the teacher will implement the prescribed program.

LEARNING DISABLED STUDENTS

Learning-disabled students will have primary difficulty in processing information. Teaching strategies should be geared to perceptual problems and movement disorders. Seaman and DePauw (1982), Geddes (1981), and Fait (1978) offer many suggestions for teaching physical education activities to learning-disabled students:

1. Remove as many distracting objects as possible from the immediate teaching environment.

2. Cratty (1980) suggests having distractable and hyperactive students perform movements as slowly as possible to establish motor control. As an example, the teacher might ask students to walk a balance beam as slowly as possible.

3. Intervene as soon as the student begins to show signs of frustration with an activity. Signs to look for are body lan-

Table 11–1 Gross-Motor Scale

Level	Item	Child's Position	Directions and Criterion
6-7 months continued	33. (B) Sitting	sitting	Release support. Observe balance.
			Criterion: Sits alone for 60 seconds; one of two trials.
	34. (D) Rolling	back	Shake *rattle*, then place at either side out of reach.
			Criterion: Rolls from back to stomach; one of two trials.
			Additional Scoring: If counter rotation, shoulder rotating in one direction and hip in the other, one of two trials, score 2 on this item and on item 45.
	35. (C) Pushing Up	stomach	Shake *rattle* above child's head three times.
			Criterion: Elevates head and stomach by pushing arms up straight. Maintains position for five seconds.
	36. (C) Lifting Head	back	Grasp wrists and hands. Pull to sitting position.
			Criterion: Holds head 15 degrees in front of midline, anterior to middle, to initiate sitting: one of two trials.
	37. (C) Flexing Body	back	Bend child's feet toward head three times, encouraging child to grasp. Say, "Get your feet," but do not place feet in child's hands.
			Criterion: Grasps feet with hands: one of three trials.
	38. (D) Pulling Forward	stomach	Place *toy* five feet in front of child. Say, "Get the toy."
			Criterion: Pulls forward a distance of three feet using arms: one of two trials.
	39. (B) Sitting	sitting	Place *toy* to grasp 12 inches in front of child. After child grasps toy, observe balance.
			Criterion: Maintains balance for 30 seconds while manipulating toy: one of two trials.
	40. (C) Extending Arm	back	Place *toy* 10 degrees to right or left of child in front of an arm. Observe support and extension.
			Criterion: Supports self on arm or elbow on one side while shifting weight to extend opposite arm to reach for toy: one of two trials.

Source: Reprinted by permission from *Peabody Developmental Motor Scales* (1983), DLM-Teaching Resources.

guage, facial gestures, and verbalizations. This allows the student to regain composure and control.

4. Show the student that you understand the frustration being experienced with a new task. This can be done by verbally giving feedback to the student about the feelings observed. For example, the teacher might say, "It was hard for you to catch the ball, but you really tried." Or "You don't seem to remember what to do. Would you like some help?" This offers support for the student and shows that the teacher is understanding.

5. Know what perceptual problems the student has. Teach to the intact perceptual system and try to let students strengthen the one/s that give some difficulty. For instance, if the student has difficulty with auditory processing, use more visual input while demonstrating a skill, but have the student practice on auditory skills by listening and repeating the instructions with some assistance.

6. Let learning-disabled students self-pace their activities. If they have difficulty with a skill, let them slow down or change the skill so that they can work at their own rate.

EMOTIONALLY DISTURBED AND BEHAVIOR-DISORDERED STUDENTS

Physical education activities for emotionally disturbed students need to meet the social, physical, and psychological needs of these individuals. Play and leisure time need to be carefully considered. Teachers should try the following strategies with disturbed students:

1. When a student misbehaves or breaks a rule, tell the student that the behavior is not approved of but the student is O.K. This avoids confrontation and an attack on the student's self-concept.

2. Provide activities that allow self-expression, such as creative movement, dance, mime, and rhythms.

3. Let withdrawn students be helpers in order to involve them in the group. This should be done with caution and in small increments.

4. Do not push withdrawn students into group activities.

5. When students have behavior under fair control, allow them to make choices of activities.

6. Competition should be avoided, emphasizing instead participation and cooperative activities.

7. Be alert to signs that a situation may be getting out of hand and intervene at that point. Problems should not be allowed to become fully developed. Prevention is much more effective than intervention. For example, if an activity is about to get out of hand to the point where the students will fight and argue if it continues, stop the activity. McDowell, Adamson, and Wood (1982) refer to this procedure as "interference technique."

8. Crowe, Auxter, and Pyfer (1981) recommend that stereotyped play activity be discouraged. For example, if the student wishes to play with the same piece of equipment in the same way each time, encourage interaction with a new item.

9. Stand nearby students for close physical proximity. This allows the teacher to sustain the student's attention.

10. Give directions and ask students to repeat them. Give out a task card with directions printed on it. Allow students to use the task card to keep them aware of the assignment during class. A picture of a drill and instructions can be included.

11. Teach students to manage situations more independently. Help them to:

- state the task, i.e., pass a football to work on accuracy.
- concentrate and try to remember the directions, i.e., get into groups of 3s, pass ball from 20 feet to others, pass ball to moving persons.
- self-pace, i.e., it's O.K. to move closer if students can't throw the ball accurately from 20 feet.
- reinforce themselves, i.e., record each other's successful attempts, cheer for each other, and congratulate each other.

12. If a student becomes verbally aggressive, never get into a verbal match with the student. Call the student aside and let feelings subside, then quietly discuss the situation with the student.

13. Be consistent with giving instructions. Use the same signal to let students know that they are going to receive directions. Have them sitting and generally in the same location. This way they will know that when the signal occurs, instructions are going to be given.

STUDENTS WITH NEUROLOGICAL AND PHYSICAL DISABILITIES

Students with neurological and physical disabilities will vary widely in ability. Methods and techniques can be modified to meet their needs, in addition to the general classroom procedures used. Students within these categories may have medical problems and require medication. Medical professionals may need to be consulted about some aspects of physical education. The following guidelines are related to instruction for students with neurological or physical disabilities:

1. Medical problems and specific impairments should be identified before initiating any physical education activities.

2. The first-aid procedures for medical problems, especially seizures, should be known. They should also be written and placed where the teacher can get access to them quickly.

3. In some cases it is wise to obtain the approval of physicians and/or physical therapists prior to beginning the program.

4. The instructional area should be uncluttered. Students who fall frequently should participate in a fall-safe area to minimize and prevent injury.

5. Equipment and playing areas should be modified. Nets can be lowered, the playing area made smaller, and lighter-weight equipment may be used.

6. Student positions in games can be substituted. Sitting can be substituted for standing.

7. Activities with high physical contact should be avoided or modified to reduce or eliminate injury that could result from contact.

VISUALLY IMPAIRED STUDENTS

Visually impaired students may not always need different teaching strategies from those used with sighted students. However, the physical educator should be aware of the following teaching strategies for use with visually impaired students whenever the impairment is severe.

1. Determine the degree of visual impairment and the amount of residual vision available to the student.

2. Ask students what they are able to see and which objects and conditions present problems.

3. Allow students to position themselves where they are able to see best.

4. Make sure that indoor areas are well lighted.

5. Use light-colored equipment whenever possible, preferably white or yellow.

6. Allow a peer to take the visually impaired student through the entire physical education area so the student can become totally familiar with it.

7. Keep the instructional area as uncluttered as possible. If major changes are made in the arrangement, the impaired students should be told and allowed to explore the new physical setting.

8. Modify activities and equipment where necessary. Use audible balls, guide ropes for running, larger equipment, and the buddy system.

9. Stand near the impaired student so that all instructions can be heard and seen.

HEARING-IMPAIRED STUDENTS

As with visual impairments, the severity of the hearing loss will determine the amount of modification needed in teaching strategies. The physical educator should keep the following strategies in mind when working with hearing-impaired students.

1. Rely on the student's visual modality for teaching skills.

2. Use whatever form of communication the hearing-impaired student uses such as total communication, or concomitant signing and verbalization.

3. Be familiar with sign language. Eichstaedt and Seiler (1978) have an excellent article on communicating with hearing-impaired students in the physical education setting.

4. Allow the hearing-impaired student to teach signs to the entire physical education class. Students seem to enjoy sign language and communicating with each other in this manner.

5. If sign language is not used a set of hand signals might be arranged.

6. Always place the hearing-impaired student in a position that allows a view of the teacher's face.

7. Never have the hearing-impaired student face the sun to view the teacher.

STUDENTS WITH COMMUNICATION DISORDERS

Students who have difficulty communicating as a result of a speech or language disorder may not need any particular modification in an activity, but a few strategies can be employed by the physical educator that will facilitate a successful and rewarding experience in physical education.

1. Be patient when the student forgets a word. Give the student time to think of it. If the student cannot think of a word, ask, "Did you mean *bat*?" if the student was trying to think of the word *bat*.

2. If the student has very poor language and speech, do not ridicule errors. Simply reply to the student with the correct form. If a student says, "Them was the winners," the teacher should respond with the phrase, "Yes, they were the winners."

3. Ask students to speak slowly.

4. Reward the student for using the correct language or speaking clearly.

5. Consult with the speech therapist in the school and ask for advice on helping the student.

STUDENTS WITH HEALTH IMPAIRMENTS

Arthritis

Arthritic students require a carefully planned teaching approach since in some cases the condition may be active or in remission. The physical educator should carefully plan strategies that will not cause further injury or trauma to affected joints. The following guidelines should be used when working with arthritic students:

1. Check to see if the student's condition is active or in remission.

2. Be aware of any side effects of medications the student may be taking.

3. Consult with a physician or physical therapist for exercises designed to stretch and strengthen muscle groups. These should be carried out on a daily basis unless movement is too painful for the student.

4. Be patient with the student when pain is being experienced. Pain can cause the student to be irritable and moody.

5. Cratty (1980) recommends quiet recreational activities when the student is unable to participate in other forms of activities.

Diabetes

The physical educator should be aware of any students who are diabetic and should understand the effects of too much or too little insulin. Exercise is important to the diabetic student for weight control and burning up glucose. The following guidelines should be used when working with diabetic students:

1. Exercise needs to be consistent.

2. Proper weight control needs to be developed with exercise and diet. The exercise program should be well rounded and offer incentives for sticking to a proper diet.

3. Be aware of mood changes and react positively and patiently to them.

4. Be ready to take appropriate action when signs of too little or too much insulin are present.

5. Be aware of signs of fatigue and offer rest periods to the student. A signal should be worked out for when a rest period is needed.

Cardiac Conditions

The strategies used with students who have cardiac disorders need to be implemented on a highly individualized basis (Cratty 1980). Some basic procedures include:

1. Consulting with a physician before beginning the physical education program.

2. Providing of a variety of activities depending on the severity of the problem: nonvigorous aquatics, mild leisure sports, and recreational activities.

3. Offering stretching, breathing, and isotonic exercises (Compton, Hill, & Sinclair 1973).

POINTS TO REMEMBER

1. Instruction of exceptional students should be approached from a general perspective, or noncategorical and categorical teaching styles. Noncategorical styles use techniques that can be applied to all disabled students, such as behavior management. Categorical teaching utilizes techniques that match the characteristics of each disabled student. Both approaches combined will be successful.

2. The teaching of motor skills should be coordinated and integrated with concepts in the academic classroom, such as addition, measurement, shape recognition.

3. Mildly retarded students need to be taught the everyday behaviors of physical education class routines such as being on time, cooperation, beginning and ending a task, and social interaction that is appropriate.

4. The more severely retarded students are, the more intense instruction will have to be on basic fundamental motor patterns and skills. Task analysis will have to be used in more detail than with other students.

5. Disturbed children will need structured-routine classroom procedures. The teacher needs to work on more independent control of behavior from students.

6. Sensory motor training will be necessary with severely mentally retarded youngsters, with much manual guidance of body parts.

7. Sensory-impaired students will have to have teaching strategies that are geared to intact senses, while coping and compensating for impaired senses.

8. Neurologically and orthopedically impaired students will require more input from medical professionals in developing a physical education program.

9. Students with cardiac and other special health problems will need highly individualized programs that do not aggravate the particular medical condition.

10. Teachers should be alert to fatigue in students with special health conditions, since fatigue can bring about difficulties that might require medical attention.

REFERENCES

Compton, D., Will, P.M., & Sinclair, T. (1973). Weight lifters blackout. *Lancet* 2, 1234–1237.

Cratty, B.J. (1980). *Adapted physical education for handicapped children and youth.* Denver: Love.

Crowe, W.C., Auxter, D., & Pyfer, J. (1981). *Principles and methods of adapted physical education and recreation* (4th ed.). St. Louis: C.V. Mosby.

Eichstaedt, C., & Seiler, P.J. (1978). Signing: Communicating with hearing impaired individuals in physical education. *Journal of Physical Education and Recreation* 49, 19–21.

Fait, H.F. (1978). *Special physical education.* Philadelphia: W.B. Saunders.

Geddes, D. (1981). *Psychomotor individualized educational programs for intellectual, learning and behavioral disabilities.* Boston: Allyn & Bacon.

McDowell, R.L., Adamson, G.W., & Wood, F.H. (1982). *Teaching emotionally disturbed children.* Boston: Little, Brown.

Seaman, J.A., & DePauw, K.P. (1982). *The new adapted physical education: A developmental approach.* Palo Alto, CA: Mayfield.

Part V

Specific Skill Areas and Modifications

Chapter 12

Games and Lead-Ups to Higher Sports Skills

Focus

- Defines the purpose and value of games for handicapped individuals.
- Offers a variety of games and teaching strategies that will be beneficial to handicapped learners.
- Discusses modification and selection of games geared to the needs and abilities of handicapped students.
- Discusses implications and implementation of games analysis, for team games in particular, so that all types of disabled students may participate.

Games provide a medium in which students can play and relate to each other in a healthy social setting. There are many reasons for playing games, including recreation, skill development, modified versions of higher sports skills, and social interaction. Games are also used to teach cognitive skills by integrating the academic and cognitive skills to be taught. Thus, games can be played for a variety of reasons and can be enjoyed by all levels and ages of people.

Games can teach many concepts when they are incorporated into the game itself. Some of the benefits of games, particularly for handicapped students, are that they:

- improve physiological functions
- increase cognitive skills
- develop social skills and interaction
- teach the concept of team work
- develop creativity
- provide emotional outlets and recreation
- teach the concept of fair play
- sharpen perceptual skills
- improve coordination and general body management
- develop self-awareness
- help establish behavior control
- teach delay of gratification
- increase independence

An important aspect of games is that for individuals to enjoy them, they must allow participation with at least some success. This chapter includes instructional methods for teaching games to handicapped students and explores four basic categories of games: (1) games that are simple and require low organization, (2) lead-up games to particular team sports, (3) games for integrating motor and cognitive learning, and (4) new games or social learning games.

SELECTING GAMES

Several points should be considered when selecting games for individuals or groups.

- The teacher needs to ask what objectives are being sought and whether they can be best met through game activities. This applies to individual or group objectives.
- The strengths and weaknesses of the group and individuals should be considered in such areas as social maturity, physical abilities, mental age, and chronological age.
- A survey of equipment should be made to ensure that it is both appropriate and sufficient to accommodate a number of skills and abilities.

- Safety is another prime factor to consider. A game needs to be as safe as possible for students to enjoy the game and not have the risk of injury.
- The amount and type of space must be adequate and appropriate.
- Whether the game will have both handicapped and non-handicapped students participating must be decided.

Matching Games to Abilities

Social Maturity

Social maturity of the students will affect how much the game will be enjoyed. It the students are too socially immature to handle the competition in a game, for example, another type of game should be chosen. A new game or partner games should be selected rather than highly competitive games.

Physical Ability

Physical abilities will also affect the amount of enjoyment the students derive. A game that involves considerable agility and speed should not be used with uncoordinated and slow students.

Mental Age

Mental age is a key factor in how successfully students will be able to participate in a game. The game should not be so simple that the students become bored with it. This is important to keep in mind for older mentally retarded students. Instead of selecting a simple game, a higher-level game might be modified.

Chronological Age

Chronological age is a factor that has to be considered along with the students' mental ages. Chronologically, students may be 13 and 14 but mentally be more like 8-year-olds. Games need to accommodate the physical development of the students but cannot be too complex for their mental and possibly social development.

Psychological Development

Psychological development of students will affect how well they do in particular games. Games, for example, that may cause a student to become angry possibly because of body contact should be avoided if the student has difficulty handling anger in a positive way. The way in which a game is organized can affect withdrawn children to the point that they are not able to participate in games involving many team players. A game that involves only two players or a smaller group might be more appropriate.

Skills

The *skills* required by the game should be matched to the motor skill ability of the group and specific individuals. When mainstreaming is in effect, more diversity of skills may be seen. However, in self-contained classes more similarities may be seen, but the skills may be on a lower level. Also, games can be modified to accommodate several levels of skills.

Rules

Young children or those with mental retardation cannot participate with a great deal of success in games with complex rules. If the rules are too complex, they can be modified or simplified to make the game less confusing.

Player Positions

Some games require more movement from certain players. For example, the forward line in soccer moves or covers much more distance on the field than the fullbacks or the goalie. Students with limited endurance may need to play in a position that does not require so much physical stamina.

The Time Element

How long the game lasts will affect how much it is enjoyed. Students with short attention spans or low physical vitality may not be able to play a game as long as it is normally played. Shorter games will have to be selected or the time elements altered.

Equipment

Students need to be able to handle or manage the equipment that is to be used in the game. Numerous modifications can be made regarding equipment such as making it lighter, bigger, smaller, or utilizing aids to help students hold the handle.

MODIFYING GAMES

Morris (1980) discusses games analysis as a process to change games so that individuals who may have difficulty can participate in the game. This model can be used quite effectively to modify games to allow participation by handicapped and nonhandicapped students, or when several levels of handicapped students are participating together. Morris suggests five steps in developing teacher skills in changing games.

Step 1

The instructor must understand the structure and components of games.

Step 2

The instructor needs to feel comfortable with finding alternatives to any one of the components of the game. Individuals who are rigid and stereotyped in their thinking, particularly about how a game should be played, will have difficulty modifying games. This may be the case when teachers get into the habit of teaching a game the same way all the time.

Step 3

Implementing some of the modifications and alternatives may require some experimentation to test out the changes. The teacher needs to be creative and even accept ideas from the students themselves.

Step 4

The instructor should decide if the alternatives meet the purpose of the game. For example, if the alternatives were geared toward the purpose of developing good sportsmanship and support for the other players, the outcome could be measured in terms of how many times players rewarded other players for a good play or for skill in the game.

Step 5

The final step requires more careful evaluation and observation of the alternatives. The teacher should evaluate if, for example, by changing the equipment, the students in fact experienced more success than if the equipment had not been changed. The teacher may then want to develop further alternatives for other components of the same game to enhance the action of the students. The skill of modifying games improves with practice. The teacher may wish to make note of ideas that are particularly successful with students who have particular types of disabilities.

Safety in Making Modifications

One of the most important points in changing a game is to make sure that it still remains safe to the maximum extent possible. Any modification of a game that risks its safety, no matter how minor, should not be used. The following are essential safety precautions:

- Modified equipment should be safe—bats free from cracks, splinters, or other unsafe features, for example.
- If the playing area is altered or changed, it needs to be free of unnecessary objects and equipment.
- Students should wear appropriate clothing to allow freedom of movement and safety. Sneakers are appropriate, never bare feet.

- If boundaries are changed the end line or goal should not be near any walls, trees, or fixtures.

SIMPLE GAMES

Games Requiring Little Movement

- *Birds Fly*
Equipment: None
Play Formation/Area: Personal space, classroom, or gym
Action: A leader is chosen and gives the name of anything that flies. When this is done, players flap their arms like they were flying. If something is named that does not fly, arms are not supposed to be flapped. Rotate the leader every few minutes. Do not eliminate those who flap their arms if a name is called and it does not fly.

- *Pass The Biscuit*
Equipment: Bean bag, tennis ball, wiffle ball, or other light object
Play Formation/Area: Even number in a circle, indoors or out
Action: Each circle of students is given a bean bag, then asked to pass the bean bag quickly around the circle from one person to the next. The group that gets the bean bag around the circle first wins a point.
Variations: Have students close their eyes and pass the object.

- *What Am I?*
Equipment: None
Play Formation/Area: Personal space, indoors or out
Action: Students are in their personal space seated on the floor or on the ground. Wheelchair students can remain in their chairs. A student is asked to think of an animal or object then try to imitate it without sound. Students take turns guessing. The one who gets it right then gets to do an imitation. If no one guesses, the teacher chooses someone else until each has had a turn.

- *Bean Bag Toss*
Equipment: Bean bags, three for each team, box for target
Play Formation/Area: Teams of three to five players each. Classroom, gym, or outdoor area can be used.
Action: Each team has three bean bags and a box for a target. The thrower stands ten feet or less, to be determined by the teacher, from the target. Each person throws the bean bag at the target three times. Each time a bean bag lands in the box, a point is scored. After everyone has thrown three bean bags, the scores are added up and then compared.
Variations: Let the students look at the box and then throw with their eyes closed. Have them toss backward facing away from the target. Specify the type of toss.

- *Flying Saucers*
Equipment: Foam circles or paper styrofoam plates, hoops
Play Formation/Area: Classroom, gym, outdoors. Teams in lines or scattered.
Action: Divide students into teams of equal numbers, from three to six players. A hula hoop can be suspended or propped up. The players try to throw the frisbee through the target. Paper plates can also be used. One point is scored if the object goes through the hoop. Players can be seated or stand at a distance specified by the teacher. Less-skilled students can be allowed to stand several feet closer.

- *Simon Says*
Equipment: None
Play Formation/Area: Personal space, room for students to move
Action: The teacher or leader calls out "Simon says blink your eyes." Students can blink their eyes. If "Simon says" is not stated before the movement to be done and the students complete the movement, they are caught. The teacher can eliminate them but, better yet, give them a point. The object is to see who can score the lowest number of points.
Variations: Substitute a favorite person for "Simon," such as "The Hulk" or "Mr. T."

Parachute Games

Parachute games require as much movement as the teacher wishes to use. These activities and games are good for integrating students with limited mobility or students with wheelchairs. The parachute can be used to develop numerous skills ranging from arm and shoulder strength, rhythmics, and cooperation. Nylon parachutes can be purchased commercially from the Preston Corporation (60 Page Road, Clifton, NJ 07012) or from Army surplus.

- *Roll The Chute*
Equipment: One parachute
Play Formation/Area: Circle on the outside of the parachute, indoors or out
Action: Students hold the parachute on the edges and stretch it out taut. When it is pulled taut, students can rock back and forth seated or standing. If several students have balance problems, sitting would be a better position.
    Ask students to roll the parachute up. This is good for developing wrist and hand strength. Ask them to go slow, then fast.

- *Mushrooms*
Equipment: Parachute
Play Formation/Area: Open space, students seated or on knees around the outside of the parachute

Action: Students are asked to grip the parachute and on a signal lift it overhead, then pull it to the floor quickly. The trapped air makes the parachute balloon and it resembles a big mushroom.

Variation: While the parachute is in the air, the teacher can call a student's name and that student must go under the parachute quickly and to the opposite side before it touches the ground as the other students begin to pull it down.

● *Cat and Mice*

Equipment: Parachute

Play Formation/Area: Circle around the outside of the parachute

Action: Four students are chosen to be the mice and are on their stomachs under the parachute. Then a cat is chosen who is on top of the parachute. The cat is blindfolded and the mice are allowed to keep their eyes open. The remaining students on the outside hold the parachute down over the mice. On a signal from the teacher, the cat tries to find the mice by feeling for them. The mice may move anywhere under the parachute. If a mouse is caught, another student takes its place. A new cat can be chosen when three mice are caught, or after a short period of time. Students love this game.

● *Ocean Waves*

Equipment: Parachute

Play Formation/Area: Students sit "Indian style" around the parachute

Action: One student stands next to the outside of the parachute. When the teacher says "Go," students begin shaking the parachute close to the floor so that it looks like ocean waves. The student standing must then walk on the parachute as if walking through the waves on the beach. This really helps with balance. After one trip around the parachute, another student may be chosen until everyone has had a turn.

Other Ideas

1. Place a ball on the parachute and roll it around the edge. Students have to concentrate and cooperate to keep the ball close to the edge.

2. Place a ball in the middle of the parachute and have the students divided into two teams, with one team on one side and the other on the opposite side. On the signal, each side tries to win a point by knocking the ball off over the other team's heads by raising and lowering the parachute.

3. Place five or six ropes of different lengths, three to five feet, on the parachute. Students raise and lower the parachute to try and knock off the snakes (ropes).

4. Have students stand in a circle around the parachute and hold it with one hand, all students facing the same direction or holding with the same hand. Then a record can

be played while the students move around in a circle; variations include changing hands all at the same time, moving three steps in and three steps out. The teacher can let the students make up a parachute dance.

RELAY GAMES

Relays are fun-type games that can be used to teach a variety of concepts including social and team skills, motor skills, sportsmanship, competition, physical fitness. Relays can sometimes be overused to stress competition. They should not be utilized in this manner.

Strategies for Using Relays

1. Avoid having too many players on a team, particularly with distractable students and those with short attention spans.

2. Geddes (1974) suggests using a walkthrough procedure when teaching the relay so that students will have a clear concept and understanding of what the relay is all about.

3. Do not let students choose the teams but let them help decide on any modifications.

4. Shorten the distance to be covered if students lack endurance and tire easily. Substitute movements such as rolling for running.

5. If students are participating who are on crutches or in wheelchairs, the movement surface should be smooth.

6. Be sure the boundaries and finish lines are clearly marked. No permanent fixtures should be near the finish line.

7. Be sure to explain all safety aspects.

8. If objects are to be used in the relay, be sure they can be easily managed by all the players.

9. Be sure to provide a rest period and watch for signs of fatigue.

10. Teach students to take turns properly and to listen and watch for all signals. Try to always use the same signal for starting and a different one for stopping. Use them consistently. Use verbal and visual signals.

11. Keep the equipment close to the teacher in a box or sack until it is needed.

12. Begin with relays that have limited movements first and gradually work up to more vigorous movements.

13. If students become confused as to which members are on their team, let the team members wear a penny, arm band, or tie a ribbon to each team member's wrist.

14. If a line is involved, tape the starting line or place a flag in the ground.

15. Some students who become easily confused may need to have the lane marked for them either by tape or flags.

16. Be sure that all students understand the skills and can execute them before including them in a relay.

Formations for Relays

Various types of formations can be used for relays. The type of formation depends on the purpose of the relay and the skills of the students.

File Formations

Schurr (1980) suggests that the file formation is the easiest for beginners to learn. This is also a good formation for distractable and lower-functioning students who are chronologically older. Students are in a line at point 1 and move a specified distance to point 2, go around an object, and return to point 1, and must tag the second person before any movement can begin to point 2 again. Any type of skill can be used in this relay. No equiment is necessary unless the skill to be developed requires it.

• *Relays Using Files*
Equipment: None
Action: Each team lines up and markers are placed 20 feet away opposite each team. Allow plenty of space between teams. Markers can be flags in the ground, weighted potato chip cans, or plastic gallon milk jugs with a flag stuck in sand or dirt in the jug. Any skill can be used for teams to move to their marker and back. These are some possibilities:

- locomotor skills without equipment
- carrying a bean bag on top of one's head
- dribbling a lightweight ball with feet or hands
- mixing different locomotor skills, such as walking down to the marker and running back
- slow students run, while skilled students walk fast
- carrying objects, such as ping pong balls in a spoon, a cup of beans, etc.
- imitating different animals while moving
- running to the marker and finding an object from among other objects, then carrying it back to the line

Competition between teams does not always have to occur. The students can compare their scores each time they repeat the relay and compete against themselves.

Circle Formations

The circle formation is good to use when there is little movement in terms of locomotion. It is also good when there is limited space or when the students do not have good locomotor skills.

• *Relays Using Circle Formations*
Circle formations can be used for passing, running, or skill development.

Equipment: May include an object or not.
Action: While the team is in a circle, objects may be passed quickly from one person to the other. Or students may pass objects with their feet around the circle.
Action: Students can have numbers. When a number is called, the person with that number runs around the outside of the circle trying to beat the person running with the same number on the other teams. A point is scored for the person who runs the circle first. It is important to keep the circles the same size. Or a slower player can run on the inside. Who will run on the inside should be designated before the relay starts.

Shuttle Formation

The shuttle formation is good to use for higher-level students and in track and field type events. Each team is divided in half. One half is a specified distance from the second half and facing the other. The first person starts and moves toward the other half of the team using whatever skill is required. When the other half of the team is reached, the first player in line is tagged and moves in the opposite direction to the other half of the team. This is continued until each half has exchanged ends or positions.

• *Relays Using a Shuttle Formation*
Equipment: None or whatever the teacher decides
Action: Students can simply move back and forth until each team has exchanged positions. Different skills may be used, with or without equipment. Some activities may use equipment such as balloons, balls, bean bags, or yarn balls and scoops.

LEAD-UP GAMES TO TEAM SPORTS

Blake and Volp (1964) define lead-up games as modified team games that involve one or several of the basic skills and rules of a standard team game. This modified approach is geared to aid students in learning the game faster and with more understanding. Lead-up games build on the similar notion of whole-part learning. Just as skills can be broken down into parts and be learned, so can team games or dual games. This approach works for all students, but particularly well for slow learners.

In adapted physical education, lead-up games can be used in several ways:

1. They may be used in mainstreamed settings as a teaching tool, keeping the interest of higher-functioning students while allowing lower-level students to participate in components of a team game.

2. They may be used in self-contained classrooms where the number of students is too small to play an entire game or the cognitive skills and behavioral deficits preclude playing a full game.

3. The games analysis procedure can be easily applied to lead-up games. Using the lead-up game and games analysis change, almost any level of student should be able to be accommodated in a game.

4. As skills and knowledge increase about the particular game, the rules can be made more complex, or other changes can be made that make the lead-up game resemble the actual game itself.

5. Skills involved in the game should be taught separately, practiced individually, then incorporated into the lead-up game.

6. The lead-up approach is also effective because those who are ready to play some form of the game can, while others who still need some skill drill can also receive individualized instruction.

In presenting the different lead-up games, it will be assumed that the adapted physical educator already knows the basic rules and concepts of the regular game the lead-ups are preparing for.

Basketball

Basketball can be played by a number of students if changes are made in the game. Some lower-level students will progress only to the lead-up level. Thus, the adapted specialist must realize the skills the student has and how they will fit into the game and at what levels.

Basketball Skills

- passing: bounce pass, chest pass, shoulder pass
- catching
- dribbling and shooting
- shots: free throw, jump shot, lay-up, set shot
- guarding and rebounding
- pivoting
- game strategies: offense and defense

Lead-Ups to Basketball

● *Center Ball*
Equipment: Two balls per team
Play Formation/Area: Circle with about six on each team. In or outdoors. Skills: passing and catching.
Action: Each team is in a circle. The leader is in the center with a ball, and a player on the circle has a ball. The leader passes the ball to the player who is to the right of the one with the ball. As the pass is started from the center, the player with the other ball passes it to the leader. This is continued all the way around the circle. Then a new leader is chosen. If the leader misses, a point is awarded. The idea is for the team to score the lowest number of points. The passers can be changed each time.

● *Guard Ball*
Equipment: One basketball per team
Play Formation/Area: Four players per team. A small court is marked off. A 10 ft. × 10 ft. square is ample.
Action: Two guards stand in the middle and two passers stand on the end lines. Passers try to pass the ball to each other but cannot pass over the guards' heads. Each time a successful pass is made without being stolen or blocked, a point is scored. When a team scores five points, team members get in the middle of the square and become the guards.
Variations: Teams switch positions after five tries, whether points are scored or not. The guards may choose the type of pass each time.

● *Shooting Relay*
Equipment: One ball per team
Play Formation/Area: Six to eight players on a team. Teams stand at the free throw line.
Action: On the signal "Go," the first person in line takes two dribbles and shoots any type of shot, then rebounds the ball. If a basket is made, two points are scored. The first player quickly passes the ball to the next player from the spot where it was rebounded. The next player repeats the procedure. The first team to score 20 points wins.
Variation: Give each team a time limit, five minutes, for example, and see who has scored the most points within the time period.

● *Spot Shot*
Equipment: One basketball for each team
Play Formation/Area: Three taped lines at different locations on the court. Each court with the taped lines should match. One line can be at the foul line and the other two to the right and left, but closer. The foul shot counts as one point, the left line counts as two points and the right-hand line counts as three points.
Action: Teams stand behind the free throw line with six to eight players per team. On the signal, "Go," the teams try to shoot from any of the three spots, but to win exactly 22 points must be scored. The team members must decide which lines to shoot from and score the 22 points first.
Variation: The teacher calls out the point line and after five minutes of shooting whichever team is ahead wins.

Basketball Adaptations

Besides lead-up games the regulation game of basketball can be modified. Some of the basic modifications include:

- allowing more than two steps to stop
- lowering the goals
- eliminating or simplifying rules
- using a smaller basketball or NeRF® ball

- substituting frequently
- using an audible ball for hearing impaired
- allowing dribbling with two hands
- allowing more time in the key on offense
- letting wheelchair students use wheelchair basketball rules

Wiseman (1982) summarizes the rule modifications in wheelchair basketball. They include the following:

1. The chair is actually counted as part of the player. The basic rules of contact in basketball apply to wheelchair basketball. So, if two wheelchairs touch, it is considered a foul. If a person not in the chair contacts the chair, it can count as a foul.

2. On a jump ball, two wheelchair players must be in the wheelchair seat and face their baskets at a 45 degree angle.

3. The three-second violation is extended to five seconds in wheelchair basketball. This can also be applied in mixed games.

4. Only two consecutive pushes with the ball in possession are allowed. Pushing and dribbling can occur at the same time.

Official rules for wheelchair basketball may be obtained from the National Wheelchair Basketball Association, 110 Seaton Building, University of Kentucky, Lexington, Kentucky.

Other adaptations include playing on only half a court following rules for half-court basketball. Also, more players per team can be used by providing them with designated spots. These players play only half-court when full-court basketball is in effect.

Volleyball

Volleyball is a team sport also played frequently for leisure. Volleyball can be adapted as easily as basketball to accommodate all levels of players. When teaching the skills for the first time to beginners, much lighter balls should be used. Large round balloons and beach balls are ideal since they are easier to control and do not travel as fast as a heavier ball.

Volleyball Skills

- passing volley
- serve: overhand and underarm
- set pass
- spike
- block at the net
- bump or dig shot or forearm pass

Lead-Ups to Volleyball

- *Balloon Volley*

Equipment: Large round balloon for each person or at least every two students

Play Formation/Area: Court or surrounding area, personal space, or, if in pairs, students face each other about five feet apart.

Action: Students try to volley the balloon in the air as long as possible. Have them count and record the number of successful volleys. More skilled students may have to count their volleys within a specified time period.

- *Beach Ball Volley*

Equipment: Small beach ball for each team.

Play Formation/Area: Teams are in a circle with a leader in the middle, eight to ten players per team.

Action: On a given signal, the leader hits the ball to a player on the circle and the player hits it back. The team to get the ball around the circle first without the ball missing a player or touching the ground wins. Only one hit is allowed per player.

- *Beach Ball Bump*

Equipment: Beach ball for each team

Play Formation/Area: Players form a line of six or seven opposite a leader.

Action: The leader begins at the left side of the line of teammates and volleys the ball to the first one in the line. A bump must be used to return the ball. Then the leader may bump or volley it to the second player, who bumps it back. This continues until the leader has gone down the line and back. The first team to finish wins. The team does not start over if the ball is missed. It is retrieved and the play begins from the person who missed it.

- *NeRF® Spike*

Equipment: 1 NeRF® ball for each team. Rope tied between two poles or standards, at least one foot higher than the tallest or average player, depending on the skills of the players.

Play Formation/Area: Two teams on one side of the rope. The other team or extras can recover the balls.

Action: The leader tosses the ball about 10 feet in the air about a foot away from the rope. The spiker tries to spike the ball. If it goes over the rope, a point is scored. If it is missed or if the ball goes under the rope, no points are scored. The team getting to 10 points first wins. Teams can rotate and compete against each other.

- *Serve Drill*

Equipment: At least two volleyballs per team. Playground balls can be used if there are not enough volleyballs. Net about five feet high and regulation size court.

Play Formation/Area: Teams of six to eight players line up on opposite sides of the court/s at a taped line 20 feet from the net. Each team member serves until a team scores 21 points. Every time a ball goes over the net and lands in bounds, it counts as a point. The team to reach 21 points first wins. A player cannot serve twice in a row. Players must alternate their serves. It is the same idea as following a batting lineup in baseball.

● *Newcomb*
Equipment: Volleyball, playground ball, or beach ball, depending on the players' skills. Volleyball court, regulation size. Net or rope about six feet high.
Play Formation/Area: Nine to twelve players cover one half of the court opposite each other on either side of the net.
Action: The ball is given to a player on one side of the court. The player tosses the ball to the other side and any player can catch it. If it hits the floor, a point is scored for the serving team, provided the ball did not touch the net when it went over. Play continues, and whoever caught the ball tosses it back. It can be tossed from anywhere on the court. At the end of five minutes, players change sides. Play continues for five more minutes. Whoever is ahead at the end of the ten-minute play period wins.

Volleyball Adaptations

Several things can be done to modify a regulation volleyball game to allow more success by lower-skilled players.
 1. The court can be made smaller as in basketball.
 2. More players per side can be allowed.
 3. The net can be lowered.
 4. A lighter-weight ball can be used.
 5. More hits per side can be allowed.
 6. The distance from the serving line to the net can be made shorter by taping a line from which to serve.
 7. Wheelchair players can play from a stationary position on the floor. Let them modify their serve.
 8. For visually impaired students, the ball may be allowed to bounce once before they hit it.

Softball

Softball can be slightly modified to allow players even with moderate disabilities to play. Students with more severe disabilities may have to play lead-ups to softball rather than a modified game.

Softball Skills

 ● throwing and catching
 ● catching and fielding
 ● batting
 ● base running
 ● playing positions and strategies

A variety of softballs are available made of softer materials than regulation balls. Handicapped children may often be afraid to field or catch a regulation softball. Sock balls or paper balls can also be easily made. Nylon softballs are also available commercially.

Lead-Ups to Softball

● *Pitching Dual*
Equipment: Softball, one glove, and one base per team
Play Formation/Area: Place teams of six a safe distance from each other. Each team should be facing the same direction. A teammate is designated as a catcher and assumes a position behind the base. Teammates are grouped 25–30 feet away, depending on their skill. Each team gets 12 throws at the plate, including the catcher. A teammate can switch when it is the catcher's turn to throw. The team with the most strikes (balls that go over the plate, in this case) at the end of 12 pitches wins.

● *Base Race*
Equipment: Four bases
Play Formation/Area: Open field. Four flags placed in a row 10 feet apart, one base placed opposite each flag about 20 feet away.
Action: Teams stand by the marker opposite a base. On the signal ''Go,'' the first person runs to the base and returns as quickly as possible. The first team to get all players to the base and back wins.

● *Kickball*
Equipment: Soccer ball, four bases, and softball diamond
Play Formation/Area: Two nine-player teams, each player playing the positions in softball
Action: The pitcher rolls the soccer ball to the batter. The batter kicks the ball and runs to first base if the ball is in fair territory. The batter may stop at a base to avoid being put out. For a runner to be put out the ball must get to the baseman and the base must be tagged before the runner gets there. Other ways of getting the runner out include tagging the runner before arrival at a base, catching a fly ball hit by the runner, or if the batter misses three well-pitched balls. Runs are scored as in softball. All players on a team bat before changing teams to bat. The team with the most runs after both teams have had an equal number of turns at bat wins.

● *Tee Ball*
Tee Ball is played like regular kickball except the players use a bat and bat from a batting tee. Various size bats should be available to meet the needs of different abilities in students.

Softball Adaptations

1. For visually impaired persons use brightly colored balls, white or yellow.

2. Reduce the distance around the bases for players who fatigue easily or who move slowly. Also the distance from the pitcher's mound to home plate may be shortened.

3. Increase the number of strikes before the person is out.

4. Allow more players in the outfield to reduce the amount of space to be covered.

5. Students who can bat but not run or move well to first base can have a designated runner.

6. Use lighter and larger bats and have students bat from a batting tee. Only students who need the batting tee will have to use it. Otherwise, let the others bat a pitched ball.

7. Use an audible ball for blind students. If the students have no residual vision, a buddy can be placed next to the blind student. The game should be modified so the ball stays on the ground, even when batted.

Soccer

Soccer can be played by many handicapped persons. The game is widely played and adaptable to meet the needs of students with limiting playing ability.

Soccer Skills

- kicking
- dribbling
- blocking and trapping
- tackling
- marking or guarding
- heaving (avoid students who have seizures, shunts, or any other risky disability)
- punting (more advanced players)

Lead-Ups to Soccer

● *Dribble The Maze*
Equipment: One soccer ball per team. Flags or other markers to make a maze.
Play Formation/Area: Teams are in lines. Place six flags five feet apart in a line to make the maze. Have a maze for each team of six to eight players. Five feet from the first flag, place a marker as the starting line. The last marker is the end line.
Action: On the starting signal the first player must dribble the ball with the feet in a weaving pattern in and out of each marker, then dribble the ball back straight to the next player. The first team to complete the maze is the winner.
Variations: Have half the team at one end of the maze and half at the other. The game ends when each half has traded ends.

● *Circle Pass and Trap*
Equipment: One soccer ball for each circle
Play Formation/Area: Teams of eight to ten make a circle with one player in the middle. This works better in a grassy area, but can be done indoors.
Action: The players on the outside of the circle try to pass the ball to one another. The player in the middle must try to block and trap the ball. If the person in the middle traps the ball, whoever kicked the ball exchanges places with the person in the middle. Lower-skilled students can have two players in the middle.

● *Take Away*
Equipment: One ball for every two teams. Three markers for every two teams.
Play Formation/Area: Three flags are placed 15 feet apart in a line. Team A stands behind one end flag and Team B stands behind the other end flag. Team A player starts dribbling the ball toward the center flag. The first player on Team B meets the person at the flag and tries to get the ball away using the feet. Player A continues dribbling toward the third flag. If the player on Team B cannot get the ball away before the A player reaches the flag, Team A scores a point, but if the ball is taken away, Team B scores a point. The team with the highest score after each player has had a turn, wins the game. The teams can then switch, with Team B becoming the dribblers and Team A the attackers. Points are scored the same way.

● *Kick for the Goal*
Equipment: One soccer ball for each team and two flags to mark the goal
Play Formation/Area: Mark the goal by placing the flags or other markers 15 feet apart. The distance can vary depending on the skill level of the students.
Action: One team stands to the outside of the marker. The other team stands 20 feet away in between the two markers. The team by the goal will be goalies. The team away from the goal will try to score a goal. On a signal to start, the team near the goal will send a player to defend the goal, while the team away from the goal will send a player dribbling the ball toward the goal. At about 5 to 10 feet from the goal, the dribbler will try to kick the ball through the flags. The goalie must try to stop the ball. If the goalie is successful, no points are scored. If the goalie misses, the kicking team gets a point. After each player has had a turn, the teams switch positions and repeat. The team with the most goals wins the game.

Soccer Adaptations

Schurr (1980) recommends a modified form of soccer that may be further adapted to handicapped students.
Equipment: One soccer ball or playground ball for each of

the two teams. The field should have a midline and the goals marked at each end.

Play Formation/Area: The field can be 100 feet long and 75 feet wide. Players assume positions as in regular soccer. Action: The ball is started at a center mark with a kickoff by one team. No one can cross the center line before the ball is kicked by the center forward. The front line or forwards try to move the ball toward the goal area. If a field goal or penalty kick is made, the ball is brought to the center and the nonscoring team gets to kick off and try to score. Free kicks are given for fouls, touching, pushing, tripping, or touching the ball with the hands. If a child is playing with crutches, a foul occurs if the crutches are touched also. Scoring is the same for regular soccer.

Other modifications include:

1. Using less air in a regular soccer ball will help students to control it better.

2. Place players who have locomotor difficulty in positions as fullbacks or halfbacks.

3. Make the goal smaller, or use two goalies.

4. Shorten the playing time.

Other Uses for Lead-Ups

Lead-ups can be used for competition, particularly the drills working on one or two skills. For example, in softball, batting and pitching can be used for students who cannot participate in a modified game. Any of the skills of the game can be modified and used in competition for students with limited abilities. Teachers will more than likely devise their own lead-up games to accommodate students and provide successful experiences for them. It would be impractical to describe all the possible lead-ups to various team sports. The best method is for the adapted physical educator to use the games analysis concept and modify until the students are successful.

NEW GAMES

Fluegelman (1976) developed the concept of New Games that allows for participation by a variety of individuals of different levels. Adults and children, young and old, or handicapped and nonhandicapped can all play. The following concepts of New Games allow this to happen:

- Individuals choose the games and modify or change rules to suit the needs of the groups, or individuals.
- The modifications can occur while the games are being played.
- Mutual trust is a theme and overriding principle.
- Another guiding principle is mutual enjoyment.
- Competition and winning are deemphasized.

Examples of New Games

- *Hug Tag*

Ten to twenty players can be accommodated. "It" is chosen and on a starting signal tries to tag the others. To avoid being tagged, players must hug another player. When a person is tagged, no elimination occurs and the tagged person becomes "It." When everyone is tagged, another game can be played.

- *Snake Tag*

Any number of players up to 25 or 30 can be accommodated. All players play this game on their stomachs and avoid being tagged by crawling on their stomachs. "It" is the snake and players must crawl to avoid being tagged. When persons are tagged, they become snakes and try to tag others. There are no winners or losers in this game, only persons having a good time. When students in Project PERMIT were playing Snake Tag one student had good control of his upper arms but little movement in his legs. Another student suggested that he be allowed to use a scooter board to play. Sure enough, it worked beautifully!

- *Getting To Know Me*

Students form a circle with a tennis ball or NeRF® ball as the equipment. The leader asks each person to go around the circle and name his or her favorite food. When this is done, the NeRF® ball is given to a player. The player has to call out someone's favorite food and toss the ball to the correct person. Then the person repeats the procedure. Students can play until they decide to name something else. If a student throws the ball to the wrong person, another turn is given. Favorite foods, hobbies, movie stars, cars, etc., can be used.

MOTOR COGNITIVE INTEGRATION GAMES

Since children enjoy moving, many academic and cognitive skills can be taught through the medium of movement. Cratty (1980) and Cratty and Breen (1972) suggest that active learning games provide the child with total involvement in the learning process. All the senses are used when children are integrating cognitive and motor processes. This approach to the development of cognitive and academic skills has been successful with mentally retarded, learning-disabled, and physically handicapped students. It works well with sensory-impaired students because their other senses are also used in the learning process. This approach will also help overactive and distractable children who have difficulty with paper and pencil tasks.

All levels of cognitive and academic skills can be incorporated into a motor activity. Very basic concepts such as letter, number, color, and shape recognition can be incorporated into a motor activity or game. More advanced concepts from memory to academics such as reading, math, and science can be taught through active learning games.

When creating motor cognitive games several considerations should be addressed by the adapted specialist.

1. The physical education teacher should consult with the special educator to determine which cognitive and academic concepts are currently being developed in the special education classes. Both resource and self-contained classroom teachers should have input.

2. The active learning games should then be designed around the academic needs of the students.

3. This approach can be used with four-, five-, and six-year-olds who are not handicapped.

4. The game needs to be arranged according to the motor ability and skill level of the students.

5. If students have decreased mobility or are in wheelchairs or on crutches, modifications will need to be considered.

6. If there is a good amount of diversity in motor and cognitive skills among the students, stations or working in similar groups a few at a time may be a more successful arrangement for the game activities.

Games for Beginning Concepts

Beginning concepts games can be used with preschoolers or older students functioning on a preschool level in terms of academics. The motor activity should not be too low a level if the older student has more skill. Remember, the game needs to coincide with both the cognitive and motor levels of the students.

• *Color Match Toss*
Equipment: Colored bean bags of basic colors. Cardboard boxes painted the same color as the bean bags.
Play Formation/Area: Place the boxes at least 5 feet from the students. Boxes can be placed in line about a foot apart or in a semicircle. Students sit about 10 feet away from the boxes. A line is taped 5 feet away from the boxes. This becomes the throwing line.
Action: Students try to match the blue bean bag by throwing it in the blue box. This continues until all the bean bags are thrown toward the appropriate box. If the bean bag goes into the box, two points are scored; if it lands near the box, within less than a foot, one point is scored. If boxes are not available, colored poster board can be used and placed flat on the floor. If the bean bag lands on the poster board of the right color, two points are scored; if it lands on the floor off the poster board but touching part of it, one point is scored. Students can have one additional try if they get the wrong

color. Students waiting their turn can tell the student if the right colors are matched.

• *Detectives*
Equipment: One sock for each student. Socks should be of basic colors: red, green, white, blue, yellow. Footprints can be made from matching color poster board. Have about five footprints for each color sock. Place the footprints scattered and mixed around the room.
Play Formation/Area: Students are in a group on one side of the room.
Action: When the teacher says "Go," students try to step on as many footprints as they can that match their sock before the teacher says stop. Have students change socks and repeat.
Adaptation: If a child is in braces, use a ribbon on the ankle. Have enough ribbons for the different colors.

• *Number Games*
Equipment: A line of numbers needs to be painted or printed with a magic marker on a piece of cardboard, oil cloth, or an outdoor concrete area. The line of numbers should be at least 1 foot wide and 10 feet long. Each number should be sectioned off into a square. Bean bags, one for each player.
Play Formation/Area: Students can work in groups of four or five.
Action: The tossing line should be about 5 feet from the number 5 if ten numbers are used. The person tossing stands or sits at the line and waits for the leader or someone in the group to call a number. The student tossing must toss the bean bag or slide it so that it touches the number space. If it does, a point is scored. This can continue until someone scores five points.
Variation: When a number is called for the student, let the student do a motor activity the number of times indicated by the called number. Thus, clap hands five times if 5 is called.

• *Toss for Points*
Equipment: Plastic coffee can lids or other plastic lids that size or larger. Yarn balls, three for each group. Mark numbers on the lids. If five lids are used they should be numbered 1 through 5 with a magic marker. Suspend the lids by yarn at eye level for the average child's height.
Action: Students toss at the lids from 5 to 10 feet away. If a lid with the number 2 on it is hit, for example, that number is recorded. If the lids are missed a zero is recorded. All the numbers hit after three trials are recorded. Thus, a student's throws may look like an addition problem after they are recorded. Then students try to add their score. The procedure can be repeated between each problem or continued until a student has five problems. Students with the highest or lowest scores can be declared winners. Students must also add their scores correctly to be winners.

Student A	Student B
2	3
3	1
+0	+4

● *Find the Shape*
Equipment: Color tape or masking tape 2 inches wide. Balls of different sizes and weights, one for each person. The ball should be matched to the student's motor skills.
Play Formation/Area: Personal space
Action: Tape different shapes, squares, triangles, rectangles, and circles on the floor. A circle can be cut from poster board or made from a rope taped to the floor. A shape should be available for every two students. Students are in partners in personal space. The teacher tells the students to find a shape. They go to a shape and must identify it correctly. They can bounce a ball in and out of the shape to themselves or to each other. The teacher then asks students to go to another shape and repeat the procedure.
Variations: Eliminate the ball and have students walk around the shape. Play "Hokey Pokey" by calling out a body part or use the song "Hokey Pokey." The student places the body part in the shape.

● *Do What You See* (Visual Memory)
Equipment: Any material can be used: bean bag, ball, hoop. Partners should have similar equipment.
Play Formation/Area: Students are in pairs scattered.
Action: The first child of each pair does two moves with the equipment. The second child watches and tries to repeat the same action as the first child. Then it becomes the second child's turn to do two moves. Any child who misses the correct sequence gets a point. The student with the lowest score wins after each one has had five trials. No verbal cues can be given.
Variation: Add more movements before the student must repeat the sequence. Eliminate the equipment and use only the child's body. Increase the size of the groups.

Reading And Memory

● *Lost Treasure*
Equipment: A simplified obstacle course with five or six different obstacles can be constructed. Use ropes, balance beams, tapes, boxes, etc., to construct the course. Make index cards with commands on them to correlate with the obstacle course.
Action: Students select a card with two, three, or four commands on it. The student reads it out loud, then tries to do what the commands say. For example, a card with two commands might say, "Take three steps on the balance beam and crawl under the rope." This will aid in both reading and memory.

Variations: Tell the student the commands instead of having them read. Have the students read each other the commands.

Word Recognition

● *Find-A-Word Relay*
Equipment: A set of identical cards for each team. The cards need to have familiar words or new words on them that have been discussed. If five players are on each team, six cards will be needed so that a student will always have to choose a card.
Play Formation/Area: Line formation for relays.
Action: Place the cards face up in a group about 10 feet from each team. Allow 3 to 5 feet between the lines. The teacher needs to have a list of the words. A word is called and on the signal "Go" the first person does a locomotor skill movement to get to the group of cards, selects the word called, and then goes back to the line with it. If it is the correct word, and the person was the first to return, a point is scored. The card is then put back in the pile. The second person waits for the next word to be called and repeats the procedure. The winner is the team with the most points after each player has had a try. If a team member finishes first but has the wrong word, no points are scored.

Problem Solving

Problem solving and creativity can be developed by presenting children with low- to high-level movement challenges.

Low-Level Movement Challenges

Low-level movement challenges for solving problems do not require equipment. The leader or teacher simply asks students to solve different problems, such as:

● How many ways can you balance on three body parts?
● Can you move without using your feet?
● Can you make circles with parts of your body while moving?
● Can you move without touching anyone?
● Can you move so that your body changes heights?

Partner Activities

● Move with your partner so only your shoulders are touching.
● Balance so that only two of your body parts touch the ground.
● Move in a circle with only your elbows touching.

Problem Solving with Balloons

Equipment: Large round balloons, one for each student
Activity: The teacher asks students to solve simple movement problems using the balloons.

- What happens if you hit the balloon with the back of your hand? Is it different from using the front?
- How do you have to hit the balloon so that you get a lot of hits in five seconds?
- What happens if you hit the balloon from the top, sides, or bottom?
- Can you hit the balloon using only your feet?
- Hit the balloon in the air so that it stays above your head. How did you have to hit it?

Higher-Level Thinking

- Divide students into groups of three and ask them to try to invent a different game using familiar equipment.
- Ask students to modify the game for a handicapped student.
- Ask students to try and predict how fast the class can run on the average and calculate the scores.
- Record jumping efforts and then compare pre- and post-measurements.

POINTS TO REMEMBER

1. If properly structured, games provide a medium for students of all abilities in which they can play and relate to each other in a healthy social setting.

2. Games can be used to teach specific teaching objectives. Games should be selected in terms of the objectives they can help achieve.

3. Games can be changed in several ways to modify them for lower-functioning students.

4. Games can be used to integrate cognitive and motor learning.

5. The New Games approach consists of modifying the game by the players to suit their needs.

6. Teachers should be flexible in thinking when trying to modify games. A stereotyped approach to formations or other aspects of a familiar game will hinder creativity and reduce maximum participation.

REFERENCES

Blake, O.W., & Volp, A.M. (1964). *Lead-up games to team sports.* Englewood Cliffs, NJ: Prentice-Hall.

Cratty, B.J. (1980). *Adapted physical education for handicapped children and youth.* Denver: Love.

Cratty, B.J., & Breen, J.E. (1972). *Educational games for physically handicapped children.* Denver: Love.

Fait, H.F. (1978). *Special physical education.* Philadelphia: W.B. Saunders.

Fluegelman, A. (Ed.). (1976). *The new games book.* San Francisco: The Headlands Press.

Geddes, D. (1974). *Physical activities for individuals with handicapping conditions.* St. Louis: C.V. Mosby.

Morris, D. (1980). *How to change the games children play* (2nd ed.). Minneapolis: Burgess.

Schurr, E.L. *Movement experiences for children: A humanistic approach to elementary school physical education* (3rd ed.). Englewood Cliffs, NJ: Prentice-Hall.

Chapter 13

Leisure Sports Skills

Focus

- Describes the kinds of leisure sports in which handicapped students are able to participate.
- Defines specific adaptations and modifications for leisure sports.
- Suggests methods of teaching leisure sports to students with specific disabilities.

Leisure sports are those sporting endeavors in which an individual participates for enjoyment during free time or for the therapeutic effect as a recreational activity. Leisure sports are more likely to consist of individual and dual sports rather than team sports. However, some sports that can be pursued individually can also be pursued as a team, such as bowling, or in a social atmosphere, such as bowling, golf, or archery.

Leisure sports can be easily adapted to individual needs. They also do not require extensive management and organization. Both handicapped and nonhandicapped individuals can be easily integrated into leisure sports. In fact, certain sports provide a "handicap," such as golf, where individuals are allowed to add strokes to their game. This particular type of "handicap" enables individuals with all types of disabilities to participate and avoids their elimination. Almost any adaptation of a leisure sport can be made so those with disabilities can participate in one form or another.

Leisure sports also provide numerous other benefits to the handicapped person that other activities may not provide. Besides physical fitness, leisure sports offer the individual a form of constructive use of leisure time as well as social interaction.

INSTRUCTIONAL ORGANIZATION

The instruction in individual and dual sports will require careful planning and individualization on the part of the instructor. Since each handicapped person will have particular needs, the equipment, space, and rules will have to be changed to meet specific abilities. Fait and Dunn (1984) recommend ample experimentation in the beginning instructional phases of the sport to determine the most feasible methods of performing the skill components. Many forms of the modified versions may have to be developed. The limit is only in the teacher's and student's imagination. It is a good idea, as we have noted, to take suggestions from students in terms of some of the modifications that might be made.

Even severely handicapped students can be taught some form of a particular sport so they may pursue it on a leisure-time basis. The pleasure derived is the important thing and not how the sport is actually played. This chapter provides ideas and methods for modifying and individualizing leisure sport skills so that the handicapped student can participate for maximum pleasure and enjoyment.

BOWLING

Bowling is an excellent leisure-time sport in which many handicapped students can participate because many modifications can be made. Most students can be grouped and all levels accommodated. Bowling is also becoming a very popular Special Olympics event held separately from the spring event.

Entry-Level Skills

Since a regular bowling alley is not usually located in a school, other teaching techniques must be employed to enable students to develop some skills of the game until they can be used in a regulation bowling alley.

Before going to an actual bowling alley, several skill practice sessions should be conducted so the students have the general concept of the game. Some students may not reach the level of being able to score a game but can at least participate at some level. The students should have some concept of the game and the objective. A film is a good way to introduce the students to the game itself. Whenever possible, the students' parents should be encouraged to expose the students to bowling by trying the game as a family activity or just visiting a bowling alley. Bowling tournaments can also be observed on television.

The skills and concepts to be taught include:

- purpose of the game
- regular and modified grips where necessary
- stance and approach
- arm swing and release of the ball

Modifications

1. All forms of lanes can be arranged in a station pattern in the gymnasium or smooth grassy area outdoors as in lawn bowling.

2. Plastic milk cartons, potato chip cans, tennis ball cans, or others can be used for pins for very beginning concepts.

3. Plastic bowling pins can also be used in the very beginning stages and may be used throughout for those who have limited strength to knock over regulation pins.

4. There are plastic bowling balls that are lighter in weight than the regulation ball.

5. Smaller NeRF® balls can be used while in the learning process.

6. Lanes can be constructed in the gymnasium by placing 2×4s that are 12 feet in length parallel to each other.

7. Bowling can be used to integrate math into the physical education curriculum by practicing game scoring.

8. Scoring can be modified by having the number of pins or cans counted after so many trials.

9. Bowling with colors can be used in scoring rather than points. Each color can be worth so many points for students who cannot grasp the idea of scoring using the standard method.

10. Stations can be arranged in a progression from very basic skill development to actual bowling and scoring using plastic pins and balls.

11. Rewards for high scores can be free games at a regulation bowling alley.

Grip Techniques

Students need to have sufficient grip strength to manage and grip the standard bowling ball. If the student lacks sufficient strength, the standard grip may have to be modified as follows:

1. Allow the student to hold the ball with two hands.

2. Metal ramps with wheels are available for use by persons with little movement in the arms and hands or by blind students if necessary. The ball is placed on top of the ramp, then little movement is needed to send it down the ramp and onto the lane.

3. Another method is to use a shuffleboard technique to give impetus to the bowling ball placed on the foul line. The long-handled pusher is used to push the ball forward as one would use it in shuffleboard.

4. A ball with a retractable handle may be used. Fait and Dunn (1984) describe the grip with this type of ball as that used for carrying a bucket. When the ball is released, the handle retracts so the ball will roll smoothly down the lane.

5. Lighter-weight bowling balls or smaller ones can be used.

Stance and Release

A backward chaining method of instruction works well in teaching the stance, backswing, and release of the ball. The technique includes letting students stand at the foul line and practice swinging the arm backward and releasing a NeRF® ball low to the floor as one would a bowling ball. A piece of tape can be placed where the ball should first touch the floor. Students should practice this until some consistency is maintained.

The second phase involves repeating the first phase, but the student takes a step before adding the first phase. Thus, the motion would be a backswing, step, and release. This should also be practiced until consistency is established. Later, more steps can be added using four steps before the release.

Once students have gained some skill in the stance and release, modified activities can be arranged.

1. Let students who have mastered the stance and release practice on milk cartons or cans using a NeRF® ball.

2. Once students have some skill at knocking over cans and plastic pins, scoring or some modification of scoring can be taught.

3. Class tournaments can be arranged as a challenge with those scoring the highest receiving a certificate for achievement. Other awards should be given for the most improved bowler, for example. Prizes can include free bowling games and passes to a bowling alley.

BADMINTON

Badminton is an excellent leisure-time sport to teach handicapped students either grouped by handicap or mainstreamed. Modifications will need to be made for students with limited movement, poor coordination, and lowered cognitive functioning. Some general modifications include:

- making the court smaller
- lowering the net
- arranging doubles play with a skilled and low-skilled player as partners
- using balloons instead of a regulation shuttlecock
- using racket modifications such as handle extensions or special fasteners for those who cannot grip the racket adequately
- having players with more ability cover the backcourt
- allowing two hits per side in doubles.

Balloon Badminton

For students who have very limited mobility or as a beginning instructional technique, balloon badminton may be played. This can be played outdoors if there is little wind. Equipment: Rope 10 feet long or badminton net, rackets made from wire coat hangers and pantyhose, round balloon weighted cans for markers

Play Formation/Area: Mark off court using the cans at each corner. The dimensions of the court can vary for the number of players. Generally, a court about 10 feet long and 6 feet wide will be ample. The net height can vary also, but about 4 feet high will do since students are seated to play. As many as six students can be placed on either side of the court, thus accommodating 12 players. Action: Player hits the balloon from the front row over the net. This first hit must be above the players' heads and cannot be a smash. Two hits are allowed to return the balloon. If the team misses, the receiving team scores a point. The serve changes sides after every two points are scored. Students are not allowed to rise up to hit the balloon; they must remain seated.

ARCHERY

Archery may be adapted in numerous ways for all types of disabilities. It also proves to be beneficial for those who cannot participate in strenuous activities.

Skills and Adaptations

Target Placement

1. The target may be placed closer for those who lack strength and skill.

2. Fait (1978) suggests that a rise behind the target be avoided for physical disabled students or those who are in wheelchairs since climbing it to retrieve missed arrows would be impossible.

3. Extra bales of hay are recommended by Fait to use with the physically disabled. These can be placed in back of and to the sides of the target.

4. A beeper or portable radio can be placed on a stand behind the target to allow blind persons to have a point of reference for the target.

5. A marker such as a block of wood should also be used with blind students to mark the stance parallel in relation to the target.

Stance

1. Wheelchairs can be turned to the side just as a standing person would have either the right or left side to the target while shooting.

2. A guide rope from the target to the shooting point should be available for blind persons to follow to and from the target. Another technique is to provide a path that is distinct enough for the blind person to feel while walking to and from the target.

Nocking the Arrow

1. Tape may be wrapped above and below the point at which the arrow should be nocked.

2. Fiberglass bows usually have a ledge on either side of the bow to rest the arrow. With these two devices, blind students should have little difficulty nocking the arrow.

3. Bows with light pull should be used until students develop sufficient strength and skill for shooting.

Aiming

1. Instinctive aiming can be used but with blind students, Fait (1978) suggests placing a pole in the ground at a point where the hand holding the bow should be placed when the proper aim occurs. Aiming can be adjusted by raising and lowering the hand along the length of the pole. Tape can also be placed around the pole where the hand should be held. By feeling the tape the blind person can adjust the aim. Trial and error will have to be used to achieve the correct aim.

2. Other adaptations can include giving the blind student two or three extra arrows to shoot and not counting these in the score. These can serve as aiming practice.

3. If an individual has restrictive use of the arms, a crossbow may be used.

Releasing the Arrow

1. Kinesthetic teaching will be helpful in letting students feel the movement and proper position for the stance and release of the arrow.

2. Practice without the bow is good for teaching the release, emphasizing that the fingers are used to release the arrow. A mirror is good for letting the student check the position.

3. Masters, Mori, and Lange (1983) suggest placing a stick at the inside of the elbow as the drawing arm is in position. If only the fingers are used to release the string and arrow, the stick should remain in place.

Hitting the Target

1. Balloons can be pinned to the center of the target so blind students will know when they have hit a bulls-eye.

2. A sighted student can be paired with a blind student to assist with arrow retrieval and for giving feedback on hits.

3. Persons with poor balance but who are not confined to wheelchairs may use a stool high enough to accommodate a semistanding position.

SHUFFLEBOARD

Shuffleboard is a good sport to learn since it can be played by family members and does not require a great deal of advanced skills. It is also good for players with low vitality since it does not require vigorous movement.

General Modifications

1. Shorten the court.

2. A yardstick can be taped in the direction of the court for visually impaired students to feel.

3. Wheelchair players can shoot from either the right or left side of the wheelchair while it faces forward.

4. Those with poor balance may play seated in a chair.

5. Doubles is more effective for those who have limited movement skills and locomotor difficulty.

6. Scoring can be modified for those with lowered mental ability by counting the disk as one point if it lands within the scoring zone.

HORSESHOES

Horseshoes is a game that can be played almost anywhere and lends itself well to family outings and social gatherings.

General Modifications

1. The distance between the stakes can be shortened.

2. Rubber horseshoes rather than metal ones can be used.

3. For students who have limited movement, the opponent can stand at the opposite end instead of the same end while pitching. This eliminates walking back and forth to retrieve the shoes.

4. The grip can be modified for those with weak or deformed hands.

5. For blind students, a person can provide a sound cue for the first throw, then another trial can be allowed before scoring any pitches so the blind person can become oriented.

6. Pitching from a wheelchair is not difficult. The chair usually faces the stake with the delivery coming from the side of the chair using a full armswing.

PING PONG

Ping pong is commonly known as table tennis and can be played by many different persons with varying degrees of handicapping conditions. Ping pong is not overly strenuous and can be made as light or vigorous as the players wish, provided the skills are developed.

General Modifications

1. Fait and Dunn (1984) suggest a modified paddle for blind players. The paddle has two handles and is rectangular.

2. The table can be made more secure by anchoring it to the floor.

3. Rails can be made for the sides to keep the ball from rolling off the table.

4. Players with one arm can serve by letting the ball drop off the paddle and hitting on the bounce.

5. The paddle can be strapped to the amputee's stump.

6. Players who cannot serve by traditional methods should be allowed to toss the ball over the net on the serve.

7. For players with limited skill, or blind players, two bounces can be allowed before the ball is hit.

8. Players with less skill and weak arms and hands may need to concentrate on form in terms of how the paddle face is held. A more open-face position will allow more height on the ball and thus carry it over the net.

OTHER CONSIDERATIONS

Some students may wish to become good spectators of many sports, particularly those who are severely limited in movement. Some handicapped students may be able to do quite well at individual and dual sports but not as well or not derive enjoyment from highly vigorous team sports. Thus, if the student desires to become a knowledgeable spectator of one or several sports, opportunities should be provided for the student to learn about players, standings, statistics, or other aspects of the game.

Many sports facilities have access ramps to enable all types of handicapped persons to visit. Winnick and Jansma (1978) offer several suggestions for helping handicapped students to become knowledgeable spectators for various team sports.

1. Games, video or other, that actually simulate a particular sport are good for learning rules, strategies, and other aspects of the game. Such activities are good for students who have restricted mobility or some other condition that would prevent them from participation.

2. Students enjoy keeping track of teams in a particular sport, such as football. Pictures of favorite players can be cut out of sports magazines with a description of their standing. Newspaper articles and televised games can be used to gain more information about players and the game itself.

3. Attending actual sports events is also a good method of learning about the game. A local high school team can be followed and scores and statistics for the game can be recorded. If the student has difficulty writing, the statistics can be tape recorded.

4. Writing short essays about the history of a sport is also beneficial.

TRACK AND FIELD EVENTS

Although track and field events may be individual or team oriented, they will be included in this chapter, since many of the events can be done on an individual basis. The events can be modified slightly or may require no modification at all for those with mild handicapping conditions. The nice aspect about track and field is that the disabled person can compete against a previous score and does not have to compete with others.

Running

Running events can be easily modified to allow all levels of students to participate. Specific events may be designed for those in wheelchairs and blind students. The major running events are

- 100-meter dash
- 200-meter dash
- 400-meter run
- one-mile run
- two-mile run
- low and high hurdles

Adaptations

1. Wheelchair participants usually do the 50- and 100-meter dashes.

2. Guidewires can be used for blind runners or someone at the end of the distance is used to make a sound to be followed.

3. Blind students who have difficulty running can jog with a sighted partner.

4. The marker for the finish line should be placed several feet beyond the finish line so that maximum speed can be maintained until the actual finish line is crossed.

5. Chalked lines may be helpful for students to follow who get lanes mixed up. The line should be white so that visually impaired students will be able to see it.

Jumping Events

Major jumping events include the standing long jump and high jump. These events are included in the Special Olympics. Prior to participating in jumping events the students should have some notion of what jumping techniques include. Also, if any competition is to be engaged in such as the Special Olympics, some notion of the particular procedures for the event should be understood.

Students can be grouped according to their skill levels. For example, a division might include those who already have some degree of jumping skill and a group consisting of those who do not know how to jump. Those with jumping skill can be instructed in the particular events themselves, while those who lack jumping skill can be instructed on jumping fundamentals.

The Standing Long Jump

The standing long jump is probably one of the most popular jumping events, particularly in the Special Olympics. The following suggestions should be used when preparing students for special track and field competition or the Special Olympics.

1. The toes need to be behind the takeoff line during the initiation of each jump. Place footprints or some other marker to indicate where the feet are to be placed.

2. Both feet must be used in the takeoff.

3. Three trials are permitted and the best distance is recorded.

4. Measuring occurs from the takeoff line to the closest impression made on the landing surface.

5. Students should be encouraged to use proper jumping techniques. Refer to Chapter 8 or other curricula explaining techniques for fundamental motor skills. Wessel (1976) includes objectives and teaching sequences of fundamental motor skills in the *I Can* series published by Hubbard Publishing Company, Northbrook, Illinois. Games and other activities are included that incorporate jumping as well as other fundamental motor skills.

6. For blind students some form of auditory signal should be used beyond the point where the student should land. A radio, beeper, or another student can provide an auditory signal to offer a challenge and indicate the direction for the jump.

7. The point where the feet should be placed should have some type of tactile cue for blind students.

The High Jump

The high jump may be the most difficult of track and field events to teach, since it requires coordination and leg strength. In the beginning, technique should be the goal, rather than height. Three types of jumps are generally used, including the scissors, straddle, and western roll.

The scissors style may be the simplest to use with beginners. The bar is approached from a slight angle, either the right or left. The takeoff leg is the one furthest from the bar while the near leg is lifted for height and clears the bar first. The takeoff leg follows by lifting it high over the bar. The leg action then forms a scissors kick.

The following are teaching suggestions:

1. Several jumps should be attempted without the bar.

2. The landing area should be well padded using foam mats or sawdust. (Foam mats are less messy than sawdust and less likely to aggravate allergic conditions.)

3. The takeoff point will differ slightly for each student. However, a chalk line or taped line may be used to mark the general takeoff point.

4. When beginning jumps with the bar, the bar should be at a low enough level for each student to clear and experience success.

5. Verbal cues such as "Kick" should be given as the student begins to take off in attempting to clear the bar.

6. Students should warm up before jumping by using stretching exercises and jumps. Running in place and lifting the legs high are helpful for warming up musculature.

THROWING EVENTS

Softball Throw

The softball throw for distance is included in the Special Olympics. Competition for distance should follow only after students are at least somewhat familiar with throwing techniques and the procedures used. Stein and Klappholz (1972) summarize the throwing rules as follows:

- A 12-inch softball is used.
- Throws occur from standing stationary or a short run of no more than 6 feet.
- Three throws are allowed with the best distance recorded.
- Throws are not recorded if the person steps over the throwing line.

The following are teaching suggestions:

1. Always have students warm up before they begin to throw for distance. Arm circles and short throws will help to warm up the arms and shoulders.

2. Concentrate on teaching the proper throwing techniques before throwing for distance is allowed.

3. Lightweight balls are better to use in the beginning since they are easier to grip and reduce the incidence of injury and muscle strain.

4. Provide motivating targets for students to hit in the beginning. Use tires placed flat on the ground at different distances. Balloons can be attached to stakes in the ground at different points. Or a net or rope tied between two standards can be used over which students must throw in order to achieve more distance and height.

5. Students in wheelchairs should be allowed to develop their own throwing style. Fait and Dunn (1984) suggest that those who cannot control the followthrough momentum be secured in the wheelchair by safety straps around the trunk.

6. Auditory signals should be placed at a distance that allows the blind student to know where to throw. A student at a safe distance with a whistle can be used.

THE SPECIAL OLYMPICS

One of the most rewarding experiences for mentally retarded students and adults is to strive to cross the finish line in a running event, or throw a ball, and receive a medal or ribbon for the attempt. While the Special Olympics goes well beyond this, the majority of events are geared toward track and field type events.

Participation in the Special Olympics provides mentally retarded individuals with opportunities to develop:

- self-confidence
- physical fitness
- a sense of achievement
- an emphasis on abilities
- a sense of belonging
- companionship
- socialization skills
- a spirit of competition and effort

Stein and Klappholz (1972) suggest several important coaching hints for training mentally retarded youngsters for the Special Olympics:

1. Activities should be geared to the students' abilities. With this in mind, the teacher should try to find an activity that each individual can participate in without fear and frustration.

2. Patience is a must since mentally retarded youngsters may need more time to achieve the fundamental skills necessary for competition.

3. Each student should be rewarded for trying.

4. Practice sessions should not be too long. It is important that the teacher watch for signs of fatigue such as breathlessness, weakness, pallor, or an overly red face.

5. New skills should be introduced early in the practice sessions.

6. Skills should be reviewed often.

7. Novel approaches should be used for motivation. Wessel (1976) provides a series of games in which fundamental skills can be used. Another example would be to use music for warmup exercises.

Conditioning and Training

Conditioning is something that many unaware teachers attempt to do a week or so before Special Olympic's competition. Conditioning is important particularly for vigorous events such as running and swimming. However, a good conditioning program should be a part of the ongoing physical education program. Overall conditioning and conditioning for particular events should be included within the scope of the physical fitness program. A guide to follow might include the following steps:

1. Begin early in the school year with mild overall conditioning and motor fitness.

2. As screening is completed for particular strengths and weaknesses, provide more individualized conditioning for the weaknesses found.

3. Begin more specialized training and conditioning for particular event/s in which the students will participate.

4. Practice the specific events as they occur in the Olympics. Also, try to take the students to the location or one similar to where the actual events will occur. Some students have difficulty generalizing from one situation to another.

The following case example will illustrate how to establish a training program for a student.

Larry

Larry is a 10-year-old Down's Syndrome boy and enjoys participating in the Special Olympics or almost any track and field day. Thus far, Larry has only completed throwing events in the Special Olympics. He is overweight but wants to run in the short running distances. Conditioning is important for Larry, even though the running distance will be short. Physical fitness tests show that Larry is weak in leg strength and endurance. In addition, throwing form needs improvement. Thus, a program for Larry should be designed to provide overall conditioning and focus on weight management and strengthening the legs. A plan for eating properly should also be included and discussed with Larry's parents. His parents send his lunch to school, but it is heavy with sugars and starches. Some of the foods included in his lunch are two cup cakes, chocolate milk, ham on white bread, candy bars several times per week. His parents should be assisted in making better selections.

A daily conditioning program should include:

- a 300-600 yard walk
- jumping activities
- modified pull-ups
- general conditioning with his class
- practice on specific events in track and field, concentrating on skill development

Small units of competition can be included within the physical education program, either including one student against another or self-competition where one student tries to improve previous performance.

GYMNASTICS

Gymnastics can provide many activities in which disabled students can compete or simply develop leisure activities. Gymnastics can be geared toward group participation or individual enjoyment. The development of a routine can challenge creativity in addition to providing self-satisfaction.

Gymnastics also lends itself well to several skill levels. The range of gymnastics skills can be included at both the elementary and secondary levels. A great deal of expensive equipment is not necessary for self-testing and small equipment activities. In addition, gymnastics can greatly contribute to physical and motor fitness. Moran and Kalakian (1974) suggest other benefits that include:

- building a new vocabulary
- planning and thinking
- group participation
- expressive communication through body gestures
- following directions
- being accepted by peers
- recreational and leisure-time pursuits

Curriculum Suggestions

Since gymnastics activities can be included at both the elementary and secondary levels, certain emphases should be developed at each level. In the early grades the program should generally focus on developmental gymnastics. This program can include younger elementary children, older elementary children with handicapping conditions, and secondary students with more severe disabilities. Developmental gymnastics would also accommodate mainstreamed students.

Developmental Gymnastics

The emphasis in developmental gymnastics is to provide a beginning broad base of fundamental gymnastics skills. In-

cluded at this level, according to Schurr (1980), are the following:

- exploration of body movements
- exploration of individual routines and challenges
- experience and exploration of a variety of small apparatus and equipment

Competitive Gymnastics

Competition can be included more fully at the secondary level. Rather than an exploration approach as in developmental gymnastics, more specified training can be included with apparatus, tumbling, and floor exercises. At this level, there are many skill options available. Many adaptations can also be made within each area to accommodate students with varying degrees of abilities. Disabled students can experience success in many gymnastics events and in competition. The goal in teaching should be to develop each student to the maximum level possible, even though the skill levels of high-level competitors may not be achieved.

Safety

One of the first points to discuss about gymnastics is safety, since it is of utmost importance. For individuals to enjoy gymnastics activities, they need to feel secure while performing and learning a particular activity or stunt. Some general guidelines for safety are listed below:

1. Know the individual's strengths and weaknesses. For instance, if a student can move fairly well in floor routines but is weak in shoulder girdle strength, activities requiring strength in the shoulders should be introduced gradually including lead-ups to the specific activity. Careful spotting is essential while students are in the initial stages of learning.

2. The practice areas for each skill should be spaced far enough apart to allow freedom of movement so that students are not in each other's way. Overcrowding can lead to injuries from accidental collisions. Also, the space allotted for each skill should not be overcrowded with equipment.

3. It may be best to begin activities without apparatus, particularly if the teacher is short of aides. Floor routines, tumbling, and simple stunts can be learned with the teacher stationed at the more complex activity area.

4. Students should not be forced to attempt an activity that appears to frighten them. Lead-ups that can build on the activity can be tried or another one may be substituted.

5. The basic safety rules should be written and illustrated on a large poster that is kept visible to students.

6. Spotting should be used for stunts where the student is inverted and on apparatus. Students should not be allowed to spot each other until they have been carefully trained.

7. Students should not be caught or lifted while doing a stunt. Spotting is designed to provide momentary support or to break a fall.

Teaching Suggestions

1. Explain safety in language that students can understand.

2. Be sure students understand the importance of spotting and are competent at it before they assist each other.

3. Always allow experimental time with an activity before asking for movement perfection.

4. Begin activities with movements the students already know and progress from that point.

5. Allow more emphasis on individual activities at first before initiating group or partner performance.

6. When movements are combined into routines, only three or four should be used at first.

7. Students with slow reaction time will need to include slower movements in routines.

8. Routines involving balls should use lightweight balls and ones that fit the ability of each student.

Visually Impaired Students

1. Visually impaired students should be oriented to the gymnasium area to provide a mental picture of how the room is set up for the program. For changing from one station to another, a sighted guide should be used to aid the blind student.

2. When using apparatus, the blind student should be given time to explore the equipment using touch. It should be explained to the student how the apparatus is used and what the different parts do. It is also wise to provide an extra spotter until the student becomes familiar with the movements to be used and somewhat proficient. A safety belt, in some instances, may be more desirable than a spotter. For example, when a blind student is on the trampoline, a safety belt would be more appropriate than an additional spotter.

3. Geddes (1974) suggests using a doll or manikin for older blind students to show body positions for a particular stunt. By tactile exploration, the blind student can more clearly understand the body positions to be assumed.

Mentally Retarded, Learning Disabled, and Physically Disabled Students

The following are some general adaptations for mentally retarded, learning-disabled, and physically disabled students:

1. Lower the height of the equipment when the student is less skilled.

2. Provide visual cues in terms of where body parts should be placed on the equipment, i.e., handprints on mats, tape lines for takeoff points, etc.

3. Display pictures of different skills using skill charts.

4. Provide apparatus that fits the size and ability of the student, i.e., balance beams with wider widths, lower heights, etc.

Behavior-Disordered Students

The following are some guidelines for teaching behavior-disordered students:

1. Place students in close proximity to the teacher, or in a highly supervised area.

2. Be sure students understand consequences for horseplay.

3. Involve some students in being the teacher's aide. Assigning such responsibility may have a positive effect on the student's self-concept.

4. Allow students to keep records of their progress including the number of stunts accomplished or performance on various apparatus. Wessel's (1976) *I Can* program provides progress charts. These can be used with older students to monitor their own progress.

5. Take Polaroid pictures of students and place them on a poster for others to use as a model. This will help motivate students.

Gymnastics Progressions

Each student will have to begin at a level that is comfortable and safe for his or her physical condition and motor ability. Considerations in evaluating the student's readiness levels for gymnastics should include a survey of:

- physical fitness, particularly strength, flexibility, and coordination
- locomotor skills
- balance skills
- manipulative skills

Moran and Kalakian (1974) provide a skill progression to be used with emotionally disturbed and mentally retarded children. The progression can also be used as a model for a general gymnastics program. They recommend the following progression as a guide. Modifications can be made where necessary since students will move along at different rates.

Mat and Floor Activities

Body positions:

- pike stand
- tuck position
- swan or layout
- straddle stand

Simple stunts:

- bridges and arches
- mule kicks, rabbit hops, etc.

Tumbling:

- log rolls
- squat forward roll to sitting position
- forward roll to standing position
- dive forward roll
- backward roll
- pyramids with partners (Schurr, 1980)

Small Apparatus and Light Equipment

Ropes:

- simple rope hangs
- simple rope swing

Wands:

- stepping over wand
- balancing wand on one hand and moving
- turning while holding wand overhead
- simple routines with the wand performed to music

Hoops:

- rolling hoop and diving through
- simple routines of movement sequences with the hoop performed to music

Balls:

- basic bouncing in rhythm
- moving and bouncing
- passing to partner
- moving ball around the body

Wands with Streamers:

- shaking wand up and down
- passing wand from hand to hand
- making small and large circles with arms
- adding body movements such as walk, skip, gallop, etc., while moving wand overhead
- developing individual routines

Wands can be made from paper sticks, broom handles, dowel rods, paint stirrers with crepe streamers attached to one end with colored tape. They should fit the hand size of each student.

Large Apparatus

Trampoline:

- walking on trampoline to get a slight bounce
- simple controlled bounce, legs straight
- tuck bounce
- straddle bounce
- pike bounce
- simple drops, hand and knee and seat
- back drop

Horizontal Bar:

- low height, simple hang (vertical)
- simple swing on bar
- knee hang
- skin the cat

Rings:

- simple hang
- bent arm hang
- hang and swing
- inverted hang
- skin the cat

Parallel Bars:

- mount and support with arms
- walk forward with hands
- swing through
- simple dismounts

Uneven Bars:

- simple mounts
- simple body positions, pike stand on low bar, supported by high bar squat stand, straddle stand
- hip balance on low bar
- kick over to high bar
- simple dismounts

Balance Beam:

- simple body positions on beam, one leg balance, tuck sit, V-sit, squat balance
- walk with dip step, backward walk, sideward
- walk stepping over objects
- walk and turn
- simple dismounts

SWIMMING ACTIVITIES FOR HANDICAPPED INDIVIDUALS

Swimming and other water activities can be some of the most adaptable activities, even for the severely handicapped person. Swimming can be a time of very exciting fun, progress, and achievement for handicapped students. However, the program must be carefully developed to ensure success.

Handicapped students may have never been exposed to a pool, lake, or other aquatic environment. Thus, the instructor will need a definite purpose in mind when beginning aquatics with such individuals. A progressive, step-by-step, program is essential for alleviating fear of the water and developing a skill sequence that is achievable.

This chapter provides ideas for establishing and implementing a swimming program for the handicapped student. Concepts and precautions about teaching swimming and aquatics to handicapped persons will be discussed.

If the aquatics program is carefully designed, many benefits may be derived by handicapped participants. The benefits include the following:

1. Once students have become adjusted to the water, it can become a good form of relaxation. It particularly allows students mobility who otherwise would not have the opportunity. The medium of water may be the only chance that students with severe forms of neuromuscular disabilities have for stretching their bodies and moving. When required to move against the weight of gravity, often their movement capacities are greatly reduced. When movement in the water is at a minimum, just wearing a life jacket and lying in the water can be relaxing.

2. Swimming provides a form of conditioning for all students in terms of basic components of physical fitness. Swimming is one of the few activities that may be used to condition the entire body.

3. Being able to participate in the activities of normal children and adults is very gratifying for disabled students.

4. Swimming is a lifetime recreational skill and an activity in which an entire family can engage with their handicapped child.

5. Swimming also provides the disabled student with a sense of self-worth and confidence, even with small achievements in aquatics activities.

6. Social benefits are derived by having the opportunity to socialize with other individuals whether they are handicapped or not.

7. Psychological benefits are achieved from the fact that students can use swimming and water play as a means for a healthy outlet for frustration and other feelings.

8. Water therapy can be used as a means for rehabilitation for handicapping conditions that can be improved or even eliminated with such measures.

Program Planning

A swimming program needs careful planning before disabled persons are involved. Several factors must be considered, such as the population to be included, facilities, staff, and equipment. How the program will be organized depends to a great extent on the type of handicapped students participating in the program.

The Population

A survey of students should be made to determine the nature of their handicapping conditions and whether there is a broad range of disabilities and levels of student capabilities. The effects of water and swimming on the type of disability must be given careful thought. Table 13–1 provides a list of some precautions that must be considered when working with specific types of handicapping conditions in aquatics activities.

Facilities

An ideal facility with appropriate architectural design and specialized equipment would be desirable for managing a swimming program for a broad range of students with particular types of handicapping conditions. In most cases, such a facility is not available. The lack of a well-designed facility, however, should not prevent a swimming program from developing.

The American National Red Cross (1977) recommends that the following be considered when examining the facilities before initiating a program for disabled youngsters:

1. The decks surrounding the pool should be wide enough to accommodate a wheelchair and another person to navigate it if necessary.

2. The deck surface should be slip resistant.

3. The bottom of the pool should also be slip resistant.

4. A shallow portion of at least 18 inches would be ideal for water orientation of all students and an area for younger students to play in and adjust to the water.

5. The water temperature should range from 78–84 degrees, but 85–88 degrees may be necessary for students with limited movement capacities, circulatory problems, and orthopedic conditions.

6. The air temperature should be, on the average, about 5 degrees higher than the water temperature.

7. Ladders should be available and secure. However, graduated steps built into the pool with a railing may be easier for students to negotiate than the ladders.

8. If a lake is being used instead of a pool, the bottom should taper off gradually and be free of sharp objects.

9. The pool bottom should be visible.

10. The pool should be clean, have a good filtering system, and the water supply should meet health regulations.

Table 13–1 Swimming Precautions

Disability	Precautions in Aquatics	Disability	Precautions in Aquatics
Cerebral Palsy Restricted movement	• Water temperature should be 80–85 degrees or higher. • Air temperature should be five degrees warmer than water.	May wear orthopedic device	• Remove all appliances before student enters the water. • Teach student to modify strokes to compensate for missing limbs. • Use a flotation device around the chest to aid balance if a limb is missing (Anderson, 1968).
Seizures and medication	• Have procedures posted for first aid during a seizure. • Know which students have seizures and the medication they take.	*Learning Disabled* Reading disability	• Be sure student can determine the shallow end from the deep end. Use colors, such as red for depth over student's head and blue for safe depths.
Poor balance and mobility	• Provide a buddy nearby at all times in case the student slips under water and cannot regain an upright position	Impulsive	• Provide close supervision or a buddy to guard against sudden movement outbursts, such as jumping in without looking or dunking another swimmer.
Poor breathing ability	• Placing the head under water may not be advisable.	Hyperactive	• Avoid long lines to enter the pool and waiting for turns on the diving board.
Hearing Impaired Susceptible to ear infections	• Avoid getting ears wet.	*Mentally Retarded* Mild cognitive disability	• Needs little modification of swimming skills. Needs close supervision.
Wears hearing aid	• Remove hearing aid before student enters water.	Poor vocabulary	• May have difficulty reading depth markers.
Problems with balance	• Provide a handrail or buddy to walk with to and from the pool area.	Physical impairments Down's Syndrome susceptible to respiratory infections	• Will need extra support on land and water. • Make sure student does not have a cold during swimming. • Keep student out of drafts. • Be sure student is dry before going outside. • Avoid swimming on cool days if pool is outdoors. • Provide rest periods to prevent undue fatigue.
Cannot communicate verbally	• Know signals or signs the student uses to communicate.		
Visually Impaired Unfamiliar with the pool area	• Provide an orientation time allowing student to learn a route to the pool. • Provide a railing or some type of auditory signal to indicate the edge of the deck. • Provide a rail or auditory cue to indicate the deep end or rope off the deep end from the shallow end.	Severe cognitive impairment	• Provide a buddy with swimming skill and extra support in the water. • Aid with dressing may be necessary. • May require more frequent medical checks before and during swimming.
Loss of direction in the pool	• Provide a lane rope to be followed while swimming. • Use a buddy to give verbal signals.	Poor locomotor skills	• Provide assistance to and from pool area. • Have buddy walk between student and the pool.
Physically Impaired Loss of sensation	• Guard against bumping body parts that may have a loss of sensation. • Use proper lifting techniques.		

11. The depth of the pool should be clearly marked.

12. The locker rooms should be uncluttered but also provide good storage space for clothing, braces, and other equipment.

13. Hair dryers should be available, either built in or portable ones.

Equipment

A minimum of safety equipment needs to be available for rescue, for emergencies, and for applying first aid. Other devices should include the following at least.

1. A safety line should be attached and supported by buoys.

2. Rescue equipment should be highly visible and within easy reach of the person responsible for lifeguard duty.

3. A first aid kit needs to be close at hand, stored in a safe dry place. Include numbers for ambulances, rescue units, hospitals, and pool maintenance personnel.

4. Kickboards and other floatation devices should be available for each swimmer. Floatation devices come in many forms. Some for the chest and some for specific body parts are available.

5. Plenty of dry towels should be on hand for those who chill easily.

6. Play and game equipment or materials are not a must, but will greatly enhance the program. Examples include plastic ball, hula hoops, bicycle inner tubes, ping pong balls, sponges, beach balls, plastic animals, toys, or objects that will sink, and corks.

7. Charts to keep records of student progress are helpful and a motivational factor.

8. A camera, although not a must, comes in handy for taking pictures of students in the water that can later be used for bulletin board displays.

Organizing the Program

Organization of the aquatics program can take place in several phases.

Preplanning Phase

Completing preliminary work will help the program run smoothly in terms of the details of getting permission and preparing the instructors. The person in charge of the program should be well trained in water safety instruction, at least a WSI with certification in adapted aquatics. Experience in teaching the handicapped in aquatics would be beneficial. The following matters must be attended to before the program begins.

1. Obtain permission, if during school hours, from appropriate school personnel to have the program.

2. Obtain permission from parents or guardians for students to participate in the swimming program. A permission form should be developed. The person responsible for organizing the program should meet with parents who may possibly participate in the program. If slides or films are available of other swimming programs for handicapped students, they may help to alleviate any fear or hesitancy parents might have about letting their child participate. Exhibit 13–1 is a sample permission form.

The format and kind of information included in the parent permission form will depend upon the conditions under which the aquatics program functions. If it is part of a regular school program, not so much information will be necessary, since the school will have most of the information already. If the aquatics program is part of a summer camp or other arrangement, more information will be needed, since the students will not be familiar to the staff. The permission form in Exhibit 13–1 is designed for an ongoing program within a school setting.

Developing a Schedule

After the number and types of students have been determined for participation, scheduling the facility will be necessary. If the school does not have a pool, usually a community will be able to provide use of a pool. The program discussed in this chapter used a nearby university pool. The physical education department at Tennessee Technological University provided a two-hour time block on Friday mornings and a trained lifeguard to be on duty during the program. Friday was chosen so that students would have something to look forward to at the end of the week.

Exhibit 13–1 Sample Parent Permission Form

Parent Permission Form—Aquatics Program

Student's Name _____ Age _____
Handicapping condition/s _____
_____

Physical Limitations
Vision _____ Hearing _____ Respiratory _____ Cardiac _____
Seizures? __ Type _____ Medication _____
Person to contact in emergency
Name _____ Relationship _____
Phone (Home) _____ Work _____
Physician's Name _____ Phone _____

Other Information
Is your child toilet trained? _____ yes _____ no
List special precautions _____
_____
Can your child be photographed for news releases?
Yes _____ No _____

I give permission for my child to participate in the aquatics program as explained by the director.

Parent Signature _____ Date _____

Training Instructors

Programs of this nature are primarily conducted by volunteers and staff. The number of instructors will depend on the number of handicapped students and the nature of their disabilities. Students with more severe disabilities will need one-on-one instruction. Some students may be grouped in twos or threes for instruction where possible. When using a university facility, college students are most willing to volunteer as instructors. The program can also be used as part of a lab assignment for physical education and special education majors. All volunteers do not need to be education majors, however. It is a good practice to recruit instructors from other disciplines since it provides exposure to handicapped persons. Parents can also be helpful in assisting with the program. There are a number of resources available from which to solicit aid and support for the program, including civic groups, boy and girl scouts, and churches.

Orientation

An orientation and training session for staff and volunteers before the program begins will enhance its chances of running smoothly. Several components should be included in an orientation session. The following are considered as minimal topics for orienting volunteers and staff to the aquatics program.

1. Provide a general overview of the goals of the program. In fact, ask the staff and volunteers to add and suggest additional goals.

2. Evaluate the swimming ability of each volunteer. Those who are more advanced swimmers may work with more advanced students. If a person wishes to volunteer but cannot swim, he or she might provide assistance on deck with dressing students and keeping track of equipment.

3. Identify those volunteers and staff who have training in first aid procedures. Have a planned drill for emergency procedures and rehearse all steps involved.

4. Provide a one-page summary of each student in the program. The summary should include the following information:

- the primary handicapping condition
- any special needs or precautions for the student
- any swimming skills already known by the student
- tips for teaching the child

5. Provide an overall organizational plan for the program. Include the following:

- arrival time of trainers
- when and where to meet each child
- responsibilities in terms of each student for toileting, dressing, undressing, etc.
- where to meet on the pool deck
- a teaching schedule that would include time for individual instruction, group activity, and free time
- procedures for leaving the pool deck and return to the locker room
- where to wait for transportation

6. Orient trainers to instructional aids and how they are to be used.

7. Provide trainers with time to learn to write reports on student progress at the end of each session. A folder should be kept on each student. Progress can be reported quickly if skill checkoff sheets are used and evaluation by the trainer is briefly summarized.

8. If enough trainers are available, the program supervisor should be a rover or consultant to the program to assist each trainer with a particular student. This also frees the supervisor to respond quickly in emergencies or to offer assistance where necessary and gives the supervisor an opportunity to spot check and evaluate student progress.

Developing Student Objectives

An individualized swimming plan should be developed for each participant. The participants will all have varying levels

Exhibit 13–2 Individual Swimming Plan

Student Name __Bobby L.__ C.A. __9__ M.A. __5__
Handicapping Condition: __Down's Syndrome__
Precautions: __Susceptible to colds, hyperactive__
Present Swimming Level: No prior experience with any swimming activities. Appears to be afraid of water.

Long-Term Goal/s

Bobby will be able to enter the water safely and return to the deck without assistance.

Short-Term Goals

1. Overcome the fear of the water
2. Adjust to the water
3. Sit on steps and play in water
4. Place face in water and hold breath
5. Float on back and stomach
6. Kick with a flutter board
7. Combine arm and leg movements with assistance
8. Push off the side and glide on stomach
9. Swim 10 yards toward the instructor without assistance
10. Enter water and return to side of pool safely

Special Instructions

Needs close supervision
Use praise and positive reinforcement.
Be sure Bobby is dry after swimming.

of skills. Trainers should be given some guidance by the supervisor in developing priority goals for their students. This will give direction to each swimming session and pinpoint particular skills on which the trainers can work with each student. The following example will illustrate how the plan can be developed. Exhibit 13–2 is a sample swim program for this case example.

After each swimming session, Bobby's instructor should briefly record the progress made and note any changes that might be necessary. Special teaching techniques that worked should be particularly noted.

Sequential Skill Development

Developing a sequence of skills for the swimming program will add additional structure to the program. For the majority of disabled students, the program can be divided into three levels.

Level 1 can include novice skills; level 2, beginner skills; and level 3, advanced beginner skills. Further skills may need to be added, as some students will surpass these levels. A catchy name for each level can be developed to motivate participants. Names such as "Tadpoles," "Turtles," "Porpoises," etc., can be used with elementary-level students.

Exhibit 13–3 Porpoise Skills I

Skill	Date	Comment
Adjusts to water		
Sits on edge of pool and kicks		
Enters pool assisted		
Enters pool unassisted		
Puts face in water and holds breath		
Bobs five times holding breath		
Bobs, inhales, and exhales		
Plays in shallow water		
Moves in water holding on to pool edge		
Floats (prone) assisted		
Kicks (prone) assisted		
Kicks (prone) with kickboard		

A sequence of skills should be developed for each level. The name "Porpoise" will be used in this example. Exhibits 13–3, 13–4, and 13–5 list the skills to be included at each level.

By using this technique, motivational charts and progress forms can be geared to the different levels. Individual goals can be developed based on the progressions.

Other skill progressions may be developed by consulting swimming curricula already established, such as *I Can Aquatics* from Hubbard Publishing Company, Northbrook, Illinois, developed by Dr. Janet Wessel. The important point is to be sure the skills are in a sequence from the least to most difficult.

Exhibit 13–4 Porpoise Skills II

Skill	Date	Comments
Bobs and breathes in rhythmical pattern		
Floats on back unassisted		
Floats on stomach unassisted and recovers		
Opens eyes under water		
Kicks on back assisted		
Kicks on back unassisted		
Prone glides 5 feet		
Recovers an object from bottom		
Combines arm and leg stroke		
Swims at least 5 yards		
Jumps in pool and recovers unassisted		

Exhibit 13–5 Porpoise Skills III

Skill	Date	Comments
Changes position from front to back and back to front		
Jumps into deep water with assistance		
Combines arm and leg stroke 10 yards and breathes		
Jumps in water and swims 5 yards out and back to pool edge		
Treads water		
Remains floating for 30 seconds		
Jumps in deep end and returns to side		
Enters water head first and swims to safety		
Plays in group games in water		

If Red Cross certificates will be issued to some students, Red Cross certified instructors must be used to teach in the program. Some disabled students will be able to earn the certificates. The skills illustrated in Exhibits 13–3 through 13–5 are simple progressions with no formal certificates to be issued. Certificates of an informal nature can be made and issued as students complete each skill sequence. Exhibit 13–6 is a certificate that may be issued for completing the Porpoise I progressions.

Related Activities

All instruction and no play makes "Bobby" a dull swimmer! There should be times for play in the water after the instructional or formal teaching has been completed. One of the goals of a good swimming program should be to develop social interaction. This goes along with the normalization concept. Most children play games in the pool, so disabled students should have the same opportunities to have as normal an experience in the water as other students.

Water games provide the opportunity for students to have fun, to learn, and to socialize. Games can range from simple

Exhibit 13–6 Sample Certificate

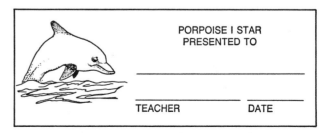

to complex and be designed for nonswimmers and swimmers as well. Students may need to be divided according to ability level to play some games. Arrangements can be made to accommodate several levels of abilities.

Individual Games and Activities

Activities can be carried out with individual students or in small groups. Games can be used to help students adjust to the water or reinforce what has been taught in the swimming lesson itself. Cognitive skills may also be integrated into simple play activities. The following are examples of activities:

1. Plastic cups or other containers can be used to pour water and teach measuring concepts; also concepts such as big, little, and shapes can be taught.

2. Washcloths can be used to let students get wet by pretending to wash. Ask them to wash their faces, legs, and arms, etc.

3. Plastic toys can be used to reinforce the notion that the water can be fun. Toy boats and plastic toys such as animals can be used to allow students to play in the shallow part of the pool.

4. Objects that sink can be used to get students to reach under the water and retrieve them. Eventually, they may go under the water and retrieve them as they pretend to be on a treasure hunt. Objects should be big enough not to pass through drain covers.

5. Tossing and catching activities can also be included in play activities while in the water. Soft objects can be used such as plastic balls, sponges, NeRF® balls, or tennis balls. They may be used in shallow water with instructor assistance. Targets can be made by placing hula hoops on top of the water. Children can toss objects that float into the hoops for points.

6. Plastic straws are good for teaching exhaling by having students place the straw in the water and blow bubbles.

7. Blowing a ping pong ball back and forth can help teach breathing and adjustment to the water.

8. Corks of different sizes can be placed on top of the water for students to retrieve.

Group Games

If the pool is shallow enough for students to stand in waist-deep water, several games can be played in a group.

1. For modified dodge ball have students form a circle with instructors between every two or three students. Using a NeRF® ball or beach ball, students try to hit each other. To avoid being hit, students must duck under the water.

2. Relays can be played in waist-deep water by having students pass objects as quickly as possible from one person to another. Objects that float should be used.

3. The regular version of the "Hokey Pokey" can be played in the water by having students stand in waist-deep

water and do the movements to a recording played with a battery-operated tape player.

4. Obstacle courses can be developed for students with swimming ability. Hula hoops, ropes, and objects placed under water may be used for students to swim around, under, and through.

POINTS TO REMEMBER

1. Individual and dual sports lend themselves well to being adapted and modified so that handicapped persons may engage them in their leisure time.

2. Participation is the key factor to consider in individual, dual, and leisure sports, rather than competition.

3. The notion of conformity to tradition has to be eliminated when modifying an activity so that handicapped persons can enjoy individual and dual sports.

4. The goal of sports for the handicapped should be similar to that for any individual: to derive pleasure and enjoyment from participating.

REFERENCES

American National Red Cross. (1977). *Adapted aquatics: Swimming for persons with physical or mental impairments*. Garden City, NY: Doubleday.

Fait, H.F. (1978). *Special physical education*. Philadelphia: W.B. Saunders.

Fait, H.F., & Dunn, J.M. (1984). *Special physical education* (5th ed.). Philadelphia: Saunders College Publishing.

Geddes, D. (1974). *Physical activities for individuals with handicapping conditions*. St. Louis: C.V. Mosby.

Masters, L.F., Mori, A.A., & Lange, E.K. (1983). *Adapted physical education: A practitioner's guide*. Rockville, MD: Aspen Systems Corporation.

Moran, J., & Kalakian, L. (1974). *Movement experiences for the mentally retarded or emotionally disturbed child*. Minneapolis: Burgess.

Schurr, E.L. (1980). Movement experiences for children: A humanistic approach to elementary school physical education. (3rd ed.). Englewood Cliffs, NJ: Prentice-Hall.

Stein, J.U., & Klappholz, L.A. (1972). *Special Olympics instructional manual*. Washington, DC: Joseph P. Kennedy, Jr. Foundation.

Wessel, J. (1976). *I Can, Fundamental skills*. Northbrook, IL: Hubbard.

Winnick, J.P., & Jansma, P. (Eds.). (1978). *Physical education inservice resources manual for the implementation of the Education for All Handicapped Children Act* (P.L. 94–142). Brockport, NY: State University of New York at Brockport.

RECOMMENDED READINGS

American National Red Cross. (1975). *Swimming for the handicapped—Instructor's manual*. Washington, DC: Author.

Grosse, S., & McGill, C. (1979). Independent swimming for children with severe physical impairments. *AAHPERD Practical Pointers*. Reston, VA: American Alliance for Health, Physical Education, Recreation and Dance.

Lawrence, C.C., & Hackett, L.C. (1973). *Water learning: A new adventure*. Palo Alto, CA: Peek Publications.

Miner, M. (1980). *Water fun*. Englewood Cliffs, NJ: Prentice-Hall.

Part VI

Therapeutic Approaches

Chapter 14

Therapeutic Activities

Focus

- Explains the therapeutic benefits of dance, play, music/rhythms, and community programs for disabled persons.
- Integrates basic elements of the concept of play therapy in the adapted physical education setting.
- Describes types of therapeutic activities that are beneficial to particular types of handicapped students.

Activities such as therapeutic recreation, dance, music, and play therapy are closely related to some of the broad-range goals of adapted physical education. One major goal of each discipline is to enhance the social, psychological, physical, and cognitive development of handicapped individuals. Another goal is to help the individual adjust and cope despite his or her disability.

The adapted physical educator will often work closely with members of the therapeutic team and may even carry out some aspects of the individualized therapeutic program as a team member. In some cases the adapted specialist will be asked to serve as a facilitator in getting recreation programs started for handicapped citizens in the community. Often, adapted specialists serve in other capacities such as members of a local community program board or sponsors of a special event. They may offer training assistance to community volunteer workers or serve as consultants to community-based programs for the handicapped.

This chapter provides an overview of three major therapeutic programs in the areas of therapeutic recreation, play therapy, and music and dance therapy. It will explore the purposes and strategies for meeting the needs of handicapped persons receiving therapeutic intervention within these disciplines.

THERAPEUTIC RECREATION

Kraus (1973) summarizes the purpose of therapeutic recreation as a service designed to provide recreation and similar activities to meet the needs of individuals with illnesses or disabilities, either long or short term. Therapeutic recreation is considered a rehabilitative process to develop mental, social, and psychological adjustment while creating methods for constructive use of leisure time.

Implementation of therapeutic recreation can occur in numerous settings such as psychiatric hospitals, community mental health centers, general hospitals with long-term patients, and mental retardation and other residential treatment facilities. With the concept of normalization and deinstitutionalization, more therapeutic recreation programs are being offered in community settings, such as group homes, sheltered workshops, and community centers.

While activities in the therapeutic recreational program may overlap with those of the adapted physical education program, their purposes may be different. The overlap occurs mostly with motor activities, sports, and active games. Included to a greater extent in the adapted program are educational goals, correctional strategies, and developmental aspects. The therapeutic program contains more outings, special events, social activity, and entertainment.

The Need for Recreational Outlets

Disabled and handicapped individuals need recreational outlets just as everyone else does. However, individuals with recreational needs who are handicapped may have fewer opportunities to engage in the variety of activities that non-handicapped individuals can experience. Fortunately, the barriers are not as numerous as they used to be. More parks are adding or making modifications so they are barrier-free, particularly those funded with federal money. Section 504 of the Rehabilitation Act specifies that all public places receiving federal money must provide access to the handicapped. The handicapped person cannot be excluded or denied the benefits of programs. Consequently, many positive changes have occurred since 1973 when the Rehabilitation Act was passed by Congress.

Still, in programs that are not receiving federal money, handicapped individuals may not be included to the extent to which they should be. In addition, individuals who are more severely disabled may need more recreational benefits than the average person, since their day may not be as filled with work and other common societal and cultural activities. Although many persons with disabilities are able to carry out everyday routines, a significant number do not work an eight-hour day, marry, or have families.

Goals of Therapeutic Recreation for the Disabled

Stein and Sessoms (1973) and Kraus (1973) discuss the major goals and purposes of recreation for specific populations with disabling conditions. Kraus (1973) suggests activities for specific disabilities.

Mentally Retarded and Learning Disabled

Goals:

- develop physical skills
- increase social maturity and adjustment to group situations
- complement vocational adjustment
- develop constructive use of leisure time
- develop an interest in hobbies
- increase independent functioning
- improve cognitive ability and independent thinking

Recommended therapeutic activities:

1. Sports and physical fitness
   - swimming
   - volleyball
   - track and field events
   - bowling
   - roller skating
2. Creative experiences
   - arts and crafts
   - dance and drama

The level of these activities depends on the mental age of the individual and the level of perceptual development.

3. Games
   - quiet games
   - lead-up games
   - new games
4. Social activities
   - club outings
   - parties and entertainment
   - special events and trips
5. Camping
   - day camps
   - wilderness camps
   - overnight camps
   - residential camps

Physically Disabled

Goals:

- provide pleasure from leisure time
- encourage personal development
- provide socially satisfying group experiences
- help person become a more productive family member
- increase participation in community life

Recommended therapeutic activities:

1. General guidelines
   - elimination of activities that cause tension and undue fatigue.
2. Specific activities
   - table and other quiet games
   - wheelchair basketball
   - arts and crafts
   - swimming
   - dance and drama
   - sports with modified equipment geared to the individual's physical needs

Blind and Partially Sighted

Goals:

- increase independence and mobility
- integrate blind individuals with sighted individuals
- develop social skills

Recommended therapeutic activities:

- dance and music
- drama
- bowling
- swimming
- hiking

Behavior Disordered and Emotionally Disturbed

Goals:

- relieve aggression and anxiety using socially acceptable outlets
- increase awareness of rules, structure, and socially acceptable behavior
- develop productive use of leisure time
- develop control of gratification
- develop an interest in hobbies
- increase tolerance of frustration

Recommended therapeutic activities:

1. Games
   - lifetime sports for adolescents
   - noncompetitive games
   - individual and dual games and sports
   - table games, cards, checkers, Monopoly, etc.
2. Hobbies
   - photography
   - painting
   - crafts
   - macrame
   - collections, coins, arrowheads, etc.
3. Creative experiences
   - dance
   - music
   - drama, plays, storytelling, puppetry
4. Camping and outdoor adventure

Program Implementation

Since activities need to be highly individualized, some form of assessment must be made before developing a program. The assessment should include several aspects such as the individual's

- physical skills
- cognitive ability
- current medical status
- interests in particular types of recreational activities
- behavioral and emotional conditions

PLAY THERAPY

Another therapeutic activity, developed by Axline (1947), includes play therapy. Axline (1947) stated that play therapy is a form of psychotherapy that enables children to gain insight into their feelings and behavior. Through this medium, insights and problem solving can occur. Ellis (1973) considers play as preparation for adulthood. It is very much instinctive in many species. Play ultimately provides children with a means for developing their arousal levels, learning, and interaction.

Elliot, Anderson, and LaBerge (1978) discuss three facets of play: learning, developmental readiness, and development of movement skills. Play serves as a means for children to engage through action with the surrounding environment and other individuals. Play also has other aspects, which include self-actualization and social and psychological development. It is a means for releasing emotions and learning to handle emotions, such as fears, tensions, and frustrations.

The Stages of Play

Children normally play spontaneously from the time of babyhood through late childhood. The first stages of play are individual and occur during the first two years. Babies will delight in looking at objects, reaching and grasping for them, and engaging in play with their own hands and feet. As the baby's motor skills increase, so do their play abilities. Babies will engage in parallel play by playing near or beside another baby, but not actually engage in an activity with another baby. After solitary and parallel play, group play eventually develops. Table 14–1 summarizes the stages of play and the characteristics of each stage.

Even though they may be older, handicapped children may still be in stages of play that are parallel or solitary. When conducting therapeutic play activities, the stage of play in which the child functions is significant. For example, if the child is in the solitary play stage, group play as a

Table 14–1 Stages and Characteristics of Play

Stage of Play	Characteristics
Solitary Play	Child plays individually by self or with object.
Parallel Play	Children play in the same location. May participate in the same or different activity.
Group Play	Play in small groups with the same activity. Generally will cooperate.

therapeutic activity will not be beneficial. The adapted physical educator should work toward developing the necessary motor skills that will enable the handicapped child to learn play skills that will eventually lead to group play. This will enable the child to participate more fully in therapeutic and recreational activities.

Implementing Play Therapy in Physical Education Settings

Reinert (1980) suggests methods that can be used to apply some of the principles of play therapy within educational settings. These will be adapted to the physical education structure.

Establishing the Structure

The physical educator may use some of the principles of play therapy but must be aware that formal training in using play therapy as a purely therapeutic method needs specialized training. First, a therapeutic environment for play to occur must be established. This enables handicapped children, particularly those with emotional conflicts and behavior disorders, to feel support through the activities provided.

Trusting relationships between the adapted specialist and the child needs to be established. This has to occur before the child will feel free to express emotions. The physical education setting provides an excellent medium for establishing rapport. One method is to engage in a favorite activity with the student. For example, if the student enjoys shooting baskets, ping pong, or some other activity, the adapted teacher can take a few minutes to engage in the activity with the student. While doing the activity, which should not be competitive, conversation can take place. This kind of interaction and dialogue between student and teacher indicates that the student is accepted, at least for the moment, by the teacher. It also establishes the individuality of the student.

While the teacher should show that the students are accepted, it should be made clear that behavior that is undesirable will not be accepted. When addressing this issue, the teacher should tell the student that it is the behavior that is not accepted and that the student is O.K. With this approach limits are set but a positive and trusting relationship can still be maintained.

Complete freedom in play is not realistic since injuries and property destruction can occur. Activities need enough structure to prevent this from happening but also should allow expression of feelings and emotions. Also, the student should feel free to explore the activity without fear or rejection. Freedom to express emotions is desirable through dance, rhythms, movement challenges, or other activities.

Some students have difficulty understanding or evaluating the consequences of their actions. The instructor can allow the student to stop and think through an action before doing it. This will still provide freedom and also include a form of structure.

Providing Opportunities for Self-Direction

Many handicapped students can be helped to learn to make decisions and become self-directed individuals. Game situations can be arranged so the students will need to make decisions. When decisions are allowed, the teacher must accept them unless, of course, they are harmful or self-destructive. Some ground rules must be established beforehand. Decision making should progress from simple to complex. Students may not be ready to make complex decisions, such as changing rules or making up new rules for a game. Some examples of less complex decisions include:

- choosing a piece of equipment
- selecting a partner
- choosing an activity
- choosing skills to practice in an activity

Complex decisions might include:

- changing the rules of a game
- developing a new game
- group decisions versus individual choices
- solving a problem related to a game, behavior, or skill

Encouraging Free Expression of Feelings

Feelings are important to individuals. Sometimes when students are sad, for example, adults may say, "Don't be sad." Actually, students should be allowed to express rather than repress such feelings. Activities should be geared to provide emotional outlets. Some of the more therapeutic activities include:

- dance and movement exploration
- mime
- exploring themes in movement
- yoga
- batting or striking objects with rackets or racket games themselves
- tether ball
- punching bag
- stunts
- gymnastics

The Let's Play To Grow Program

In 1979 the Kennedy Foundation began a new program called Let's Play To Grow Clubs. The purpose of the program is to

- develop the excitement and delight of play and other related experiences for developmentally disabled persons and their families and friends.
- experience the joy of play through the play guides developed in the Let's Play To Grow Kits.
- develop cooperative family partnership in play.

The exciting aspect of this program is the focus on the family. Children, both handicapped and nonhandicapped, who have difficulties or disabilities have a profound effect on the family. Often the entire family needs to be a part of the treatment effort. They need to have their needs as well as the handicapped child's needs met. Let's Play To Grow focuses on the family and community in offering support and recreational or developmental activities in which the entire family can be involved. The program has many therapeutic features:

1. The family learns to cooperate and share in the play experience.
2. A broad age span is covered so the family can choose and arrange activities according to the developmental level of each child.
3. Success and achievement can be documented.
4. Parents and siblings can feel a sense of being a significant part of the child's play skills, learning, and development. Relatives may also receive the same benefits.
5. Parents and siblings can improve their perceptions of each member's worth. Often the nonhandicapped sibling is excluded and left out when a handicapped child comes into the family.
6. Healthy recreation and leisure skills can be developed.
7. Family relationships can be improved. Other families with similar needs can offer support.
8. Family members of disabled persons are able to share close and creative experiences through the medium of play.
9. Parents and disabled children through adults can feel a sense of community support.

The adapted physical education specialist should act as a catalyst to begin a Let's Play To Grow program in the community. The program is built around 12 play guides that include sequentially arranged activities with teaching strategies and adaptations for the physically and severely handicapped. The following is an overview of each guide.

Guide 1: Activities geared to the very young child or one who is severely handicapped and sensory motor activities

- touching objects
- body management
- body utilization

- beginning locomotor skills
- play skills

Guide 2: Rhythmic movements and dance

- basic rhythmic skills
- exercise to music
- moving to music
- musical games

Guide 3: Seeing and creativity

- expression of ideas
- drawing
- colors, shapes
- painting
- constructing
- writing poetry
- hobby development

Guide 4: Locomotor skills and rope activities

- jogging and running
- jumping and skill variations
- rope activities

Guide 5: Outdoor fun

- hiking
- camping
- picnics and outings

Guide 6: Water fun

- adjustment to the water
- fundamental swimming skills
- water games

Guide 7: Basic skills

- rolling a ball
- beginning throwing
- catching
- kicking
- batting

Guide 8: Bowling fun

- bowling lead-up skills at home
- hints for skill development
- bowling at bowling lanes

Guide 9: Volleyball

- basic volleyball skills
- modified volleyball
- adaptations for wheelchairs

Guide 10: Basketball

- basic fundamental skills
- lead-up games
- modifications for physically disabled

Guide 11: Soccer and kickball

- fundamental skills
- lead-up games for soccer and kickball
- adaptations for physically disabled

Guide 12: Softball

- fundamental skill development
- modified softball and lead-up games
- adaptations for wheelchair players

Five more guides are included with specialized activities related to topics and cultural aspects.

Guide 13: Fun with kites

- making and flying kites

Guide 14: Winter fun

- activities that can be done in the winter in the snow and indoors

Guide 15: Desert fun

- geared toward those who live in the desert regions
- activities and fun while traveling through the desert

Guide 16: Pueblo games

- games and crafts related to the culture of the Pueblo Indians of New Mexico

Guide 17: Mini games

- games that can be used as ice-breakers in the beginning of a club meeting
- relaxation games
- get-acquainted games

Progress is kept on each handicapped individual belonging to a Let's Play To Grow Club by documenting the number of hours spent in any activity on a progress chart included with the kit. When a family has completed 30 hours of play, a patch with a picture of a famous person can be earned and a certificate of achievement is awarded.

If a community wishes to begin a local club, information may be obtained by writing Let's Play To Grow, 1701 K Street, N.W., Suite 205, Washington, DC 20006. While the clubs and programs are designed for use in a community setting, they may also be used in schools, camps, and residential settings.

DEVELOPMENTAL THERAPY

Developmental therapy was primarily developed by Wood (1975) as a psychoeducational curriculum for severely emotionally disturbed and behavior-disordered children who range in age from three to sixteen years. The approach has also been used with children having other types of handicapping conditions, particularly young children.

The major idea of developmental therapy is to use the normal changes that occur in development as a component of the therapeutic process. The feature of developmental therapy is that it does not isolate the handicapped, particularly the disturbed, child from normal experiences. Basic developmental therapy teaches the child to cope using inner resources of movement skills, sensory and perceptual abilities, and communication. Developmental progressions are used to eliminate inappropriate behavior and stimulate constructive behaviors in children with maladaptive behaviors. These may include mentally retarded, emotionally disturbed, or other children with poor or inappropriate coping skills.

Major Components

McDowell, Adamson, and Wood (1982) describe the four basic curriculum areas of behavior, communications, feelings, and pre-academics that are included in developmental therapy:

Behavior refers to movement and adaptive skills the child makes in response to the environment. Behavior objectives in the developmental therapy curriculum might include:

- stimulus awareness
- simple motor reactions to stimuli
- body management
- controlling impulses and involvement with rules and expectations

Communication refers to all the verbal and nonverbal methods of interaction with others. Wood (1975) emphasizes

the importance of developing communication, since it is needed to express feelings and emotions.

Socialization is a phase in the curriculum that concerns the development of affective components, including positive group activity, cooperative play, caring for others, self-confidence, sharing, and valuing others.

Pre-academics are the tools for building thinking skills and eventually problem solving. Components include:

- perceptual skills
- body coordination
- eye-hand coordination
- memory and discrimination
- concept development
- generalization of information
- problem solving

Wood (1975) explains that in each of the four major components of the developmental therapy curriculum there are sequenced hierarchical objectives. The curriculum specifies the procedures, activities, and general approaches to be used to teach the specific objectives.

Developmental Therapy in Adapted Physical Education

The physical education curriculum lends itself as a means for implementing developmental therapy concepts and components. The curriculum is designed for a variety of personnel working with children who have poor or maladaptive responses to the environment and others. It is highly suited for use with recreation specialists, special education teachers, parents, regular classroom teachers, and a variety of personnel in treatment centers for more severely disturbed individuals.

There are five stages in developmental therapy. The implications for the adapted physical educator using this model will be illustrated within the context of the five stages. Table 14–2 illustrates the examples.

By keeping in mind the five sequential stages of developmental therapy, the proper physical education activities can be geared to the needs of the handicapped individual with adjustment difficulties or other types of emotional and behavioral problems. For more information on developmental therapy, the books by Purvis and Samet (1976), Williams and Wood (1977), and Wood (1979) are recommended.

MUSIC AND DANCE THERAPY

Music is considered one of the most beneficial therapeutic activities for handicapped individuals. While music therapists complete a highly specialized degree, a program of

Table 14–2 Implications of Developmental Therapy for Adapted Physical Education

Stage	Implications for Adapted Physical Education
Stage 1 Responds to the environment with pleasure	• Provide pleasant sensory motor experiences: rocking, swinging, holding, etc. • Begin exploration of body parts and their movements. • Introduce vestibular boards.
Stage 2 Responds successfully to environment	• Begin basic fundamental motor skills. • Begin exploration of movement and imitation of animals. • Begin simple rhythm skills.
Stage 3 Learns skills to participate in groups	• Let child demonstrate a simple motor skill and provide peer reinforcement. • Try simple movement challenges. • Include simple stunt and partner activities. • Introduce simple equipment used with a partner: balloons, bean bags, hoops, wands, etc. • Introduce New Games. • Teach sharing equipment. • Refine development of basic fundamental motor skills.
Stage 4 Participates in group process	• Introduce lead up-games to sports. • Simplify rules for games. • Discuss why rules are necessary. • Use dance and exercise groups.
Stage 5 Applies individual and group skills to new situations	• Introduce conditioning and fitness activities. • Use social, folk, and square dance. • Provide coed experiences, and more leisure-time sports and games. • Involve in peer teaching or being a student assistant in P.E. • Provide intramural sports or after-school sports clubs. • Include Special Olympics bowling. • Allow evaluation of own performance and of others. • Develop and create new games with different equipment.

music and related rhythmic activities can be successfully developed and implemented by the adapted physical education specialist. These activities will aid the student in expression of emotions and feelings and expand communication abilities. Masters, Mori, and Lange (1983) note that even severely and profoundly handicapped students respond well to music and that it often reduces self-stimulation, which these groups often exhibit.

Music, according to Kraus (1973), has been used to relate to severely disturbed individuals by allowing the disturbed person to express feelings in a nonthreatening form and environment. Music and dance therapy have similar purposes and are closely interrelated. In dance therapy, the main goal is to use the medium of dance and rhythmic movement to develop nonverbal communication. This ultimately leads to the ability to relate to others. Dance therapy uses very simplified forms of unstructured movement. Individuals are allowed a great deal of freedom of movement expression. Music may or may not be used as a rhythmic accompaniment.

Dance therapy can also help students become aware of their own bodies. Positive changes in social behavior may result from students increasing their ability to control their impulses and release emotions and tensions.

Fitt and Riordan (1980) distinguish between dance therapy and creative dance. As a therapeutic procedure, dance therapy develops or attempts to build a trusting relationship between the child and therapist. Self-expression is encouraged so that the therapist can gain emotional insight into the persons's difficulties. On the other hand, while creative dance and movement also include self-expression, performance standards are involved. Themes in dance therapy center on the individual's behavior, emotions, and needs in perceptual development. In creative dance the themes may be more generalized and less individually centered. Dance therapy focuses on the individual's movements as expressions of psychological, cognitive, and motor development.

Fitt and Riordan (1980) explain the benefits of dance and music therapy for specific handicapped populations. Table 14–3 describes the benefits directly related to specific disabilities.

Many of the benefits may overlap since the needs of each disability may be similar. The table focuses on the major emphasis for each disability.

Creative Movement and Music in the Adapted Physical Education Classroom

Using the concepts of dance and music therapy may be more advantageous with mild to moderately handicapped students. The personal satisfaction that the students achieve is really the final goal. Some students may not move with grace and rhythm but the important benefits are the exploration and satisfaction derived.

Table 14–3 Benefits of Dance and Music Therapy for Specific Disabilities

Disability	Benefits
Sensory Impaired	• reduces inappropriate self-stimulating behaviors • provides movement alternatives • helps overcome fear of moving • reduces make believe through active movement and role play • develops trust • develops posture and good body alignment • facilitates the use of other senses • reinforces abstract concepts • develops spatial awareness
Emotionally Disturbed	• helps increase socialization • encourages control of isolated body movements • teaches positive behavioral responses • develops awareness of self in relation to surrounding objects in space • facilitates development of more flexibility in movement choices • aids in keeping the person more reality oriented
Learning Disabled	• develops movement control • increases perceptual awareness • improves time and spatial relationships • may reduce hyperactivity by moving slowly • improves self-concept
Mentally Retarded	• provides an outlet for frustration • aids in developing a vocabulary • aids in communication • teaches abstract concepts
Physically Impaired	• allows group participation • provides a sense of accomplishment • provides an opportunity to share feelings with others • provides relaxation

Presenting Creative Movement

During the normal course of development children are generally uninhibited in expressing themselves through movement. Handicapped students, however, may not have had the opportunity to experience movement the way their nonhandicapped peers did through the normal course of development. According to Elliot, Anderson, and LaBerge (1978), several guidelines should be followed when conducting creative movement experiences for handicapped students:

1. Lead up to the idea of creative movement rather than beginning immediately, particularly for those students who are new to this form of experience.

2. Use some type of rhythmic accompaniment. It need not be sophisticated and can range from a simple hand clap to drums, piano, or records and tapes.

3. To get students used to the idea of moving to music, allow them to play simple types of instruments and move in rhythm with the instrument. Instruments can be homemade such as tambourines, sand blocks, shakers, bells, triangles, rhythm sticks, or drums.

4. Be accepting of the students' movements and the desire to move. Quality of movement is not the objective at this point.

5. Begin by having students seated and moving only one or two body parts.

6. The first experiences should be light and lively and enjoyable for the students. This should leave them with a desire to continue similar activities.

7. Reinforce the students with positive statements and gestures when any attempt to move is made.

Lead-In Activities to Creative Movement

Once the teacher feels comfortable with the idea and the students begin responding positively to the notion of moving in an uninhibited form, some lead-in activities may be used. These will help students who are inhibited feel more comfortable with moving.

1. Ask students to listen to music and tell if it is slow or fast. To save time short segments can be recorded and played.

2. Play the music again and ask students to clap their hands to the beat. Some may follow a leader if they are having difficulty but the idea is for the students to be creative.

3. Give students an instrument to keep time to the instructor's hand clapping. Let students try to experiment with the instrument for a period of time.

4. Let students make up their own beat with the instruments.

5. Have students get into a personal space and move around the room to slow and then fast music. No particular form of movement should be asked for; students should just move in their own way.

Movement Challenges

Once students feel less inhibited about moving, more structure may be added to the movement experiences. Movement challenges involve asking the student to move in a certain way, though the student is still free to use self-interpretation for the solution. This develops creativity and is a therapeutic activity in itself. Movement challenges also enable the student to discover movement and skill ability. By making the challenges more difficult, more skill can be gained.

Knoblock (1982) suggests that creative movement and exploration can use other therapeutic media such as stories, music, poems, and dramatics. Using partners enables individuals to relate their creativity to one another. It is the general idea of sharing through movement that enhances students' awareness and acceptance of others. Challenges also encourage freedom and nonrestrictive expression. The following are some guidelines for movement challenges:

1. The teacher should have some basic rules. These might include:

- Students should make only positive comments about others.
- Each person can feel free to work at individual rates.
- Students may encourage other students or help only if the student asks for help.

2. The teacher should use terms such as "How can you . . . ?" "How many different ways . . . ?" etc. A statement or request might be "How many different ways can you move across the room?" Solutions to a challenge should not be given by the teacher.

3. If a student constantly copies another student, ask the student if he or she can think of another solution.

4. If students become out of control or disruptive in some way, simply remove them from the activity for five minutes, then permit them to return.

5. The challenges must be geared to the intellectual level of the students.

These are some examples of challenges using feelings:

1. Talk about a feeling such as sadness. Ask students what makes them sad and let them respond. Ask them if they can hold their bodies so they appear sad. Ask them how they would move if they were sad.

2. Talk about anger. Anger is a difficult feeling to manage. Many times parents and teachers do not let students express their anger. They tell them not to be angry or that it is not nice to be angry. Thus, students may not learn to handle their anger appropriately. It may be held within and finally turned or directed to one's self. This can lead to psychological difficulties and eventually more serious emotional problems. Angry students may be hostile, aggressive, or depressed. Have students role play a scene in which they were angry, then ask them to move their body like they would if they were angry. Some may grit their teeth, clench their fists, or use other facial gestures.

4. Aggression is sometimes handled in nonacceptable ways by students. Provide experiences in which students are able to kick a ball or try mime movements that may be aggressive. Students with aggressive tendencies may be allowed to beat a drum during the rhythm section.

POINTS TO REMEMBER

1. Therapeutic disciplines generally have similar goals for the handicapped individuals they serve. The major difference in the disciplines is the form in which the therapeutic approach is applied.

2. The adapted physical educator has a major role in developing skills in handicapped students so they will be able to derive the benefits of therapeutic activities.

3. The physical education service provider, while not necessarily a certified therapeutic specialist, will often be involved in cooperative programs with the therapeutic specialist.

4. By understanding the goals of therapeutic activities the physical educator can participate as a team member with these specialists and integrate activities into each student's physical education program.

5. Therapeutic activities need to be provided in a trusting and nonthreatening environment.

REFERENCES

Axline, V.M. (1947). *Play therapy.* Boston: Houghton Mifflin.

Elliot, M.E., Anderson, M.H., LaBerge, J. (1978). *Play with a purpose: A movement program for children* (3rd ed.). New York: Harper & Row.

Ellis, M.J. (1973). *Why people play.* Englewood Cliffs, NJ: Prentice-Hall.

Fitt, S., & Riordan, A. (1980). *Dance for the handicapped.* Reston, VA: American Alliance for Health, Physical Education, Recreation and Dance.

Kennedy Foundation. (1979). *Let's Play To Grow—Club leader manual.* Washington, DC: Author.

Knoblock, P. (1982). *Teaching and mainstreaming autistic children.* Denver: Love.

Kraus, R. (1973). *Therapeutic recreation services: Principles and practices.* Philadelphia: W.B. Saunders.

Masters, L.F., Mori, A.A., Lange, E.K. (1983). *Adapted physical education: A practitioner's guide.* Rockville, MD: Aspen Systems.

McDowell, R.L., Adamson, G.W., and Wood, F.H. (1982). *Teaching emotionally disturbed children.* Boston: Little, Brown.

Purvis, J., & Samet, S. (1976). *Music in developmental therapy.* Baltimore: University Park Press.

Stein, T.A., & Sessoms, H.D. (Eds.). (1973). *Recreation and special populations.* Boston: Holbrook Press.

Reinert, H. (1980). Children in conflict: Educational strategies. St. Louis: C.V. Mosby.

Williams, G., & Wood, M.M. (1977). *Developmental art therapy.* Baltimore: University Park Press.

Wood, M.M. (Ed.). (1975). *Developmental therapy.* Baltimore: University Park Press.

Wood, M.M. (Ed.). (1979). *The developmental therapy objectives: A self-instructional workbook,* (3rd ed.) Baltimore: University Park Press.

Chapter 15

Camping and Outdoor Experiences for the Handicapped

Focus

- Explains the values and benefits of camping and outdoor adventure for handicapped students.
- Discusses various types of camps and their purposes for handicapped campers.
- Discusses and develops methods for establishing camps, including staffing, scheduling, and organizing a schedule of activities.
- Defines other types of outdoor adventure and learning experiences for handicapped students.

Camping and outdoor adventure programs can be some of the most exciting experiences that disabled students will have. Camping has been shown to be a therapeutic and productive experience for most individuals. Shea (1977) explains that exceptional persons can be provided with the benefits of learning, growth, skill attainment, recreation, social development, cooperation, and emotional development through camping and other outdoor activities.

THE BENEFITS OF CAMPING

Camping and Learning

Many cognitive skills can be developed through the camping experience. Examples include measuring, reading maps, identifying trees, animals, rocks, and planning a day's hike. Writing skills can be developed by having campers keep a daily log or weekly newspaper. All types of learning experiences can be developed through the camping experience itself.

Camping and Growth

Physical development can be maintained by having campers participate in a series of vigorous activities each day. The experience of hiking and climbing can also be included, though not on a daily basis.

Camping and Motor Skills

Motor skills can be developed or enhanced through the camp experience. Arts and crafts help to develop fine motor skills, the use of hand tools, painting and drawing techniques, to name a few. Gross motor skills that are involved in games can be developed in activities scheduled to target the special needs of each student.

Camping and Recreation

Besides camping, which can be a leisure-time skill throughout adulthood, other recreational outlets can be explored and developed in the camp setting. Skills such as those related to fishing, hiking, photography, and crafts may also be included within the camp program.

Camping and Social Development

Camping requires a group effort and cooperation when several campers are involved. The teamwork to set up the camp and participate in the activities lends itself well to developing the social interaction skills of each individual. Camps have been known to bring some very withdrawn campers into the group process. A model of companionship

and cooperation can quickly be established in the camp setting.

Camping and Emotional Development

Camps that are residential, in particular, can aid in the emotional growth of each individual by participation in the various activities. Students who become campers in a residential setting are able to develop emotional relationships within the camp setting. Counselors may also be helpful in aiding campers in their emotional growth by offering group and individual guidance.

THE CAMP SETTING

Many of these areas of development can be aided through a variety of camp settings, which may or may not integrate handicapped and nonhandicapped campers. Moreover, outdoor experiences may not necessarily involve camping. Fait (1978) defines outdoor experiences as educational experiences that are directly taught by using the natural environment. Mainstreaming should certainly be involved in both camping and outdoor experiences. Integrated outdoor experiences that involve mainstreaming offer many positive benefits.

- Individuals can learn to accept differences in others.
- Both handicapped and nonhandicapped campers can gain a sense of accomplishment.
- Activities can provide each person with opportunities to see the worth of other individuals.
- The outdoor experience provides a means for campers to grow together through acceptance and understanding.

This chapter will discuss various methods of providing camping and outdoor adventure activities for handicapped youngsters. The emphasis is on mainstreaming. Various types of camps will be discussed as well as methods for organizing camp activities.

Camping experiences can be conducted according to the type of camp. However, whatever type of camp is used, the experiences should be geared to the individual needs of the camper as much as possible. The three types of camps to be discussed are day camps, residential camps, and specialized camps.

DAY CAMPS

Shea (1977) explains that the major goal of the day camp is to provide an activity program geared toward the recreation and socialization of children and adolescents based on their needs. Day camping is just what it implies. Campers attend the setting during the day and then return home that same day. No overnight stays are generally involved. Day camps are most often held during the summer months for a week or two weeks at a time. They may be offered or sponsored by civic organizations, schools, public recreation agencies, or agencies supporting a particular type of handicapped group.

Day camps lend themselves well to implementing a mainstreaming approach. No overnight accommodations need to be arranged and no great numbers of meals prepared.

Number of Campers

The number of campers to be accommodated depends on the space, the size of the staff, and the nature of the handicapping conditions. If mainstreaming will occur, a one-to-one ratio is essential. One nonhandicapped camper should accompany a handicapped camper. Shea (1977) recommends that one counselor be available for every five campers when mild to moderately handicapped youngsters participate in the day camp setting. A smaller counselor-to-camper ratio is required if more severely handicapped campers are involved.

Mainstreaming in Day Camps

Mainstreaming in day camps seems to have been on the increase during the last decade. Since Project PERMIT was so successful in mainstreaming handicapped students into physical education settings, some of the same principles were adopted by the Cookeville, Tennessee, YMCA. This particular YMCA is one of the few to offer an integrated summer day camp for handicapped and nonhandicapped youngsters.

Some of the concepts used by the day camp director to mainstream youngsters had proven successful in Project PERMIT. These included:

1. peer camper concept derived from the peer teacher concept
2. more noncompetitive activities to accommodate all levels of students

   - parachute games
   - new games
   - swimming
   - frisbee
   - arts and crafts
   - challenge courses
   - lead-up games
   - physical fitness activities
   - picnics

   - movies
   - playground activities
   - field day events
   - special field trips
   - fishing

Choosing a Location

Mainstreamed day camps can be held in a variety of settings. The particular camp described below was held on the large grounds of a community swim center. The setting was ideal for several reasons.

1. It had ideal facilities, including a large swimming pool with ample room, large open grassy areas, and a playground.
2. A challenge course was also constructed to accommodate all levels of skills and abilities.
3. Restrooms were easily accessible and a good shelter area was available.
4. An indoor area for arts, crafts, and rainy day events was also provided.
5. The location was convenient so that travel and transportation were easily arranged. This allowed for easy access in case of emergencies. Field trips were also easily arranged because of nearby attractions such as state parks, lakes, farms, bowling lanes, petting zoos, etc.
6. Several acres of wooded and pasture land were nearby for hiking and exploring.
7. Shade trees and picnic tables provided ideal lunch settings.

Numerous settings are available to have good summer day camps with mainstreaming as a major feature. Several summers before, the camp was held at one of the local county elementary school gymnasiums. All of the outdoor facilities adjacent to the school were also available.

Staff

The camp director should have a good working knowledge of a variety of handicapping conditions and experience in organizing camp activities. He or she should be able to organize and train the staff and direct planning.

The day camp may employ a full-time paid staff or volunteers who serve as counselors. Counselors should be in charge of five or six handicapped and nonhandicapped students. The paid staff should have some background in providing camping experiences to handicapped youngsters. The counselors should also have the skills to provide and lead the activities included in the camp program.

Volunteers may be used in capacities other than that of counselor. Numerous volunteers may be available to help with or lead certain activities. Volunteers may range from children to adults. Some resources that might be considered include:

- an elderly person good at storytelling
- persons good at a particular art or craft who could lead the activity or assist with counselor training
- students good in gymnastics who could provide demonstrations or assist with basic students and tumbling
- individuals with music ability who could offer time to provide rhythmics or sing-a-longs at picnics or other occasions
- individuals with carpentry skills who could help with building equipment

Organization/Staff Development

The way in which the camp is organized will greatly affect how successful it really is. Preplanning and comprehensive staff orientation will save much time during the actual camp time for the campers. AAHPERD (1976) recommends that staff training should be the first priority and that it should include:

- orientation to the camp facility
- involvement in making the camp schedule
- discussion of teaching methods and practices to be employed
- staffing of each camper

Orientation to the Camp Facility

All staff members, including volunteers who will participate for more than one activity, need to be included in the portion of staff training that includes orientation to the camp. Everyone should be totally familiar with the camp setting and specific facilities.

Scheduling

The staff should be involved in helping to make the camp schedule. The director should solicit ideas and suggestions from the staff. This approach allows the staff to feel involved in the camp process. In addition, they are more apt to follow the schedule with fewer problems when they have been involved in its development.

Teaching Methods and Practices

Some camps may be geared to students who have to have particular structure and teaching strategies to provide a successful camping experience. If particular teaching strategies are to be used, they need to be consistent among the staff. Inconsistency can be very confusing to campers and can only lead to problems in the management of the campers. Any particular type of behavior management program should be fully understood by the staff and they should be capable of implementing it.

Staffing Needs

Before campers arrive, a staffing conference on each camper should occur. Information on the camper should be provided so that each staff member has some idea of the needs of that particular student. Any special activities that should be avoided must be noted. Generally, in a day camp, concern about medications is not as much a priority as in residential camps. However, the staff should know which campers require medication and the problems resulting if the parents forget to give the medication.

Behavioral and teaching strategies should be developed for each camper. The camper's particular strengths and weaknesses should also be discussed. After the camper has been reviewed, some basic goals and objectives should be delineated. These can be changed after the arrival of the campers if necessary.

Daily Schedule

A daily schedule for the number of weeks the campers will attend should be developed. Before specific activities are used in a daily schedule, arrangements for the proper equipment, supervision, and space need to be made.

Generally, in a day camp, the schedule will cover the time period from 9:00 A.M. to 2:00 P.M. for the campers. The schedule can be made to include a variety of activities. Some time periods will be devoted to the same activity each day, such as lunch and arrival and departure of the campers. Shea (1977) recommends that no more than 30 to 40 campers be included in a day camp. Table 15–1 is an example of a schedule for a day's activities.

Alternative activities need to be planned. In case of rain, for example, swimming would have to be canceled. Special events, such as a track and field day or a field trip, may take up a half day at the camp. Schedules will more than likely have to be adjusted from time to time. Thus, the staff needs to be flexible.

Table 15–1 Sample Schedule

Time	Activity	Location
8:30– 9:00	arrival	shelter
9:00– 9:30	rhythms	gymnasium
10:00–10:30	stunts/gymnastics	gymnasium
10:45–12:00	swimming	pool
12:00– 1:00	lunch/rest	picnic shelter
1:00– 1:30	parachute games	open field
1:30– 2:00	finger painting or other craft	shelter/indoors
2:00– 2:30	departure	shelter
2:30– 3:00	clean up/evaluation	indoors

Criteria for Selecting Activities

Activities cannot be haphazardly assigned to the day camp schedule. The following should be kept in mind when scheduling an activity:

- developmental levels of campers
- activities that challenge both the handicapped and non-handicapped camper
- availability of space for the activity
- necessary adaptations of the activity to accommodate the handicapped camper
- grouping of campers for particular activities
- availability of equipment for the activity

Modifying Activities

The following is an example of modifying an activity so that several levels of individuals can participate. The activity is frisbee toss. Several students are capable of tossing the frisbee using the standard procedure. Since there are others who cannot move fast enough to catch the frisbee or who cannot throw the frisbee correctly, several options need to be developed. Three basic stations can be formed to include skills at different levels.

Station I. Frisbee Toss (Regular Format)

Experienced frisbee players may toss at this station choosing whatever format they wish.

Station II. Frisbee Target Toss

Targets are set up using potato chip cans on cones. Students stand 5 to 10 feet away and try to knock the cans off the cones by tossing the frisbee. Another target can be developed by hanging a hula hoop from a tree limb. The students are required to toss the frisbee to each other through the hoop.

Station III. Frisbee Pass

This station can be used for campers who have had no experience with the frisbee. A peer camper can help with this group. Campers sit or stand in a circle and pass the frisbee around the circle as quickly as possible using a grip that is normally used to toss the frisbee. Also, potato chip cans can be placed in the middle of the circle and the frisbee can be tossed at the cans. Figure 15–1 depicts how to set up the frisbee stations.

Nature Activities

Kraus (1973) suggests the following nature activities:

- exploring the natural settings that surround the camp
- hiking
- practicing camping skills such as cooking, putting up a tent, rock collecting, building a camp fire, leaf pressing, bird watching

Figure 15–1 Frisbee Modifications

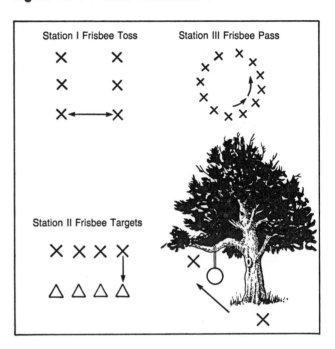

AAHPERD (1976) suggests the following considerations when hiking and other nature activities are involved:

- Allow slower groups to start out earlier.
- Provide rest periods if fatigue is observed.
- Pair campers according to abilities: blind camper with a sighted camper, physically disabled camper with a camper who is not physically disabled.
- All trails should be clearly marked.
- A counselor should always be the last person in a line of hikers.

Games

Games can be modified in the following manner:
Net and Court Games

- Use a smaller court.
- Allow more players on the court.
- Lower the net.
- Use lighter weight balls.
- Allow more hits or modify hits.
- Decrease time to be played.

Striking Implements

- Use lighter weight bats or other implements.
- Use rackets with big heads.

- Shorten the racket.
- Use a batting tee.
- Increase the number of strikes, swings, etc.
- Allow crutches to be used as striking implements.
- Use playing surfaces that can accommodate wheelchairs.
- Substitute frequently.
- Simplify the rules.

RESIDENTIAL CAMPS

A residential camp requires much more money and staff to operate and may serve several purposes different from those of a day camp. Residential camps are often sponsored by large organizations or are associated with special schools for particular types of handicapped individuals. Campers stay overnight for a period of at least one week or two weeks in residential camps. The advantage to sending handicapped campers to a residential camp is that the experience is more intense than in a day camp setting. More goals can be defined for the residential camper than for the day camper. In addition, residential camps may provide more independence for the camper. For some, a residential camp experience may be the first time the child has ever been away from home.

SPECIALIZED CAMPS

Specialized camps may be camps organized for a single purpose. For example, computer camps are becoming popular and include both gifted and handicapped students. Computer skills may be studied in the morning with recreation provided in the afternoon. Evening time is devoted to practice on the computer. Generally, a physical education specialist is employed to provide the recreation program.

Another example of a specialized camp is the vocational competition camp. Secondary students who are handicapped go to a camp setting for one week and display their vocational work from vocational instructional and awareness programs. At these camps, too, physical education specialists are employed to provide the recreational program for the students.

PARENT-CHILD TRAINING CAMPS

Some camps are structured for parents and children with handicapping conditions. The major purpose of such camps is to assess the handicapped child and train the parents to work with their child. Recreation is used to teach the parents that these kinds of activities can be enlisted to develop a variety of skills in which the child may be deficient.

This type of camp is usually located on the grounds of a residential facility that is geared toward the type of handicapped child being served. For example, a residential facility for the severely retarded or multihandicapped may sponsor this type of camp. The major objectives are to:

- provide diagnostic/prescriptive programming for each child
- determine the needs of the parents for working with their child
- provide the concept of a structured teaching routine using recreational settings as the means for achieving these goals
- conduct parent training and parent groups to enable parents to express their needs
- provide activities in which parents work directly with their children

Staff

The staff for this type of camp needs to be adequately trained to deal with the particular type of child being served. The following section provides an example of this type of camp. The adapted physical educator will have very specific roles in this camp setting:

- assess motor skills of each handicapped child
- set up the teaching stations and activities
- demonstrate to parents how to teach motor activities
- plan an individualized program for each child
- conduct group motor and recreational activities
- serve on the team to work with parents in parent group sessions
- evaluate parent and child progress in motor training sessions
- plan recreational activities in the daily schedule.

Daily Schedule

The schedule should have built into it the training activities themselves and continue throughout the day and in each activity. (See Table 15–2.)

These camps are very effective in providing parents with skills to work with their children for an intensive five-day period. Parents generally leave with a feeling that they have developed skills and new relationships with their handicapped children. The advantage of this type of camp is that parents can gain the skills they need to manage their handicapped child in an informal setting. Also, much support is provided by other parents. Thus, both the parents' and the child's needs are met in this setting.

Table 15–2 Sample Schedule

Time	Activity	Objective
8:00–9:00 A.M.	Breakfast	Parents learn to teach feeding skills.
9:15–9:45 A.M.	Group Activity	Parents work with their child on a particular activity: rhythmics, etc.
9:45–11:45 A.M.	Stations Self-help skills Motor (Gross) Motor (Fine) Language	Parents rotate to each station for a 30-minute training session.
11:45 A.M.–1:00 P.M.	Break Lunch	Parents again practice teaching feeding skills and eat lunch.
1:00–1:30 P.M.	Free-Time Recreational activity	Parents may take a walk or choose a free-time activity with their child.
1:30–2:00 P.M.	Arts/Crafts	Parents work with their child on an arts and crafts project.
2:00–3:30 P.M.	Swimming	Parent works with child on swimming skills.
3:30–4:30 P.M.	Parent Group Session	Parents discuss and evaluate the day's progress.
4:30–5:00 P.M.	Break	Children play under staff supervision. Parent's free time.
5:00–6:00 P.M.	Dinner	Parents work with child on feeding.
6:00–7:30 P.M.	Parent Goal Planning	Goals are planned for the next day using the same structure. Parents have time to share feelings and discuss their needs.

DISABILITY CONSIDERATIONS

Table 15–3 presents a summary of the general range of considerations for camping required of each disability type.

EVALUATION

All camp experiences should be evaluated at the session's end. Evaluation should focus on the staff, the camper gains, and the activities. The following points should be covered:

Staff

- effectiveness with campers
- motivation
- leadership and direction offered by director

Table 15–3 Disability Considerations

Disability	Considerations for Camping
Mildly Retarded	• can participate in most camp activities, needs few modifications.
Moderately Retarded	• needs closer supervision than mildly retarded or regular camper • needs more modifications in games • needs activities geared to mental age • functions better in small groups and with a buddy system
Severely Retarded	• may have limited locomotion • may have difficulty with self-help skills • needs one-on-one supervision • needs sensory motor stimulation • needs much modification of an activity • needs rest periods
Emotionally Disturbed	• will benefit from dual and noncompetitive activities • will benefit from more therapeutic activities: dance, art, music, story telling, and dramatics. • needs consistency • can use a buddy to serve as a good role model • needs relaxation time • needs to be able to talk and express feelings
Physically Disabled	• needs more time to complete an activity • requires camp area to be as barrier-free as possible • needs frequent rest periods • will benefit from partner activities • should not have too many overly exciting activities
Learning Disabilities	• functions best when playing areas are uncluttered • will benefit from a distinct schedule, though different activities can be used • will benefit when perceptual training is integrated in as many activities as possible • needs crafts geared to perceptual strengths • can use peer helpers as models

Camper (see Burnes, 1966)

- change in camper's skills
- improvement in group activities
- new friends, hobbies developed

Activities and Schedule

- effectiveness of activities
- good and bad points of the schedule
- needs for next camp experience
- recommended changes in activities or schedule

POINTS TO REMEMBER

1. Camping and outdoor adventure can provide a multitude of wholesome, stimulating activities for handicapped children and their families.

2. The camp experience, particularly the day camp, lends itself well to implementing the mainstreaming concept.

3. Camps have a variety of purposes ranging from day settings to specific teaching camps to train parents in working with their handicapped child.

4. Preplanning seems to be the most effective method of ensuring that the camp experience is both enjoyable and productive.

5. The adapted physical educator can be an invaluable staff member at a camp or serve as a catalyst in starting/directing summer day camps for handicapped youngsters.

6. There are a number of resources in terms of both volunteers and locations for beginning a day camp. The only limits are the imaginations of those who wish to embark on the undertaking. The rewards are far too many not to begin at least a community day camp.

REFERENCES

American Alliance for Health, Physical Education, Recreation and Dance (AAHPERD). (1976). *Involving impaired, disabled, and handicapped persons in regular camp programs.* Reston, VA: IRUC Publications.

Burnes, A.J. (1966). A pilot study in evaluating camping experiences for the mentally retarded. *Mental Retardation, 4,* 15–17.

Fait, H.F. (1978). *Special physical education.* Philadelphia: W.B. Saunders.

Kraus, R. (1973). *Therapeutic recreation services: Principles and practices.* Philadelphia: W.B. Saunders.

Shea, T.M. (1977). *Camping for special children.* St. Louis: C.V. Mosby.

Index

About the Author

M. Rhonda Folio is currently a professor of special education and physical education at Tennessee Technological University, Cookeville, Tennessee. Her Ed.D. degree was earned at George Peabody College of Vanderbilt University in 1975. She has four years of public school teaching experience. Since her position in higher education, Dr. Folio has coordinated, co-directed, and directed several federally and privately funded projects including Project PERMIT, a model demonstration program in physical education emphasizing mainstreaming and peer teaching; Project SSAVE, an inservice training project for mainstreaming in vocational settings; Project ETIPS, Educational Television Intervention Programs for high risk and handicapped infants, toddlers, and their families; and Project LEAP, a research project on nutritional problems of handicapped children. Dr. Folio is the co-author of the *Peabody Developmental Motor Scales and Activity Cards,* has published in professional journals, and conducted extensive inservice training on physical education program development for handicapped children.